SECOND EDITION

Public Health Nursing

Practicing Population-Based Care

The Pedagogy

Public Health Nursing: Practicing Population-Based Care, Second Edition drives comprehension through various strategies that meet the learning needs of students, while also generating enthusiasm about the topic. This interactive approach addresses different learning styles, making this the ideal text to ensure mastery of key concepts. The pedagogical aids that appear in most chapters include the following:

Learning Objectives

These objectives provide instructors and students with a snapshot of the key information they will encounter in each chapter. They serve as a checklist to help guide and focus study. Objectives can also be found on the companion website at **http://go.jblearning.com/londrigan**

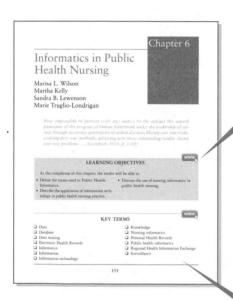

Key Terms

Found in a list at the beginning of each chapter, these terms will create an expanded vocabulary. The "www" icon directs students to the companion website **http://go.jblearning.com/londrigan** to see these terms in an interactive glossary and use flashcards and word puzzles to nail the definitions.

Case Studies

Read and analyze real-life vignettes dealing with public health nursing and use your critical thinking skills to apply what you have learned from the text. Answer questions to these case studies on the companion website at **http:// go.jblearning.com/londrigan**

www.

CASE STUDY (3)
VIGNETTE OF ADAPTING A COMPUTERIZED SCHEDULING SYSTEM
Martha Kelly, EdD, RN

My introduction into the world of nursing informatics started with the implementation of a computerized scheduling system in a large medical center in 1980. Very few hospitals had a computerized scheduling system at that time. From an informatics standpoint, the software package that was purchased allowed us to use our current staffing patterns; however, the concept of taking the control away from the role of the head nurse was a major paradigm shift. Until that time nurses did not typically have control of their unit's budget and subsequently used the time sheets as part of their reward system. The real issue was how to show nurses they still retained the decision-making portion of the schedule. The computerized system generated the first draft of the schedule, but the final decision was made by the head nurse who knew the staff and what the staffing mix should be for the unit to run well.

During this period I attended what was the first national nursing conference engaged in computer technology, entitled "Computer Technology and Nursing," that was hosted by the Clinical Center at the National Institutes of Health and held in Bethesda, Maryland. Many of the speakers at that conference addressed what we see today. Computerized patient records and computerized care plans were discussed at the conference. To my chagrin some of those in attendance seemed quite resistant to these new computer applications for nursing. For example, some were not supportive and others were critical of the concept of computerized care plans. Although the speakers were innovative, there was reluctance for early adoption on the part of some in the audience. Their reluctance was most likely reflective of this new field and the role of nursing informatics that was still being carved out. It was a time when there were mainframes but few desktop computers in a clinical setting. Even as a novice informatics nurse, it was clear that a merger of computer technology and nursing would soon come together.

technology to be supported by the very people who use it and benefit from it, adaptation to various settings may be required. Rural settings versus urban environments create different challenges for nurses using technology.

Connections

Information technology is used in a variety of settings, including hospitals, private practices, voluntary visiting nurse services, and municipal health departments. Currently, many institutions have their own data systems; however, many of the systems do not talk to each other within or between institutions. The lack of interfaces and compatibility is related to the inability to share information. The integration of systems is costly but critical for a comprehensive model of care. This is an area where focused attention will be directed in the coming years. How to develop systems that

The Integrated Teaching and Learning Package

W elcome to *Public Health Nursing: Practicing Population-Based Care, Second Edition*. To help meet the changing needs of today's faculty and students, this text has been fully integrated with a full suite of instructor and student ancillaries, helping instructors teach more efficiently and students learn more effectively.

STUDENT RESOURCES

The companion website, specifically designed to complement *Public Health Nursing: Practicing Population-Based Care, Second Edition*, offers students a valuable integration of the text and online study tools, including:

- Interactive Glossary
- Interactive Flashcards
- Crossword Puzzle
- Chapter Objectives
- Case Studies
- Nursing Assessment Tool

Learn more about Student Resources Online:
http://go.jblearning.com/londrigan

INSTRUCTOR RESOURCES

- **Test Bank** – Customize quizzes and tests that can be printed or administered online.

- **PowerPoint Presentations** – Modify pre-made classroom presentations and use them in your course.

- **Exercises, Reflections, Suggested Readings, and Web Links** – Promote student discussion and critical thinking with these additional activities, or use as a homework assignment or in-class quiz.

SECOND EDITION

Public Health Nursing

Practicing Population-Based Care

Edited by

Marie Truglio-Londrigan, PhD, RN
Professor
Pace University, College of Health Professions
Lienhard School of Nursing
Pleasantville, New York

Sandra B. Lewenson, EdD, RN, FAAN
Professor
Pace University, College of Health Professions
Lienhard School of Nursing
Pleasantville, New York

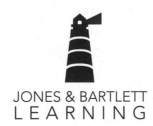

JONES & BARTLETT
LEARNING

World Headquarters
Jones & Bartlett Learning
5 Wall Street
Burlington, MA 01803
978-443-5000
info@jblearning.com
www.jblearning.com

Jones & Bartlett Learning books and products are available through most bookstores and online booksellers. To contact Jones & Bartlett Learning directly, call 800-832-0034, fax 978-443-8000, or visit our website, www.jblearning.com

Substantial discounts on bulk quantities of Jones & Bartlett Learning publications are available to corporations, professional associations, and other qualified organizations. For details and specific discount information, contact the special sales department at Jones & Bartlett Learning via the above contact information or send an email to specialsales@jblearning.com.

Production Credits
Publisher: Kevin Sullivan
Acquisitions Editor: Amanda Harvey
Editorial Assistant: Sara Bempkins
Associate Production Editor: Cindie Bryan
Senior Marketing Manager: Elena McAnespie
V.P., Manufacturing and Inventory Control: Therese Connell
Composition: Circle Graphics, Inc.
Cover Design: Scott Moden
Cover Images: Clockwise from top left: Courtesy of the American Red Cross Cornhusker Chapter, © iStockphoto/Thinkstock, Courtesy of the Visiting Nurse Service of New York, © BananaStock/Thinkstock, Courtesy of the Visiting Nurse Association of Community Services of Abington, PA, © VStock/Thinkstock
Printing and Binding: Edwards Brothers Malloy
Cover Printing: Edwards Brothers Malloy

To order this product, use ISBN: 1-978-1-4496-8358-0

Library of Congress Cataloging-in-Publication Data
Public health nursing : practicing population-based care / [edited by] Marie Truglio-Londrigan, Sandra B. Lewenson. — 2nd ed.
    p. ; cm.
  Includes bibliographical references and index.
  ISBN 978-1-4496-4660-8 (pbk.) — ISBN 1-4496-4660-3 (pbk.)
  I. Truglio-Londrigan, Marie. II. Lewenson, Sandra.
  [DNLM: 1. Public Health Nursing—United States. 2. Evidence-Based Nursing—United States. 3. Models, Organizational—United States. WY 108]

  610.73'4—dc23
                            2012004585
6048
Printed in the United States of America
16 15 14 13 12   10 9 8 7 6 5 4 3 2 1

Contents

FOREWORD   xiii
PREFACE   xv
ACKNOWLEDGMENTS   xxiii
CONTRIBUTORS   xxv
REVIEWERS   xxix

1   What Is Public Health and Public Health Nursing? 3

Learning Objectives 3
Key Terms 3
Public Health Defined 4
Public Health Nursing 10
Public Health Now 11
Conclusion 21
References 21

2   Public Health Nursing in the United States: A History 25

Learning Objectives 25
Key Terms 25
What Is a Public Health Nurse? 26
Evolution of the Public Health Nurse 27
Education of Public Health Nurses 47
Conclusion 49
References 49

3   Assessment: Using the Public Health Nursing Assessment Tool 53

Learning Objectives 53
Key Terms 53

Overview of the Unique Qualities of the PHNAT 55
PHNAT Four Foundational Health Measures 58
Analysis of Health 62
Prioritize Public Health Issues 62
Plan and Implementation:
    Applying the Minnesota Intervention Wheel Strategies 62
Tracking and Evaluation 63
Reflection 64
Conclusion 65
References 65
Appendix: Public Health Nursing Assessment Tool 67

4 Fundamentals of Epidemiology and Social Epidemiology 103

Learning Objectives 103
Key Terms 104
Epidemiology 104
Social Epidemiology 117
Conclusion 127
References 127

5 Evidence-Based Practice From a Public Health Perspective 131

Learning Objectives 131
Key Terms 131
Introduction to Evidence-Based Practice and Public Health 131
What Is an Evidence-Based Practice Lens for Viewing
    Population-Based Health Issues? 132
Healthy People 2020—Public Health Conditions:
    An Evidence-Based Perspective 134
References 146

6 Informatics in Public Health Nursing 151

Learning Objectives 151
Key Terms 151
Role of Technology in Public Health Nursing Practice 153
Information Technology 154
Information Technology in Public Health Nursing 161
Conclusion 176
References 176

7 Considerations of Culture in the Health of the Public 179

Learning Objectives 179
Key Terms 179
Culture 180
Case Studies 189
Conclusion 196
Acknowledgments 196
References 197

8 Healthcare Policy and Politics: The Risk and Rewards for Public Health Nurses 201

Learning Objectives 201
Key Terms 202
Why Care About Federal Policy? 202
What's Wrong With the Current U.S. Healthcare System? 206
How Does the Affordable Care Act Address Our Health System's Problems? 208
What Is the Impact of the Affordable Care Act on Public Health? 210
What Is the Federal Government's Role in American Society:
    Is Health Care a Right? 211
How Does History Shape Health Care? 213
The Economy, Polarization, Public Confusion, and Misinformation:
    Will the Affordable Care Act Survive? 214
State Responses to the Affordable Care Act 216
Understanding Policy Making and Public Health Nursing 217
Public Health Nurses and Political Engagement 217
Conclusion 219
References 219

9 Hitting the Pavement: Intervention of Case Finding: Outreach, Screening, Surveillance, and Disease and Health Event Investigation 223

Learning Objectives 223
Key Terms 224
Minnesota Department of Health Population-Based
    Public Health Nursing Practice Intervention Wheel Strategies 224
Public Health Issues in Practice 237
Case Study Application: When Time Is of Importance 244

Minnesota Department of Health Population-Based Public Health Nursing
   Practice Intervention Wheel: Levels of Practice 246
Conclusion 247
References 247

10 Running the Show: Referral and Follow-up, Case Management,
   and Delegated Functions 251

Learning Objectives 251
Key Terms 251
Minnesota Department of Health Population-Based Public Health Nursing
   Practice Intervention Wheel Strategies and Levels of Practice 252
Minnesota Department of Health Population-Based Public Health Nursing
   Practice Intervention Wheel: Application to Practice 269
Conclusion 273
References 274

11 Working It Out: Consultation, Counseling, and Health Teaching 277

Learning Objectives 277
Key Terms 277
Minnesota Department of Health Population-Based Public Health Nursing
   Practice Intervention Wheel Interventions 278
The Case/Issue 287
Minnesota Department of Health Population-Based Public Health Nursing
   Practice Intervention Wheel: Applying and Doing 290
Conclusion 293
References 294

12 Working Together: Collaboration, Coalition Building,
   and Community Organizing 297

Learning Objectives 297
Key Terms 297
Issue: Physical Inactivity Is a Major 21st Century Public Health Concern 298
Minnesota Department of Health Population-Based Public Health Nursing
   Practice Intervention Wheel Strategies and Levels of Practice 300
Minnesota Department of Health Population-Based Public Health Nursing
   Practice Intervention Wheel: Application to Practice 309
Conclusion 311
References 311

13 Getting the Word Out: Advocacy, Social Marketing, and Policy Development and Enforcement 315

Learning Objectives 315
Key Terms 315
Issue: Overweight and Obesity Are Major 21st Century Public Health
    Concerns 316
Minnesota Department of Health Population-Based Public Health Nursing
    Practice Intervention Wheel Strategies and Levels of Practice 320
Conclusion 330
References 331

14 Protecting, Sustaining, and Empowering: A Historical Perspective on the Control of Epidemics 335

Learning Objectives 335
Key Terms 336
Protecting the People Against God's Wrath: Bubonic Plague
    in Early Modern Italy 336
Serving and Sustaining a Desperate Population: Influenza in the Modern
    United States 341
Empowering the Vulnerable: AIDS in Contemporary Britain 344
Conclusion 347
References 349

15 Historical Highlights in Disaster Nursing 353

Learning Objectives 353
Key Terms 353
Yellow Fever and the Johnstown Flood 354
The Galveston Hurricane, 1900 355
The Flu Pandemic, 1918–1919 356
1947 Texas City Ship Explosion 358
The Alaska Earthquake of 1964 362
Conclusion 365
References 366

16 Emergency Preparedness in the 21st Century: Two Post-9/11 Case Studies 369

Learning Objectives 369
Key Terms 369
Push Point of Dispensing and Pull Point of Dispensing Defined 370

The Pull POD: Smallpox Initiative 370
The Push POD: The Influenza Vaccine Initiative 372
Thoughts, Reflections, and Lessons Learned 373
Summary 374
References 375

17 **Nursing Education and Public Health Nursing** 377

Learning Objectives 377
Key Terms 377
Challenges to Nurse Educators 378
Responding to the Public Health Needs 379
Integrating Learner Knowledge, Skills, and Aptitudes
    to Develop Public Health–Focused Nursing Care 381
Public Health Clinical Experiences 382
Paradigm Shift From Local to Global Worldview 389
Nurse Educators: Embracing Public Health in Teaching, Learning,
    and Evaluation 393
Conclusion 394
References 396

18 **Conversation About Primary Health Care** 399

Learning Objectives 399
Key Terms 399
The Declaration of Alma-Ata 400
Primary Health Care 400
What Has Been Our Progress? 404
Why the Struggle? 407
The Teaching of a Philosophy 409
References 413

APPENDIX 414
GLOSSARY 415
INDEX 423

Foreword

In 2010, the Institute of Medicine (IOM), in partnership with the Robert Wood Johnson Foundation, released a landmark report: *The Future of Nursing: Leading Change, Advancing Health*. This remarkable report, the first major broad report on nursing at the IOM since 1983, set forward a blueprint for improving access, quality, and value of healthcare services through a transformation of the nursing profession. Public health nursing as a way of practicing and thinking, as well as a way to fundamentally structure the care of individuals, families, and populations within communities, is an essential part of the transformation supported by the IOM report. As evidence of its critical position, public health nursing is highlighted throughout the report by case studies and narrative content.

The second edition of *Public Health Nursing: Practicing Population-Based Care* provides the historical context, skills, and knowledge for public health nurses to participate in the transformation and to practice to the fullest extent of their knowledge and skills. Just as important, it provides a broader perspective of patient care for nurses practicing across all specialties and places of practice. This is a critical attribute because The Affordable Care Act of 2010 directed attention to new care delivery models such as accountable care organizations and medical homes. The successful implementation of these models depends upon the seamless movement of the public across healthcare settings and a supply of knowledgeable providers to plan and prioritize services by placing the individual, family, and population within the social, economic, and cultural context of community. These models will not work unless there is a strong cross-professional understanding and integration of public health nursing.

The second edition of this cutting-edge text reflects the editors' immersion in the healthcare arena and facility with historical evidence and includes many updates that reflect the constantly changing healthcare milieu. The cornerstone of the book, the public health nursing assessment tool, has been revised to reflect the goals and determinants of *Healthy People 2020,* and each chapter has been refined to parallel the new content of this extraordinary policy-formulating document. The editors also included new content on emergency preparedness, much of it historically based, to both highlight the new threat potential we face as a nation and to ready the healthcare workforce for current and future infectious diseases. The final chapter focuses on the constantly evolving healthcare needs of our nation and brings our attention to primary care and its changing conceptualization. As the editors note, our healthcare needs are too great to provide care in specialty silos or to focus only on disease and medical care, and the Affordable Care Act provided an opportunity for highlighting the synergistic nature of public health and primary care. As the historiographical integration found in the book tells us, most of the public's healthcare needs across various times and places have not been met by acute care institutions, but in the community through a population focus. From this perspective, when public health nurses can "see" patients in their own homes, with their families, or in the community, they are more likely to analyze strengths and weaknesses (including housing, transportation, and cultural issues), identify health promotion and disease prevention needs, and respond accordingly.

In a very real, practical, and authoritative way, through its case studies, content, and historical integration, the second edition of *Public Health Nursing* situates public health nursing as the linchpin of the nation's health. Public health nursing *is* the future of nursing. This text provides students and practitioners across all levels with the skills and knowledge to bridge public health nurses' historical place with their capabilities to shape the future and transform patient care.

Julie Fairman
Nightingale Professor of Nursing
Director, Barbara Bates Center for the Study of the History of Nursing
School of Nursing
University of Pennsylvania
Philadelphia, PA

Preface

That morning's experience was a baptism of fire...On my way from the sick-room to my comfortable student quarters my mind was intent on my own responsibility. To my inexperience it seemed certain that conditions such as these were allowed because people did not know*, and for me there was a challenge to know and to tell. (Wald, 1915, p. 8)*

Truglio-Londrigan and Lewenson, both public health nurses and educators, conceived of the first edition of this text as a way of exploring what it means to practice population-based public health nursing. The questions they raised about public health nursing at curriculum meetings, in the classroom, and in clinical settings led to the writing of the first edition. For example, they asked, "How do you provide clinical experiences in public health? Do students only need 'carry the bag'-type experiences usually found in voluntary visiting nurses service associations, or should they also have surveillance-type activities found in publicly funded health departments? Or, should they have both?" Often, they argued that students could learn public health nursing by offering blood pressure screenings at social service-type agencies, such as the Henry Street Settlement in New York City or at a recycling bottling plant near a homeless shelter, or even in a local shopping center. Other questions emerged that expanded their thinking, such as "How can evidence-based practice and technology be integrated into the work of public health nurses and how can we use history to explain how public health nursing has been defined over the past hundred years?" Questions about diversity and cultural competence became relevant as the authors further explored ways to convey the concepts of public health to students, faculty, and other healthcare professionals. How can we speak to diversity and relate this to students and nurses engaged in the practice of public health nursing? And, finally, they wanted to understand what so many nurses have already asked: "What is public health nursing?" The first edition used *Healthy People 2010* as a framework that supported the answers generated to some of these questions. In the second edition, the editors of this text revisited these same questions, only this time using the newly published *Healthy People 2020* to guide them. In addition, new questions arose that facilitated a broader worldview that permitted exploring primary health care. These new questions include: What is the meaning of primary health care and how is it different than primary care? Where does public health nursing fit into primary health care and primary care?

Public Health Nursing: Practicing Population-Based Care offers a variety of different perspectives on community and public health nursing from other texts already being used. For example, the authors address the relevance of historical evidence in coming to know the meaning of the terms used to describe public health nursing, disaster nursing, and global perspectives; they explore the use of technology in public health; they provide the meaning of social epidemiology as well as the traditional content on epidemiology; and they offer an innovatively designed assessment tool that now uses *Healthy People 2020* as its framework. Another highlight of this text is the focus on the 17 intervention strategies identified in the *Population-Based Public Health Nursing Practice Intervention Wheel* developed by the Minnesota Department of Health in the mid-1990s. In addition, they examine how these interventions may be applied throughout the three levels of practice: individual/family, community, and systems levels (Minnesota Department of Health, 2001; Keller, Strohschein, & Briske, 2008). *Public Health Nursing: Practicing Population-Based Care* aims to add greater clarity to the body of public health nursing literature, inclusive of primary health care, and serve as a useful tool for educators, students, and practitioners of public health nursing. While the editors have revised chapters and developed several new ones, they would like to include the caveat that knowledge is ever evolving, and they urge the reader to continually support this work with additional sources as they become available. Finally, the final chapter of this new edition provides a conversation about the place of primary health care and primary care within the healthcare delivery system.

Audience for Text

This text can be used by nursing students in both baccalaureate and graduate degree programs. In addition, all nurses, whether practicing in public health, community health, or home care settings, would benefit from this book because it offers a way to understand how care of the individual, family, and population relates to larger systems and the care of communities. Nurses in all healthcare delivery systems already practice population-based care; this text simply provides nurses with the information they need to provide this care.

Organization and Pedagogical Features of Text

Each chapter begins with a quotation and a photograph from nursing history that resonates with the content of the chapter. Objectives and key terms for each chapter offer direction to the reader as to what can be expected. Those chapters that address public health intervention strategies contain case studies. The use of history as evidence is threaded throughout the chapters, where it illuminates the didactic content and case studies. Noted historians from around the world participated in the writing of several chapters that provide this historical evidence. To aid the reader further, a glossary defining the various key terms used in the text can be found at the end of the text. Although the editors wrote several chapters, they also turned to experts to write many of the chapters throughout the text. These contributing authors represent a cadre of outstanding nursing professionals who were willing to rethink the way they practice and share their thoughts with the reader. Another unique feature of this book is that each contributor's "voice" can be heard in his or her own chapter. This means that consistency of style and pedagogy was purposely avoided by the authors so they could showcase a diversity of ideas in how to approach public health nursing.

The first chapter, "What Is Public Health and Public Health Nursing?" explores the ideas of health promotion and disease prevention and refers the reader to the evolutionary nature of nursing activities in primary, secondary, and tertiary prevention. Nursing care, Truglio-Londrigan and Lewenson point out, especially public health nursing, is not a linear process. Using a nonlinear approach encourages us to think about providing care for disease while simultaneously promoting health. This first chapter includes definitions of public health and public health nursing, the three core functions of public health, ten essential public health services, and an explanation of *Healthy People 2020*. Truglio-Londrigan and Lewenson use these various documents and meanings of public health to help explain the work of public health nurses.

The reader finds an unusual approach to public health nursing history in Chapter 2, "Public Health Nursing in the United States: A History." Lewenson approaches this chapter from the standpoint of how changing definitions show the social, political, and economic influences that altered the work of nurses in the home setting. The author turns to past nursing leaders in public health nursing and examines how they defined public health nursing. Instead of writing a traditional history of public health nursing, Lewenson uses the past to explain the tensions that exist between and among the various titles nurses have used to delineate care provided in the community, including district nurse, health visitor, public health nurse, community health nurse, and home care nurse. These changing definitions and titles show the evolutionary nature of public health nursing and the response of these nurses to the social, political, and economic environment. The use of historical evidence also offers insight into the questions Truglio-Londrigan and Lewenson asked, including "What is public health nursing?", "How is public health nursing different from community health nursing or home care nursing?", and "How do we educate students about the role of public health nursing when the names and contextual meanings change over time?"

Chapter 3, "Assessment: Using the Public Health Nursing Assessment Tool," presents the innovative public health nursing assessment tool (PHNAT) designed by Lewenson and Truglio-Londrigan. The PHNAT engages nurses, nursing students, and public health nurses in an assessment process that applies the newly published Process Model for *Healthy People 2020* (U.S. Department of Health and Human Services, 2010) with specific emphasis placed on the determinants of health and health status. In addition, the PHNAT directs the reader to use the intervention wheel strategies in their work. This chapter sees assessment as a fluid process, and the PHNAT offers the user a kaleidoscopic view of this process.

In Chapter 4, "Fundamentals of Epidemiology and Social Epidemiology," Susan Moscou presents the science of epidemiology. Moscou begins the chapter with a discussion of the history of epidemiology that highlights two epidemiological revolutions. The chapter covers the terms descriptive epidemiology, analytical epidemiology, the epidemiological triad, and the chain of infection. The author then introduces social epidemiology and the social determinants of health in the second part of the chapter. Comparisons between epidemiology and social epidemiology provide the reader with an understanding between the two and allows for greater application of the concepts.

Joanne K. Singleton and Renee McLeod-Sordjan contribute their expertise to Chapter 5, "Evidenced-Based Practice From a Public Health Perspective." This chapter defines the meaning of evidence-based practice, specifically focusing on public health nurses. Through the examples and case study, the authors describe a systematic approach to finding best available evidence. Specifically, they explore the application of evidence-based practice to the public health issues of health literacy and tobacco use. The case study allows the reader to gain insight into how a public health nurse can use an evidence-based approach to improve the health of a local community.

Chapter 6, "Informatics in Public Health Nursing," approaches technology in public health nursing from the perspective of how public health nurses use technology in their practice. Marisa Wilson with Martha Kelly, Lewenson, and Truglio-Londrigan begin the chapter with the rationale for including technology in practice. They define the various concepts needed to understand nursing informatics and explore the use and acceptance of technology in public health nursing practice. The authors use case studies from nurses who work in public health and have firsthand experience adapting to technology in the workplace. The case studies highlight issues related to introducing laptops, pagers, nursing informatics systems, and other forms of technology into practice. Their case studies give insight into how technology can be incorporated into practice.

Astrid Hellier Wilson and Mary de Chesnay contributed Chapter 7, "Considerations of Culture in the Health of the Public." In this chapter, Wilson and de Chesnay define the subconcepts associated with culture. They compare and contrast public health issues in terms of cultural influences and provide analysis of public health nursing interventions for selected cases in terms of cultural competence. Wilson and de Chesnay explore the meaning of culture, ethnocentrism, xenophobia, and ritual and what it means to be a participant observer, and then relate these to the meaning of culturally competent care in public health. Throughout this chapter they ask the reader to participate in "field observations" that allow for active learning and self-reflection.

Chapter 8, "Healthcare Policy and Politics: The Risk and Rewards for Public Health Nurses," is a new chapter written by Donna M. Nickitas and Deborah Gardner. In this chapter these authors present issues facing the U.S. healthcare system including: rising costs, reduction in employer-based contributions, the growing ranks of the uninsured, inadequate supply of health providers, a healthcare system that is hierarchical, complex and not well coordinated, and a system that is interdependent with the politics and policies of this country. The authors talk of the professional obligations of public health nurses as strong "influencers" and "advocates" for the population, particularly within the context of an environment ripe with debate surrounding the Affordable Care Act. These authors discuss many of the concepts inherent in other chapters of this text, again demonstrating the interconnectedness of heathcare reform, population health and protection while improving quality and controlling costs, as well as increasing access to care. Nickitas and Gardner suggest that nurses look to their history and reflect on what our past leaders did during their time of practice and, at the same time, look toward our challenging future.

The next five chapters address the strategies found on the intervention wheel. These intervention strategies have been separated out into five themes: Hitting the Pavement, Running the Show, Working It Out, Working Together, and Getting the Word Out. One of the assumptions of the intervention wheel includes the idea that public health nurses apply the nursing process to the multiple levels of practice, including the individual/family, community, and systems levels (Keller et al., 2008). Each intervention chapter explains a particular portion of the wheel and includes a vignette or case study that highlights the interventions and levels of practice.

Chapter 9, "Hitting the Pavement," refers to the outreach, case finding, screening, surveillance, and disease and health event investigation strategies that are found on the red wedge of the intervention wheel. The authors of this chapter, Margaret Macali and Truglio-Londrigan, divide the chapter into several sections. The first section describes the key intervention strategies. The second section demonstrates the application of these intervention strategies within the context of several public health issues. The third provides a case study to help the reader understand the process of these interventions as they are applied to the various levels of practice including individual/family, community, and system.

In Chapter 10, "Running the Show," Janna Dieckmann addresses three important public health interventions found in the green wedge of the intervention wheel: referral and follow-up, case management, and delegated functions. Dieckmann writes that these interventions have similarities, may overlap, and may be addressed toward similar working objectives. All three interventions draw the public health nurse to stretch beyond the nurse–client dyad, as the nurse seeks to add the contributions of other community services and health providers to improve the system for client support and change. At the community practice level, this means the public health nurse participates in initiating services or expanding availability/access to meet an identified need. At the systems practice level, the public health nurse modifies organizations and policies that shape systems of care. At the individual/family practice level, the public health nurse uses interventions designed to change knowledge, attitudes, beliefs, practices, and behaviors (Rippke, Briske, Keller, Strohschein, & Simonetti, 2001).

In Lin Drury's Chapter 11, "Working It Out," the reader returns to the modern-day Henry Street Settlement where Lillian Wald first introduced the idea of public health nursing in 1893. Drury focuses on the blue wedge of the intervention wheel, specifically focusing on intervention strategies that include counseling, consultation, and health teaching. The chapter defines and describes these strategies, then identifies an issue in public health practice, and finally demonstrates via a case study the "applying" and the "doing" of these interventions. The case study refers to the Henry Street Settlement, now a not-for-profit social service institution located on the Lower East Side of Manhattan in New York City. This settlement supports the needs of the vulnerable populations who live in the community, expanding over the years to include 19 sites such as day care centers, youth groups, workforce training, homeless shelters, mental health centers, summer camps, senior centers, and in the performing arts. Drury uses the Henry Street Settlement and the multicultural community it serves as a case study for public health nursing interventions that she and her students at Pace University in New York City have brought back to Henry Street.

In Chapter 12, "Working Together," author Adrienne Wald presents the strategies found in the orange wedge of the intervention wheel. The chapter explores the interventions of collaboration, coalition building, and community organizing. This chapter devotes a separate section to each of the three interventions and then one that discusses them as a collective action. As in all the chapters, this chapter describes the best evidence-based practices that address the issue of physical inactivity. The application of these interventions to this important 21st century public health crisis illustrates how each intervention strategy works and reinforces key concepts.

In Chapter 13, "Getting the Word Out," Susan Moscou addresses the interventions found on the yellow wedge of the intervention wheel. These strategies include advocacy, social marketing, and policy development and enforcement of public health nursing interventions. Moscou identifies obesity as one of the major public health issues in the United States, with a specific focus on obesity in children, primarily in junior high school, using a case study that highlights this public health issue. The case study depicts how the public health nurse engages in the application and the doing of the three interventions—advocacy, social marketing, and policy development—and enforcement through the three levels of public health practice.

The final chapters move the reader from the intervention wheel to issues reflecting global perspectives, disaster nursing, economic issues, and public health nursing education. Here the text draws from history, economics, and education to provide a unique way of presenting the content to the reader. The use of history provides an understanding of how public health nurses responded to public health issues in the past, which can be used to inform the work that public health nurses do today. In addition, the authors include a chapter that asks the reader to reflect on primary health care and primary care and their relationship to public health nursing.

Christine Hallett, in Chapter 14, "Protecting, Sustaining, and Empowering: A Historical Perspective on the Control of Epidemics," traces the means by which humans have attempted to eradicate certain of those "bugs" they consider harmful: the bacteria and viruses that cause epidemic and endemic infections. Hallett uses three case studies showcasing specific diseases appearing at specific historical moments: bubonic plague, as it appeared in the Early Modern Italian city states during the 16th and 17th centuries; Spanish influenza as it appeared in the cities of the United States in 1918 and 1919; and AIDS as it appeared in the United Kingdom during the 1980s. From this historical perspective, the reader explores the ways in which human societies have attempted to combat global epidemics. They learn the role the nurse has played working alongside governments, doctors, and scientists in the prevention of epidemic diseases. In addition, Hallett explores the nurse's role in the treatment and care of patients with life-threatening infectious diseases at different historical moments and in different places.

In Chapter 15, "Historical Highlights in Disaster Nursing," Barbara Mann Wall and Arlene Keeling continue to use a historical perspective as they examine the role of public health nurses in disasters. Wall and Keeling state that "evidence for practice for disaster management logically comes from history." They turn to history to gain an understanding of what has worked in the past and recognize that nurses' contributions in the past are "often overlooked" and seen as "routine." Wall and Keeling present nurses' responses to several late 19th and 20th century disasters, including the yellow fever epidemic of 1888, the Johnstown flood of 1889, the 1900 Galveston hurricane, the 1918 influenza pandemic, the 1947 Texas City ship explosion, and the 1964 Alaskan earthquake. The experiences learned during these disasters become a rich source of evidence for nurses today addressing modern-day disasters.

Lucille Ferrara, Keith Veltri, and Michela Catalano authored this new Chapter 16, "Emergency Preparedness in the 21st Century: Two Post 9/11 Case Studies." This chapter mirrors some of the historical highlights of disaster nursing while offering the reader a contemporary view of two initiatives that demonstrate emergency preparedness in acute care settings: the "push POD model" and the "pull POD model." The authors discuss and analyze these models and offer suggestions for enhancing emergency preparedness initiatives by bringing public health strategies to acute care settings.

Cathleen Shultz and Karen Kelley address the need to include public health in nursing curricula. Chapter 17, "Nursing Education and Public Health Nursing," challenges nurse educators to respond to the public health needs of society both locally and globally. Shultz and Kelley use their own institution, Hardy University in Searcy, Arkansas, as an example where faculty must create the clinical experiences that integrate public health nursing concepts into the curriculum. Some of the student clinical experiences that Shultz and Kelley present include wellness screening, simulation experiences, disaster drills, mass immunization drill, service learning, faith-based clinic, and school health screening. The chapter explores the shift from a local to a global worldview and looks at concepts of social justice and the culture of poverty. This chapter shows how the various issues and intervention strategies found throughout *Public Health Nursing: Practicing Population-Based Care* can be brought into the classroom to create the nurses we need in the future.

In the final chapter, Truglio-Londrigan, Joanne Singleton, Lewenson, and Liliana Lopez reflect on primary health care and primary care as they relate to the health of the public and public health nursing. Chapter 18, "Conversation About Primary Health Care," speaks to the challenges faced by public health nurses and other public health practitioners. The Declaration of Alma-Ata, with consideration of what this document means in today's world, serves as the centerpiece for this chapter. Discussion of the progress made, as well as of the progress that has yet to be made, takes shape as the reader explores successful international Primary Health Care Initiatives.

Public Health Nursing: Practicing Population-Based Care offers the reader a broad view of public health nursing, encouraging all nurses to consider themselves public health nurses. It is only through the applying and doing of public health nursing that society may attain the goal expressed in the historic 1978 Declaration of Alma-Ata of "Health for All" (International Conference on Primary Health Care, 1978). This call to action reverberates throughout nursing's rich history then and now. An early public health nursing leader, Edna Foley wrote the following in 1921:

Public Health means health for all. . . . Good health is the inalienable right of every citizen, man, woman, or child, and since this vague, almost unknown quality is the right of every citizen, should not good public health nursing be the concern of the laity, as well as of the handful of nurses who are struggling with this big problem? (1991/1922, p. 135)

References

Foley, E. L. (1991/1922). Main issues in public health nursing. In N. Birnbach & S. B. Lewenson (Eds.), *First words: Selected addresses from the National League for Nursing 1894–1933* (pp. 133–137). New York, NY: National League for Nursing.

International Conference on Primary Health Care. (1978). *Declaration of Alma-Ata*. Retrieved from www.who.int/hpr/NPH/docs/declaration_almaata.pdf

Keller, L., Strohschein, S., & Briske, L. (2008). Population-based public health nursing practice: The intervention wheel. In M. Stanhope & J. Lancaster (Eds.), *Public health nursing: Population-centered health care in the community* (pp. 186–214). St. Louis, MO: Mosby-Elsevier.

Minnesota Department of Health, Division of Community Health Services, Public Health Nursing Section. (2001). *Public health interventions: Applications for public health nursing practice*. St. Paul, MN: Minnesota Department of Health.

Rippke, M., Briske, L., Keller, L. O., Strohschein, S., & Simonetti, J. (2001). Public health interventions: Applications for public health nursing practice. *Public Health Nursing Section, Division of Community Health Services, Minnesota Department of Health*. Retrieved from http://www.health.state.mn.us/divs/cfh/ophp/resources/docs/phinterventions_manual2001.pdf

U.S. Department of Health and Human Services. (2010). *About Healthy People*. Retrieved from www.healthypeople.gov/.2020/about/default.aspx

Wald, L. D. (1915). *The house on Henry Street*. New York, NY: Henry Holt & Company.

Acknowledgments

We want to thank the contributors, educators, public health nurses, and students who showed enthusiasm and support for this work. We want to thank our families, too, for giving us the love and support for us to grow! We also want to acknowledge our friendship that thrived throughout the process of editing this exciting second edition. And, finally, we want to thank our publishers who believed in this work and gave it another chance. Thank you all!

Contributors

Carole A. Baraldi, MS, RN
Consultant, Public Health Nurse Educator
New York, NY

Madeline R. Cafiero, MS, RN, FNP, CWOCN
Assistant Professor
The Sage Colleges–Nursing
Troy, NY

Lois O. Carnochan, MS, RN
Coordinator Clinical Undergraduate Programs
School of Nursing
The College of New Rochelle
New Rochelle, NY

Michela Catalano, MD
Director, Occupational Health Services
Montefiore Medical Center
Bronx, NY
Professor of Clinical Medicine
The Albert Einstein College of Medicine
Bronx, NY

Marisa A. Cortese-Peske, RN, MS, PNP
Lienhard School of Nursing
Pace University, College of Health Professions
New York, NY

Mary de Chesnay, DSN, RN, PMHCNS-BC,
  FAAN
Professor, WellStar School of Nursing
Kennesaw State University
Kennesaw, GA

Janna L. Dieckmann, PhD, RN
Clinical Associate Professor
School of Nursing
University of North Carolina at Chapel Hill
Chapel Hill, NC

Lin Drury, PhD, RN
Associate Professor
Co-Chair, Institutional Review Board
Lienhard School of Nursing
Pace University, College of Health Professions
New York, NY

Julie Fairman, PhD, RN, FAAN
Nightingale Professor of Nursing
Director, Barbara Bates Center for the Study of
  the History of Nursing
Robert Wood Johnson Investigator in Health
  Policy Research
University of Pennsylvania School of Nursing
Philadelphia, PA

Lucille Ferrara, EdD, MBA, RN, FNP-BC
Assistant Professor and Program Director,
  Family Nurse Practitioner Program
Pace University, College of Health Professions
Lienhard School of Nursing
Pleasantville, NY
Family Nurse Practitioner, provider
Montefiore FHC
Bronx, NY

Shirley Franco, MSN, FNP
President
NP in Family Health, PC
Mahopac, NY

Deborah Gardner, PhD, RN, FAAN
Senior Advisor, Bureau of Health Professions,
  HRSA
Member of Nursing Economic Editorial Board
Lead for the Policy Column for *Nursing
  Economic$*

Teresa M. Haines, DNP, RN, FNP-BC
Assistant Professor of Nursing
Pace University, College of Health
  Professions
Lienhard School of Nursing
Pleasantville, NY

Christine Hallett, PhD
Professor of Nursing History
The University of Manchester
Manchester, England

Arlene Keeling, PhD, RN, FAAN
Centennial Professor of Nursing
Director for the Center of Historical Nursing
  Inquiry
University of Virginia
Charlottesville, VA

Karen Kelley, MSN, RN
Assistant Professor
College of Nursing
Harding University
Searcy, AR

Martha Kelly, EdD, RN
Associate Professor
Pace University, College of Health Professions
Lienhard School of Nursing
Pleasantville, NY

Sandra B. Lewenson, EdD, RN, FAAN
Professor
Pace University, College of Health
  Professions
Lienhard School of Nursing
Pleasantville, NY

Liliana Lopez, MSN, RN, FNP
Promesa, Inc./Basics, Inc.
Primary Health Care
Former Program Director and Health Provider
Detox/Rehab Promesa "Amanecer"

Margaret Macali, RN, PHCNS-BC
Clinical Assistant Professor
St. Peter's College School of Nursing
Jersey City, NJ
Former Director of Public Health Nursing,
  Bergen County Department of Health
  Services
Bergen County, NJ

Rene McLeod-Sordjan, DNP, CCRN, FNP,
  BC: AAHIVM Board Certified
Assistant Clinical Professor
Pace University, College of Health Professions
Lienhard School of Nursing
New York, NY

Susan Moscou, FNP, MPH, PhD
Associate Professor
Mercy College
Dobbs Ferry, NY

Donna M. Nickitas, PhD, RN, NEA-BC, CNE
Professor
Hunter College, City University of New York
Hunter Bellevue School of Nursing
Deputy Executive Officer
Doctor of Nursing Science
Graduate Center, City of University of New York
Editor, *Nursing Economic$, The Journal for Health Care Leaders*

Irene S. Rempel, BS, RN, LMSW
Instructor
School of Nursing
Long Island College Hospital
Brooklyn, NY

Lisa Seiff, RN, BSN
Prime Care
New York, NY

Cathleen M. Shultz, PhD, CNE, FAAN
Dean
College of Nursing
Harding University
Searcy, AR

Joanne K. Singleton, PhD, RN, FNP, BC
Professor
Chairperson, Department of Graduate Studies
Director, FNP-Doctor of Nursing Practice Program
Pace University, College of Health Professions
Lienhard School of Nursing
New York, NY

Marie Truglio-Londrigan, PhD, RN
Professor
Pace University, College of Health Professions
Lienhard School of Nursing
Pleasantville, NY

Keith Veltri, PharmD
Assistant Professor
Touro College of Pharmacy
New York, NY
Clinical Pharmacy Manager, Family Medicine
   Montefiore Medical Center
Bronx, NY

Adrienne Wald, EdD, MBA, RN, CHES
Director, Wellness Education & Programs
The College of New Rochelle
New Rochelle, NY

Barbara Mann Wall, PhD, RN, FAAN
Associate Professor and Associate Director,
   Barbara Bates Center for the Study of
   History of Nursing
University of Pennsylvania School of Nursing
Philadelphia, PA

Doreen Gallagher Wall, MS, RN, BC
Psychiatric Nurse
Assertive Community Treatment Team
Visiting Nurse Service of New York
New York, NY

Astrid Hellier Wilson, DSN, RN
Professor of Nursing
WellStar School of Nursing
Kennesaw State University
Kennesaw, GA
Member and Secretary, Board of
   Directors, International Honor Society of
   Nursing Building Corporation

Marisa L. Wilson, DNS, MHS, RN-BC
Director, Masters Programs
Assistant Professor, Nursing Informatics
University of Maryland School of Nursing
Baltimore, MD

Reviewers

Kimberly Balko, MS, RN
Empire State College
Saratoga Springs, NY

Emily Barey, MSN, RN
Epic Systems Corporation
Verona, WI

Angeline Bushy
University of Central Florida College of
   Nursing, Daytona Campus
Daytona Beach, FL

Jennell P. Charles, PhD, RN
Clayton State University
Morrow, GA

Kim Clevenger, MSN, RN, BC
Assistant Professor of Nursing
Morehead State University
Morehead, KY

Arlene Rosen, EdD, RN
Assistant Professor
The College of New Rochelle
New Rochelle, NY

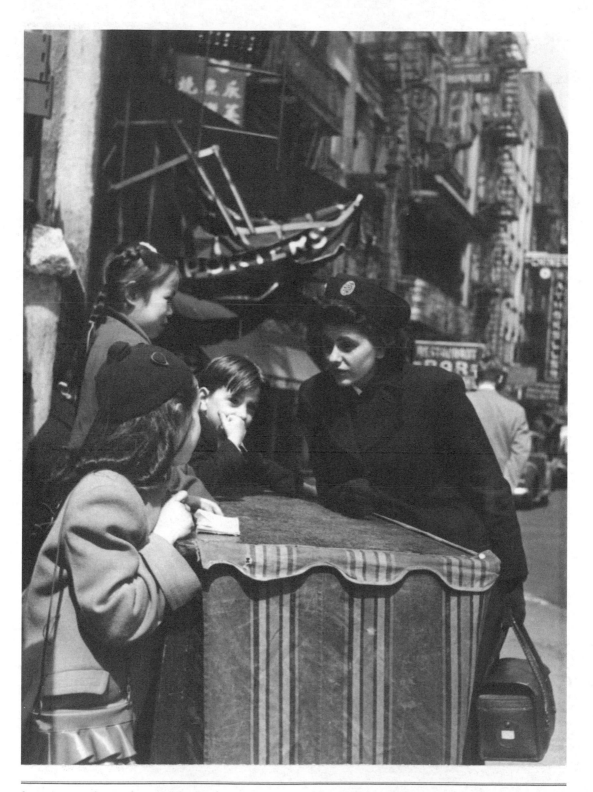

Source: Courtesy of the Visiting Nurse Service of New York.

Chapter 1

What Is Public Health and Public Health Nursing?

Marie Truglio-Londrigan
Sandra B. Lewenson

Recognizing limits to what the health service professions can now do, in relation to common health problems faced everyday, by no means negates the fact that as conditions essential for health are more fully known and are provided and used by individuals and communities, more and more individuals will be enabled to experience greater health (Peplau, 1952, p. 15).

www

LEARNING OBJECTIVES

At the completion of this chapter, the reader will be able to

- Define the meaning of public health and public health nursing.
- Describe what is meant by the terms "care of the public" and "population-based care."
- Describe the vision, mission, overarching goals, topics, and objectives of Healthy People 2020.

- Examine the 10 essential public health services in relation to the core functions of public health practice.
- Examine the role of the public health nurse within the larger context of public health.

www

KEY TERMS

- ❏ Assurance
- ❏ Core functions of public health
- ❏ Essentials of public health
- ❏ Health promotion
- ❏ *Healthy People 2020*

- ❏ Maintaining health
- ❏ Preventing disease
- ❏ Public health
- ❏ Public health nursing
- ❏ Risk reduction

It never fails. Sit around a table and discuss the health of the public or population-based care and one frequently receives blank stares. What is **public health**? What does it mean when one speaks about the health of the "public" or "population-based care"? What is the role of the public health nurse within this larger framework? And who pays for public health? These questions need to be answered for those in practice, and this chapter provides answers to these questions, thus enhancing practitioners' working knowledge of the scientific discipline known as public health. Creating a professional nursing workforce that demonstrates a vigorous practice of integrating culturally congruent nursing actions based on evidence and recognizing the funding streams lay the groundwork for a strong public health infrastructure that will ultimately enhance and sustain the public's health.

Public Health Defined

To fully understand the concept of public health, it is important to review the definitions put forth over time by those in practice. This exercise will assist the reader in knowing and understanding the important characteristics and features of this discipline.

"Public health work is as old as history," wrote J. Howard Beard in 1922. Beard's article, published in *The Scientific Monthly,* charts the early progress of public health starting with the early Egyptians, who filtered mud from the Nile River to create a safer water source for citizens. Throughout history the health of the public has been a concern for local and national governments and all members of society. The public health movement in the United States originated in Boston, Massachusetts, in the mid 1800s when Lemuel Shattuck's noted reports on the healthcare needs of the community became the "blueprint for American health organization"

(Beard, 1922; Scheele, 1949, p. 293). A noted public health leader in the early 20th century, C. E. Winslow (1920), defined public health as follows:

{T}he science and the art of preventing disease, prolonging life, and promoting physical health and efficiency through organized community efforts for the sanitation of the environment, the control of community infections, the education of the individual in principles of personal hygiene, the organization of medical and nursing service for the early diagnosis and preventive treatment of disease, and the development of the social machinery which will ensure to every individual in the community a standard of living adequate for the maintenance of health. (p. 30)

The definition of public health has changed over time to accommodate the needs of American society.

In 1988, the Institute of Medicine (IOM) defined public health as "what we, as a society, do collectively to assure the conditions in which people can be healthy" (IOM, 1988, p. 1). Society collectively works together to provide services generally to a population to prevent disease and to maintain health (Buttery, 1992). The Association of Schools of Public Health's website defines public health as "the science and art of protecting and improving the health of communities through education, promotion of healthy life styles, and research for disease and injury prevention" (n.d., para. 1). In 2003, the IOM published *The Future of the Public's Health in the 21st Century*. This report was comprehensive in nature and spoke to partnerships; intersectoral collaboration; the strengthening of the public health infrastructure, including the building of our nation's public health workforce; and an enhanced understanding of what we mean when we speak of community and population, along with an awareness of the shifting of our demographics (the aging of our population and the shift from acute to chronic care). Another IOM report, titled *For the Public's Health: The Role of Measurement in Action and Accountability* (2010), looks at the critical importance of measurements in summarizing the impact that the health system has on the population, thus emphasizing the importance of outcomes. Although brief, this information serves as a template to remind us of the progressive steps we have taken over the decades.

Populations

When one considers the preceding definitions of public health, one comes to understand that the discussion of health moves beyond the health of the individual, family, and community to the health of the population. For example, Hurricane Katrina hit the U.S. Gulf Coast, with particular destruction in Louisiana, on August 29, 2005. In the weeks that followed, healthcare professionals cared for individuals and their family members who were evacuees without shelter and who had suffered from physical and emotional distress. Brodie, Weltzien, Altman, Blendon, and Benson (2006) surveyed the experiences of the Hurricane Katrina evacuees. Their results provide valuable information for public health professionals, "highlighting challenges of effectively evacuating cities' most at-risk residents during a disaster and providing for long-term health needs of vulnerable populations in the aftermath" (p. 1407). The outcomes of this research also provided important guidelines for public health officials as they planned for future evacuations when disasters hit and discussed how to ensure the protection of the public during this evacuation. **Table 1-1** gives additional examples of how a specific public health intervention, such as education, may vary depending on whether the focus is on individuals, families, populations, or communities.

The concept of caring for populations can be difficult to understand and perhaps serves as a barrier to the way nurses or other healthcare workers are educated and approach care. The noted 20th-century nursing leader Virginia Henderson, when questioned on how one could nurse an aggregate, said, "I think it impossible to nurse an aggregate effectively until you have effectively nursed individuals and acquired considerable judgment as to what helps clients or patients prevent disease, cope with it, or die with dignity when death is inevitable" (Abrams, 2007, p. 384). This question has been raised many times in hopes of understanding what a population means and what it means to care for a population. Definitions of "populations" illustrate characteristics and features specific to public health. Williams and Stanhope (2008) define a population or aggregate as "a collection of individuals who have one or more personal or environmental characteristics in common" (p. 11). The Association of Community Health Nursing Educators, as demonstrated in Levin et al. (2007), uses the same definition as Williams and Stanhope. The American Nurses Association (2007) builds on the definition of population as "those living in a specific geographic area (e.g., a neighborhood, community, city, or county) or those in a particular group (e.g., racial, ethnic, age, disease) who experience a disproportionate burden of poor health care outcomes" (p. 5).

Henderson's concern about nursing populations versus nursing individuals may stem from her concern about the division in health care that separates the care of populations from the care of individuals. Henderson asked, "Should we have one category of health workers treating disease and another preventing it? Or should we all be trying primarily to prevent disease, and, even while treating it, to be helping the victim to prevent a recurrence?" (Abrams, 2007, p. 384). Changing definitions of **public health**

Table 1-1 Examples of the "Educational" Interventions for Individuals, Families, Populations, and Communities

	Individual	Family	Population	Community
	Refers to individual clients, who may be part of a family, a population, and live in a community.	Refers to a family system, which may be defined as any or all individuals who live in what they consider a family system.	Refers to a defined number of people.	Refers to individuals, families, populations, and organizations (for-profit and not-for-profit) that may or may not share the same ideas, values, beliefs, and/or physical location, but do intervene and network with each other.
Lyme disease prevention and early detection programs	Target the client (e.g., young adult gardeners) and provide education about Lyme disease, its cause, and methods of prevention, such as pulling socks over pants and wearing repellent. This education can be provided in a pamphlet and placed in areas where individuals may pick it up and read it, such as pharmacies and gardening supply stores.	Target families and provide education for caretakers of children about the cause of Lyme disease and methods of prevention. This information may be developed and delivered in magazines available in primary care practitioner offices or at organizations such as Boys and Girls Clubs of America.	Target the population and provide education for the public about Lyme disease. This information may be developed and delivered on signs in high risk areas (such as hiking trails) or in special service announcements on the radio.	A healthy community ensures that a hiking trail in their geographical area is clear of brush and that appropriate signs are posted warning of high risk areas. A healthy community will also ensure that funding is available to sustain these endeavors.
Child car seat prevention programs	Target the child, using developmentally appropriate play strategies that illustrate use of child car seats and booster seats.	Target caretakers (e.g., parents, grandparents, day care workers), educating them about the importance of using child car seats, with pamphlets and videos in preschools.	Target populations through the use of billboards highlighting the importance of appropriate use of child car seats.	A healthy community will have strong organizations that provide programs to support use of child car seats. For example: a local hospital may stage a "drive through" child car seat safety check; a fire department may install safety car seats for newborns.

nursing explore the dichotomy between care of the individual and the aggregate.

Preventing Disease and Maintaining Health

Other important characteristics of public health are **preventing disease** and **maintaining health**. Care is the main focus of public health nurses and practitioners, with an emphasis on **health promotion** and **risk reduction**. To understand these concepts fully, public health nurses can turn to the historic work of Leavell and Clark (1965), who note, "The ultimate objectives of all medical, dental, and public health practice, whether carried out in the office, the clinic, the laboratory, or the community-at-large, are the promotion of health, the prevention of disease, and the prolongation of life" (p. 14).

According to Leavell and Clark's (1965) seminal work, there are three levels of prevention. The first level, primary prevention, includes interventions designed to promote health via health promotion strategies and to specifically protect the individual from disease "by providing immunizations and reducing exposure to occupational hazards, carcinogens, and other environmental health risks" (Greiner & Edelman, 2006, p. 17). These interventions take place before the presence of disease and disability, in the period known as the prepathogenesis period. The second level of prevention, which occurs in the period of pathogenesis, takes place once disease is present. Interventions include screening activities and early treatment to prevent the consequences of advanced disease, such as disabilities. Finally, the third level of prevention includes rehabilitation intervention strategies; "This is more than stopping a disease process; it is also the prevention of complete disability. . . . Its positive objective is to return the affected individual to a useful place in society and make maximum use of his remain-ing capacities" (Leavell & Clark, 1965, p. 26). **Figure 1-1** offers a pictorial view of the natural history of any disease.

Today, public health nursing activities in primary, secondary, and tertiary prevention have evolved and take into consideration the idea that health is not linear; in fact, if a person requires tertiary rehabilitative services, health promotion strategies are still important. The question Henderson raised earlier speaks to this nonlinear approach and encourages public health nurses to think about providing care for disease while simultaneously promoting health.

Multiple Disciplines

The definitions of public health thus far given demonstrate the collective nature of public health and the need for multiple disciplines to work together in ensuring the health of the public. **Figure 1-2** is a visual depiction of this.

The IOM speaks to this collective endeavor as a process that must involve multiple individuals and multiple organizations: "The concept of a public health system describes a complex network of individuals and organizations that have the potential to play critical roles in creating the conditions for health. They can act for health individually, but when they work together toward a health goal, they act as a system—a public health system" (2003, p. 28). The IOM further describes participants as "actors" in the public health system. Actors include the governmental public health infrastructure, such as local and state departments of health; the healthcare delivery system; academia; and communities; in turn, communities may include schools, religious organizations, and other not-for-profit organizations, just to name a few. In addition, businesses and corporations are considered important actors because they too play a role in influencing population health with regard to the working conditions and healthcare

Figure 1-1 Levels of prevention.

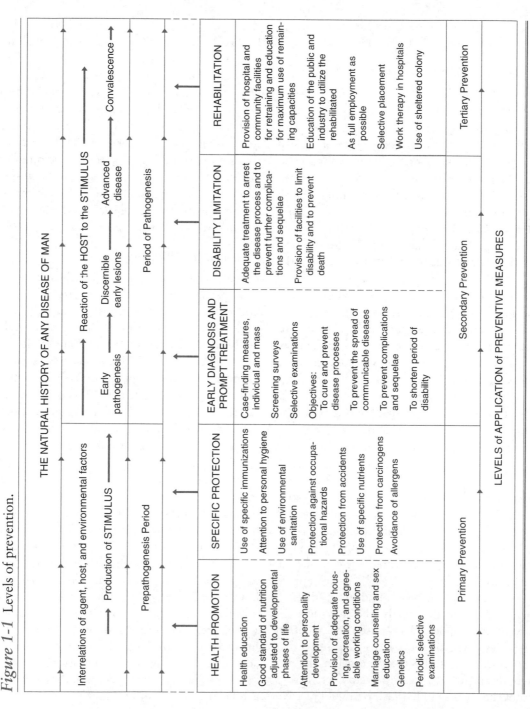

THE NATURAL HISTORY OF ANY DISEASE OF MAN

Interrelations of agent, host, and environmental factors

→ Production of STIMULUS →   → Reaction of the HOST to the STIMULUS →

Prepathogenesis Period

Early pathogenesis → Discernible early lesions → Advanced disease → Convalescence

Period of Pathogenesis

HEALTH PROMOTION	SPECIFIC PROTECTION	EARLY DIAGNOSIS AND PROMPT TREATMENT	DISABILITY LIMITATION	REHABILITATION
Health education	Use of specific immunizations	Case-finding measures, individual and mass	Adequate treatment to arrest the disease process and to prevent further complications and sequelae	Provision of hospital and community facilities for retraining and education for maximum use of remaining capacities
Good standard of nutrition adjusted to developmental phases of life	Attention to personal hygiene	Screening surveys	Provision of facilities to limit disability and to prevent death	Education of the public and industry to utilize the rehabilitated
Attention to personality development	Use of environmental sanitation	Selective examinations		As full employment as possible
Provision of adequate housing, recreation, and agreeable working conditions	Protection against occupational hazards	Objectives: To cure and prevent disease processes		Selective placement
Marriage counseling and sex education	Protection from accidents	To prevent the spread of communicable diseases		Work therapy in hospitals
Genetics	Use of specific nutrients	To prevent complications and sequelae		Use of sheltered colony
Periodic selective examinations	Protection from carcinogens	To shorten period of disability		
	Avoidance of allergens			

Primary Prevention		Secondary Prevention		Tertiary Prevention

LEVELS of APPLICATION of PREVENTIVE MEASURES

Source: Leavell, H., & Clark, A. E. (1965). Preventive medicine for doctors in the community (3rd ed.). New York: McGraw-Hill, p. 21. Reproduced with permission.

Figure 1-2 The intersectorial public health system.

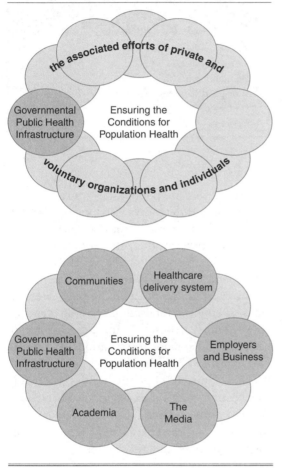

Source: Institute of Medicine, 2003.

benefits they provide. Finally, the IOM identifies the media as important actors in the public healthcare system. Consider the impact that the media can have with their ability to reach populations through the various media streams. Ultimately, public health system actors, with their integrative and participatory roles, serve as a reminder of the historic Declaration of Alma-Ata International Conference (1978) that

recognized primary health care as a major strategy for achieving health for all. At this historic international conference, participants expressed a need for all governments and other international organizations to engage in actions that would ensure the implementation of primary health care around the world. The Declaration of Alma-Ata International Conference (1978) described and explained primary health care as follows:

> {R}equires and promotes maximum community and individual selfreliance and participation in the planning, organization, operation and control of primary health care, making fullest use of local, national and other available resources; and to this end develops through appropriate education the ability of communities to participate. (para. 12)

Ensure the Public's Health

Working together as actors is important, but the ability to ensure the health of the public is critical. How does one ensure the health of the public? The involvement and role of the government are important in this regard. The IOM (2003) speaks to this very issue:

> In the United States, the government's responsibility for the health of its citizens stems, in part, from the nature of democracy itself. Health officials are either directly elected or appointed by democratically-elected officials. To the extent, therefore, that citizens place a high priority on health, these elected officials are held accountable to ensure that the government is able to monitor the population's health and intervene when necessary through laws, policies, regulations, and expenditure of the resources necessary for the health and safety of the public. (p. 101)

The public cannot be healthy without strong governmental support of the services that keep the public healthy. Late-19th and early-20th-century public health nursing leaders—such as Lillian Wald and Mary Brewster, who began the Henry Street Settlement in the Lower East Side of New York City—recognized the need to garner government support for their efforts to improve the health of the immigrant population that flooded the streets of New York during this period. As they visited the homes of the families in the community, Wald and Brewster's public health nurses wore official badges showing endorsement by the New York Board of Health (Buhler-Wilkerson, 2001). Wald, along with the other public health nurses, continued to advocate for playgrounds for children in the community, school nurses in the public schools, and votes for women as a means of ensuring the public's health (Lewenson, 2007). Suffragist and public health nurse Lavinia Dock equated the ability to vote with the ability to improve health. In an early issue of the *American Journal of Nursing,* Dock (1908) asks nurses to consider the value of the women's vote, saying, "[T]ake the present question of the underfed school children in New York. How many of them will have tuberculosis? If mothers and nurses had votes there might be school lunches for all those children" (p. 926).

Service

Finally, the definitions of public health mention the types of services to be provided—for example, the importance of education as a service. Providing services, which can be of various types, to a population can be approached in many ways, and it is for the readers and practitioners of public health to define the types of services. This text, for example, features the application of the Minnesota Department of Health Population-Based Public Health Nursing Practice Intervention Wheel Strategies. This wheel contains 17 intervention strategies

> **BOX 1-1 OVERVIEW OF KEY CHARACTERISTICS AND FEATURES OF PUBLIC HEALTH**
>
> Population-based
> Preventing disease
> Maintaining health
> Multiple disciplines
> Assurance
> Services

or services that are population-focused and can be applied to different levels of practice, including individuals, families, communities, and systems. Most recently, this intervention wheel was noted to be the basis for the SPHERE system framework, which (1) suggests that case finding be included as one of the individual interventions, raising the total number of interventions to 18, and (2) presents subinterventions for each of the 18 major interventions (Wisconsin Department of Health, 2011).

The definitions of public health presented in this chapter highlight certain key characteristics and features. **Box 1-1** presents an overview of these key characteristics and features that are further explained in later chapters.

Public Health Nursing

Public health nurses play a central role in supporting the health of the public. Chapter 2 is dedicated to the history of public health nursing, showing the development of this role over time. Public health nursing, a term first coined in the late 19th century by nursing leader Lillian Wald (Buhler-Wilkerson, 1993), included the roles of "health visitor, health teacher, social worker and even health inspector" (Crandall, 1922, p. 645).

Crandall wrote that these roles evolved based on the rich foundation of nursing (Crandall, 1922). This strong nursing background continues today as public health nursing serves the health of the public.

In a statement originally published in 1996, the American Public Health Association, Public Health Nursing Section (2011) defined public health nursing as a practice that is affected by ". . . biological, cultural, environmental, economic, social, and political factors. As part of the healthcare system public health nursing practice is responsive to these factors through working with the community to promote health and prevent disease, injury, and disability" (para. 2). The Missouri Department of Health and Senior Services (2006) uses the following contemporary definition of public health nursing as:

> *the practice of promoting and protecting the health of populations using knowledge from nursing, social, and public health sciences. Public health nursing is a systematic process by which the health and the health care needs of a population are: 1) assessed in order to identify individuals, families, and populations health care needs, 2) a plan for intervention is developed with the community to meet the identified needs, 3) evaluations are conducted to determine the extent to which the intervention has an impact on the health status of the individual, family, and the population, and 4) the results of the process are used to influence and direct the current delivery of care. (p. 8)*

What the reader may glean from this is that public health nursing by definition mirrors the general definitions of public health, with an emphasis on the systematic process that nurses use to "do" their work. This process is the nursing process. Therefore, throughout this text the reader will note that the nursing process is the guiding framework for assessing the needs of the population, diagnosing the needs of the population, planning interventions based in evidence using the intervention wheel, implementing those strategies, and ultimately evaluating outcomes of the population. The preceding definition of public health nursing also notes how results of the process are used to influence and direct the current healthcare delivery system, therefore making assurances to the public when results and outcomes are positive that these outcomes will be sustained over time. The readers of this text will find it useful to access *The Public Health Nursing: Scope and Standards of Practice* (American Nurses Association, 2007). This document serves as a detailed outline of the role and expectations of the public health nurse. This document is also helpful in that is serves as a guide and offers direction for the public health nurse's professional and noble practice.

Public Health Now

For centuries, diseases such as the Black Death, leprosy, smallpox, tuberculosis, and influenza terrorized the population with extraordinary death tolls. Similarly, for centuries it was assumed that nothing could be done about these little-understood outbreaks because they were a message from the supernatural that was, in some way, dissatisfied with humans. Since these earlier times, the scientific discipline of public health has made remarkable strides, noted by the decrease in communicable diseases along with the marked improvements in sanitation efforts (Beard, 1922).

In recent years, communicable and infectious diseases such as H1N1 have experienced a resurgence, along with a renewed cry to strengthen the public health infrastructure in the United States. Problems such as chronic illnesses; obesity; a healthcare system in which cost of care is out of control, coupled with populations with no or limited health insurance; health disparities; the stripping of the environment; rising mental health issues; and violence and terrorism clearly inform public health professionals of the need for a call to action. The Institute of Medicine (2003) spoke about the IOM 1988 report and stated that the earlier report "presented strong evidence to indicate that the governmental public health infrastructure was in disarray" (IOM, 2003, p. xi).

Ten Essential Public Health Services

Historically, public health professionals have responded to the call to action by making changes and progress in meeting the needs of the public. One outcome was the development of the 10 essential public health services by the Public Health Functions Steering Committee (U.S. Department of Health and Human Services [DHHS] Public Health Service, 1994a). This steering committee included representatives from U.S. Public Health Service agencies and other major public health organizations. The 10 **essentials of public health** provide a guiding framework for the responsibilities of local public health systems and the foundation for strategy-building toward a healthy, integrated public health system capable of ensuring the health of the public. **Box 1-2** presents these 10 essential public health services, which include the key characteristics and features noted in the previous definitions of public health.

Three Core Functions

Each of these 10 essential services falls under one of the three **core functions of public health**: assessment, policy development, and **assurance** (IOM, 1988). To assess the health of the population for early identification of health problems and/or other potential problems, a public health agency must collect and analyze data systematically. The policy devel-

---

BOX 1-2 THE TEN ESSENTIAL PUBLIC HEALTH SERVICES

1. Monitor health status to identify community health problems.
2. Diagnose and investigate health problems and health hazards in the community.
3. Inform, educate, and empower people about health issues.
4. Mobilize community partnerships to identify and solve health problems.
5. Develop policies and plans that support individual and community health efforts.
6. Enforce laws and regulations that protect health and ensure safety.
7. Link people to needed personal health services and ensure the provision of health care when otherwise unavailable.
8. Ensure a competent public health and personal healthcare workforce.
9. Evaluate effectiveness, accessibility, and quality of personal and population-based health services.
10. Conduct research to attain new insights and innovative solutions to health problems.

Source: U.S. Department of Health and Human Services Public Health Service, 1994a.

---

opment function means that public health agencies serve the public by developing public health policies, based on evidence, for the correction of issues or problems. Finally, assurance requires that public health agencies provide services directly or through other private or public agencies. In addition, assurance guarantees services for those unable to afford them. These three core functions guide the public health professional in the development, implementation, and evaluation of various public processes that assist in meeting the healthcare needs of the public (**Figure 1-3**).

Figure 1-3 Three core functions of public health.

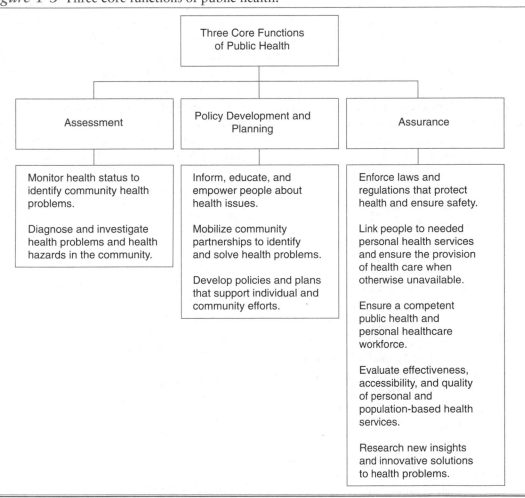

Source: Adapted from Institute of Medicine, 1988. U.S. Department of Health and Human Services, 1994b.

Healthy People 2020

The three core functions of public health and the 10 essential public health services provide the foundation for the health agenda for the nation, known as **Healthy People 2020**. *Healthy People 2020* is a continuation of previous initiatives that began in 1979 when the report *Healthy People: The Surgeon General's Report on Health Promotion and Disease Prevention* was released, which provided national goals for reducing premature deaths and preserving independence for older adults. *Healthy People 2020* was unveiled on December 2, 2010, and this ongoing work documents the evolving nature of public health through the systematic use of overarching goals, topics, and objectives that facilitate action. *Healthy People 2020* "provides science-based, 10-year national objectives for improving the health of all Americans" (U.S. DHHS, 2010a, para. 1). This document serves as a guide for healthcare professionals and their partners as they decide collectively what types of health initiatives to engage in and how to implement and evaluate these initiatives. These partners are central to the success of the *Healthy People 2020* agenda: "Addressing the challenge of health improvement is a shared responsibility that requires the active participation and leadership of the Federal Government, States, local governments, policy makers, healthcare providers, professionals, business executives, educators, community leaders, and the American public itself" (U.S. DHHS, 2000, p. 4).

This resonates with the need mentioned earlier for intersectoral and collective work of public health practitioners. Public health nurses are important actors in this collective work and have historically been present in public health initiatives. The *Healthy People 2020* website is interactive and a powerful tool for all stakeholders. Readers can find more information on this initiative at http://www.healthypeople.gov/2020/default.aspx.

The Graphic Model for *Healthy People 2020* is shown in **Figure** 1-4. This depiction of the determinants of health includes physical environment, health services, social environment, individual behavior, and biology and genetics. Although this model does not show policymaking as one of the concentric circles, policymaking is described as a determinant of health on the website (U.S. DHHS, 2010b). The authors of this text expanded the Graphic Model for *Healthy People 2020,* including this additional determinant of policymaking. They developed the visual depiction called the Process Model for *Healthy People 2020* (Process Model) that readers can view on the inside cover of this text. This visual depiction was developed as a broader representa-

tion of the work in which health professionals must engage if they are to achieve the overarching goals of *Healthy People 2020.* In addition, as a comparison, the authors of this text include in the appendix the earlier representation of this model, which was titled Systematic Approach to Health Improvement.

The multiple components of the Process Model depict the entire process, not just the determinants of health. The outcome of this model is the promotion and improvement of the health of the general public. Following is a list of these important components:

- Vision
- Mission
- Overarching goals
- Topics and objectives
- Four foundation health measures
- General health status
- Health-related quality of life
- Determinants of health
- Physical environment
- Health services
- Social environment
- Individual behavior
- Biology and genetics
- Policymaking
- Disparities

VISION AND MISSION

Box 1-3 includes the vision and mission of *Healthy People 2020.* The vision statement is critical because it creates the point on the horizon to which all stakeholders set their sights in their combined efforts to achieve public health. The mission of *Healthy People 2020* is to identify how the vision is realized. It essentially guides the action of the stakeholders.

OVERARCHING GOALS

The earlier *Healthy People 2010* included two goals: (1) to increase the quality of years of

Figure 1-4 Screenshot of the Graphic Model for Healthy People 2020.

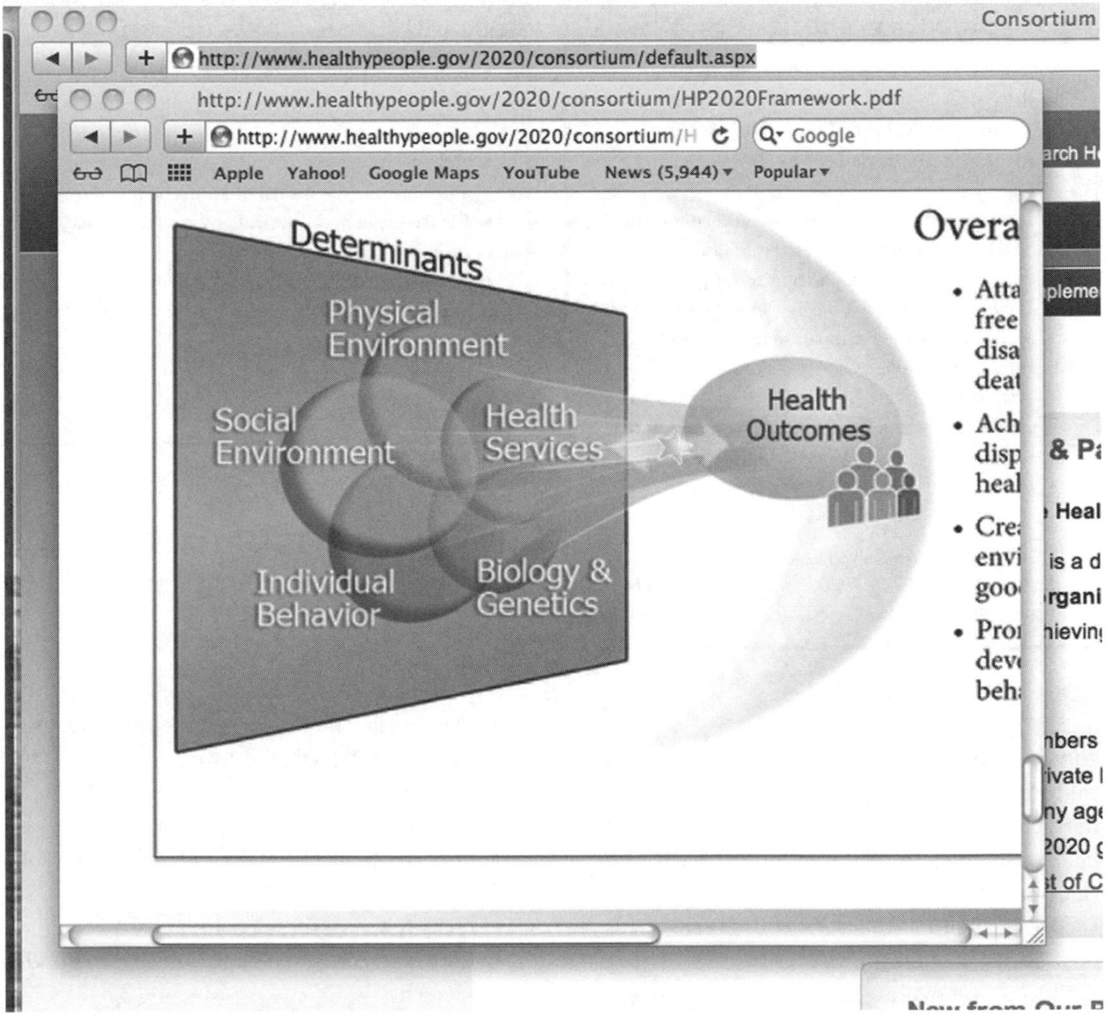

Source: U.S. Department of Health and Human Services. (2010a). *About Healthy People.* Retrieved from www.healthypeople.gov/2020/Consortium/HP2020Framework.pdf

healthy life, and (2) to eliminate health disparities. The first goal also addressed life expectancy, defined as "the average number of years people born in a given year [were] expected to live based on a set of age-specific death rates" (U.S. DHHS, 2000, p. 8). This goal speaks to the need for not only extending life, but also for improving the quality of those years lived. The second goal addressed the health disparities evident among various U.S. demographic groups, including groups based on "gender, race or ethnicity, education or income, disability, geographic location, or sexual orientation" (U.S. DHHS, 2000, p. 11). An awareness of the existence of these disparities

BOX 1-3 *HEALTHY PEOPLE 2020* VISION AND MISSION

Vision: A society in which all people live long, healthy lives.

Mission: *Healthy People 2020* strives to:

- Identify nationwide health-improvement priorities
- Increase public awareness and understanding of the determinants of health, disease, and disability and the opportunities for progress
- Provide measurable objectives and goals that are applicable at the national, state, and local levels
- Engage multiple sectors to take actions to strengthen policies and improve practices that are driven by the best available evidence and knowledge
- Identify critical research, evaluation, and data collection needs

Source: U.S. Department of Health and Human Services. (2010b). *Healthy People 2020 framework.* Retrieved from http://www.healthypeople.gov/2020/about/default.aspx

BOX 1-4 *HEALTHY PEOPLE 2020:* OVERARCHING GOALS

- Attain high-quality, longer lives free of preventable disease, disability, injury, and premature death.
- Achieve health equity, eliminate disparities, and improve the health of all groups.
- Create social and physical environments that promote good health for all.
- Promote quality of life, healthy development, and healthy behaviors across all life stages.

Source: U.S. Department of Health and Human Services. (2010b). *Healthy People 2020 framework.* Retrieved from http://www.healthypeople.gov/2020/about/default.aspx

and an understanding of their etiology are critical for public health professionals and their partners to develop initiatives to create a balanced healthcare system in which health parity rather than health disparity is the rule.

Presently, in *Healthy People 2020* the goals are now termed overarching goals, of which there are four. The overarching goals were developed with a twofold purpose: to develop the objectives and to assist the stakeholders in their work to achieve the stated objectives. See **Box 1-4** for the new overarching goals.

TOPICS AND OBJECTIVES

In *Healthy People 2010,* the nation's progress in achieving the two goals was measured through 467 objectives in 28 focus areas. *Healthy People 2020* includes 39 topic areas with objectives,

and others are still evolving (U.S. DHHS, 2010c, para. 8). The current initiative includes the following new topic areas:

- Adolescent Health
- Blood Disorders and Blood Safety
- Dementias, including Alzheimer's Disease
- Early and Middle Childhood
- Genomics
- Global Health
- Health-Related Quality of Life and Well-Being
- Healthcare Associated Infections
- Lesbian, Gay, Bisexual, and Transgender Health
- Older Adults
- Preparedness
- Sleep Health
- Social Determinants of Health

Public health nurses can use *Healthy People 2020* as a tool to create health initiatives to address public health goals. Suppose a public health nurse conducts an assessment and identifies tobacco smoking as a major problem in a population of adolescents in a particular community. The public health nurse identifies the topic area as "Tobacco Use." On the home page of the *Healthy People 2020* interactive website (see **Figure 1-5**), in the row of tabs across the top of the page, is a tab labeled 2020 Topics and Objectives. By clicking the tab, the public health nurse can view a list of the 39 topics, one of which is "Tobacco Use." Once the public health nurse clicks into the "Tobacco Use" topic area, he or she will note three tabs along the top: Overview, Objective, and Interventions. The Overview tab includes links to the following topics: goal, overview, related topic areas, why preventing tobacco use is important, and

a framework for ending tobacco use, as well as other important information (see **Figure 1-6**). It also includes a reference list that offers evidence to support this particular topic area and objective.

The Objective tab presents the 20 objectives (see **Figure 1-7**). One of the objectives is directed toward adolescents and is presented as follows:

- TU-2 Reduce tobacco use by adolescents.

Directly underneath this major objective are four subobjectives. These include:

- TU-2.1 Tobacco products (past 30 days)
- TU-2.2 Cigarettes (past 30 days)

Figure 1-5 Main page of *Healthy People 2020*.

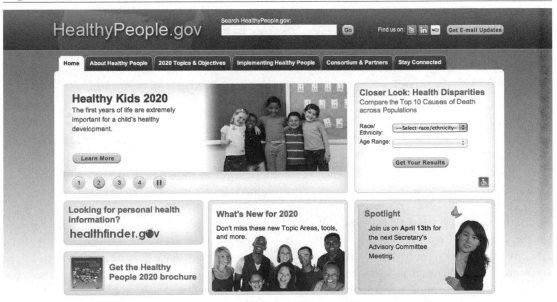

Source: U.S. Department of Health and Human Services. (2010d). *Healthy People.* Retrieved from www.healthypeople.gov/2020/default.aspx

Figure 1-6 Healthy People 2020 topics and objectives: Overview.

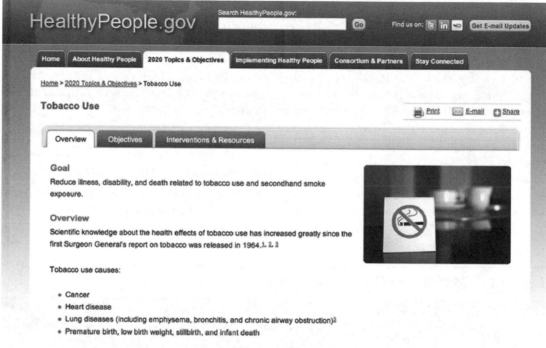

Source: U.S. Department of Health and Human Services. (2010e). *2020 topics & objectives: Tobacco use: Overview.* Retrieved from www.healthypeople.gov/2020/topicsobjectives2020/overview.aspx?topicid=41

- TU-2.3 Smokeless tobacco products (past 30 days)
- TU-2.4 Cigars (past 30 days)

Each of these four subobjectives includes a baseline, a target, a target-setting method, and a data source. It is important for the reader to note that *Healthy People 2020* is a living document and as such changes continually with new evidence, stakeholder interest, and participants.

Finally, the Interventions and Resources tab offers the public health nurse direct links to clinical recommendations for evidence-based community intervention strategies and consumer information (see **Figure 1-8**).

FOUR FOUNDATIONAL HEALTH MEASURES

The final component is the Four Foundational Health Measures found in *Healthy People 2020* and the Process Model. These foundational measures include General Health Status, Health-Related Quality of Life and Well-Being, Determinants of Health, and Disparities. Each of these health measures forms the basis of the Public Health Nursing Assessment Tool that is introduced and discussed in great detail in Chapter 3 of this text.

Application to Communities

How do public health nurses apply and use *Healthy People 2020* for a community of interest?

Figure 1-7 *Healthy People 2020* topics and objectives: Objective.

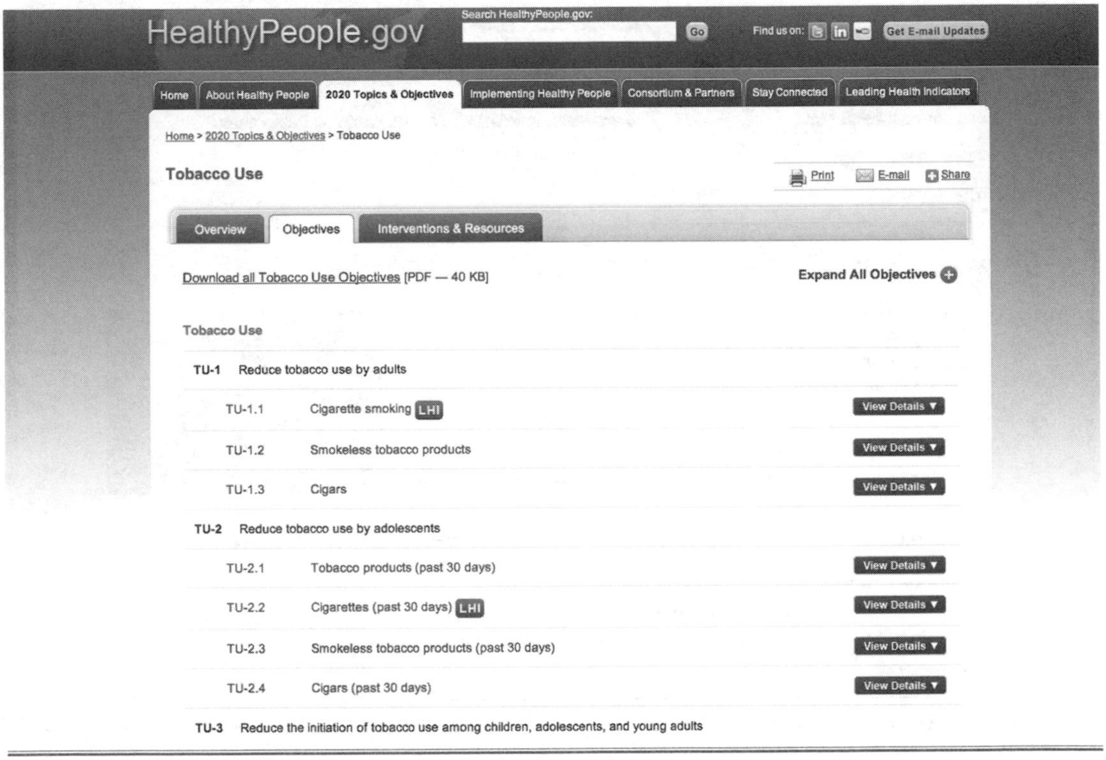

Source: U.S. Department of Health and Human Services. (2010f). *2020 topics & objectives: Tobacco use: Objectives.* Retrieved from www.healthypeople.gov/2020/topicsobjectives2020/objectiveslist.aspx?topicid=41

Public health nurses and their partners can apply *Healthy People in Healthy Communities.* The U.S. DHHS (2001) presented this document in an attempt to enlist communities to use *Healthy People 2020* as a tool to ensure a healthy population locally. A healthy community is defined as "one that embraces the belief that health is more than merely an absence of disease; a healthy community includes those elements that enable people to maintain a high quality of life and productivity" (U.S. DHHS, 2001, p. 1).

To become a healthy community and to implement *Healthy People 2020,* the public health nurse and members of the community must work together using multiple strategies. One such strategy is to use MAPIT, a mnemonic for Mobilize, Assess, Plan, Implement, and Track (U.S. DHHS, 2001, 2010h). MAPIT is a broader application of the nursing process. In addition to assessment, diagnosis, planning, implementation, and evaluation, the MAPIT process includes the critical step of mobilization, which sets the stage for coalition, collaboration, and group decision making to occur. The Process Model depicted on the inside front cover of this text also presents the MAPIT process and demonstrates how it is aligned with the entire Process Model. The first step in MAPIT

Figure 1-8 *Healthy People 2020* topics and objectives: Interventions and resources.

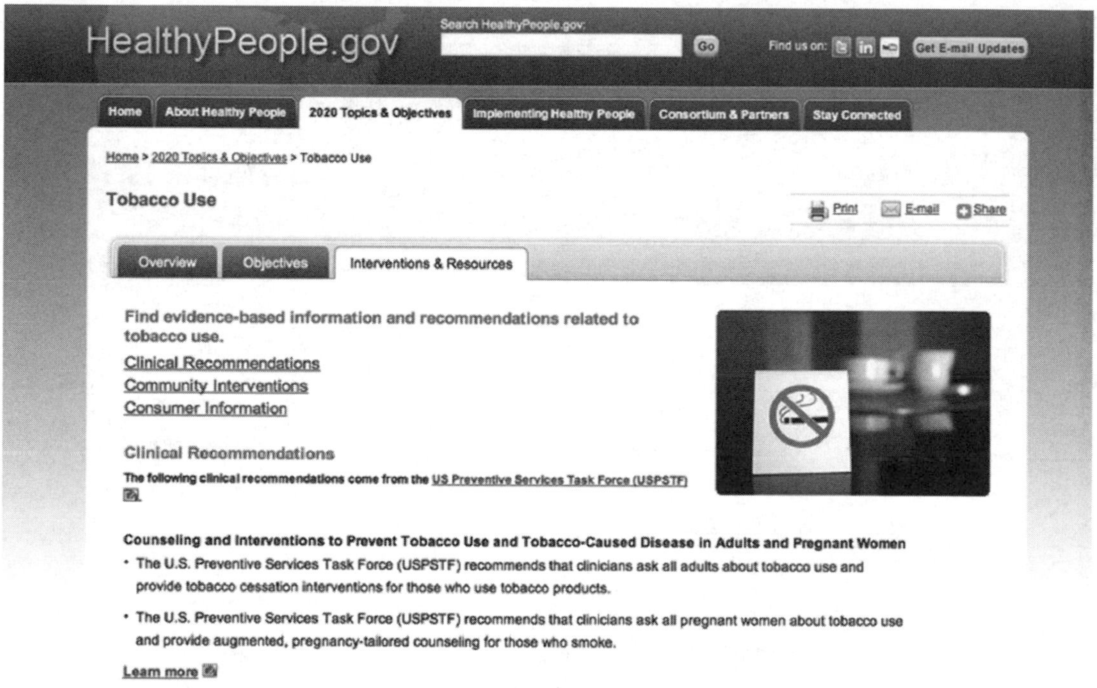

Source: U.S. Department of Health and Human Services. (2010g). *2020 topics & objectives: Tobacco use: Interventions and Resources.* Retrieved from www.healthypeople.gov/2020/topicsobjectives2020/ebr.aspx?topicid=41

is to mobilize. One way to mobilize a group is through partnering with others and developing a coalition. Truglio-Londrigan (2008) notes, "This coming together to work together brings the notion of making decisions together. Group decision making, therefore, allows individual [sic] to come together in a partnership to work toward a goal and ultimately achieve their vision" (p. 131). In this case, the vision is a healthier community.

The next step in the MAPIT technique is to assess the community of interest. Chapter 3 contains detailed information on assessment of a community and population. There are a number of ways to assess a community, both quantitatively and qualitatively. What is important is

that assessment is the collection of data to identify the priority needs of the community. Those who have been mobilized, including the community participants, must look at the data collected and identify whether the issues are in line with one or more of the topic areas listed in *Healthy People 2020*. If yes, the community members can then use *Healthy People 2020* as a guide for the development of initiatives.

Once an issue is identified, the mobilized group moves on to the third step, the development of the plan. The plan takes into consideration resources such as funding, people, technology, methods of communication, and time. It is critical that those involved work with the topic areas and the objectives, with particular emphasis on the baseline, target, target-setting method, and data source for the identified topic area of need. Specific steps need to be developed, along with time frames and the clear identification of who is responsible for which portions of the plan. It is very important to remember that the community participants must be included in the development of this plan, as being inclusive accounts for the various social, political, economic, and cultural factors that affect the plan. Successful plans are culturally congruent with the values, beliefs, and needs of the population and are based in evidence. Plan development uses the intervention strategies found on the Minnesota Department of Health Population-Based Public Health Nursing Practice Intervention Wheel Strategies.

Once the plan is identified, the next step in the MAPIT technique is to implement the plan. Again, clear communication between and among all members is important so that every member knows who is responsible for which activities. For this communication to be effective, one must remember, "There is no 'power over' in a coalition, only 'power with.' . . . This requires equal empowerment of all members of the coalition in order for the members to communicate and work together" (Truglio-Londrigan, 2008, p. 135). The application of technology to reach populations is critical to consider in the implementation phase, and the technology applied must be appropriate for the population in question. Methods for tracking progress during the implementation process are also important to consider.

The final step in the MAPIT technique is to track progress and evaluate movement toward the outcomes. What was the original baseline? Was the target reached? Sharing success is critical. If there is a need to improve, then all members of the group, including community members, must analyze what transpired. Were the initial data collected correctly? Was the plan accessible and appropriate? What changes need to be made? How will the new plan be implemented and evaluated? These are just some questions that should be asked. As mentioned earlier, the MAPIT strategy is presented in the *Healthy People 2020* Process Model located on the inside front cover of this text. It is placed there to enhance clarity for users.

Public health nurses must become familiar with the *Healthy People 2020* website, especially the Implementing *Healthy People 2020* tab, which offers guidelines and resources for the MAPIT process.

Conclusion

This chapter serves as a guiding framework. It discusses public health and the nation's agenda to achieve a society in which people live long and healthy lives (U.S. DHHS, 2010a). This framework demonstrates how to incorporate the public health nursing agenda into the nation's agenda. Chapter 3 uses this guiding framework to design the Public Health Nursing Assessment Tool. Later chapters are based on the Minnesota Department of Health Population-Based Public Health Nursing Practice Intervention Wheel Strategies, which serve as a template for action for the profession and are models by which public health nurses can guide their own practice.

References

Abrams, S. E. (2007). Nursing the community, a look back at the 1984 dialogue between Virginia Henderson and Sherry L. Shamansky. *Public Health Nursing, 24*(4), 382–386.

American Nurses Association. (2007). *Public health nursing: Scope and standards of practice.* Silver Springs, MD: American Nurses Association.

American Public Health Association, Public Health Nursing Section. (2011). *A statement of APHA public health nursing section (1996) definition and background.* Retrieved from http://www.apha.org/membergroups/sections/aphasections/phn/about/defbackground.htm

Association of Schools of Public Health. (n.d.). *What is public health?* Retrieved from http://www.whatispublichealth.org/what/index.html

Beard, J. H. (1922). Progress of public health work. *Scientific Monthly, 14*(2), 140–152.

Brodie, M., Weltzien, E., Altman, D., Blendon, R., & Benson, J. (2006). Experiences of hurricane Katrina evacuees in Houston shelters: Implications for future planning. *American Journal of Public Health, 96*(8), 1402–1408.

Buhler-Wilkerson, K. (1993). Bringing care to the people: Lillian Wald's legacy to public health nursing. *American Journal of Public Health, 83*(12), 1778–1786.

Buhler-Wilkerson, K. (2001). *No place like home: A history of nursing and home care in the United States.* Baltimore, MD: Johns Hopkins University Press.

Buttery, C. M. G. (1992). Provision of public health services. In J. M. Last & R. B. Wallace (Eds.), *Public health and preventive medicine* (13th ed., pp. 1113–1128). Norwalk, CT: Appleton & Lange.

Crandall, E. P. (1922). An historical sketch of public health nursing. *American Journal of Nursing, 22*(8), 641–645.

Declaration of Alma-Ata International Conference on Primary Care. (1978). *Primary health care.* Retrieved from http://www. who.int/hpr/NPH/docs/declaration_almaata.pdf

Dock, L. (1908). The suffrage question. *American Journal of Nursing, 8*(11), 925–927.

Greiner, P., & Edelman, C. (2006). Health defined: Objectives for promotion and prevention. In C. Edelman & C. Mandle (Eds.), *Health promotion throughout the life span* (pp. 3–22). St. Louis, MO: Elsevier Mosby.

Institute of Medicine. (1988). *The future of public health.* Washington, DC: National Academies Press.

Institute of Medicine. (2003). *The future of the public's health in the 21st century.* Washington, DC: National Academies Press.

Institute of Medicine. (2010). *For the public's health: The role of measurement in action and accountability.* Washington, DC: National Academies Press.

Leavell, H., & Clark, A. E. (1965). *Preventive medicine for doctors in the community* (3rd ed.). New York, NY: McGraw-Hill.

Levin, P., Cary, A., Kulbok, P., Leffers, J. Molle, M., & Polivka, B. (2007). Graduate education for advanced practice public health nursing: At the crossroads. *Association of Community Health Nursing Educators (ACHNE),* 1–24. Retrieved from http://www.achne.org/files/public/GraduateEducationDocument.pdf

Lewenson, S. B. (2007). A historical perspective on policy, politics and nursing. In D. J. Mason, J. K. Leavitt, & M. W. Chaffee (Eds.), *Policy and politics in nursing and health care* (5th ed., pp. 21–33). St. Louis, MO: Saunders Elsevier.

Missouri Department of Health and Senior Services. (2006). *Public health nursing manual.* Retrieved from http://health.mo.gov/living/lpha/phnursing/manual.pdf

Peplau, H. (1952). *Interpersonal relations in nursing.* New York, NY: G. P. Putnam's Sons.

Scheele, L. A. (1949). Anniversary program—150th year U.S. Public Health Service. *American Journal of Public Health and the Nation's Health, 39*(3), 293–302.

Truglio-Londrigan, M. (2008). Flattening the field: Group decision-making. In S. B. Lewenson & M. T. Truglio-Londrigan (Eds.), *Decision-making in nursing: Thoughtful approaches for practice* (pp. 131–144). Sudbury, MA: Jones and Bartlett.

U.S. Department of Health and Human Services Public Health Service. (1994a). *The public health workforce: An agenda for the 21st century. A report of the Public Health Functions Project.* Retrieved from http://www.health.gov/phfunctions/pubhlth.pdf

U.S. Department of Health and Human Services—Public Health Functions Steering Committee. (1994b). *The public health workforce: An agenda for the 21st Century.* Washington, DC: U.S. Government Printing Office.

U.S. Department of Health and Human Services. (2000). *Healthy People 2010 (Vol. 1).* Washington, DC: U.S. Government Printing Office.

U.S. Department of Health and Human Services. (2001). *Healthy people in healthy communities.* Washington, DC: U.S. Government Printing Office.

U.S. Department of Health and Human Services. (2010a). *About Healthy People.* Retrieved from http://www.healthypeople.gov/2020/about/default.aspx

U.S. Department of Health and Human Services. (2010b). *Healthy People 2020 framework.* Retrieved from http://www.healthypeople.gov/2020/Consortium/HP2020Framework.pdf

U.S. Department of Health and Human Services. (2010c). *HHS news.* Retrieved from http://www.healthypeople.gov/2020/about/DefaultPressRelease.pdf

U.S. Department of Health and Human Services. (2010d). *Healthy People.* Retrieved from http://www.healthypeople.gov/2020/default.aspx

U.S. Department of Health and Human Services. (2010e). *2020 topics & objectives: Tobacco use: Overview.* Retrieved from http://www.healthypeople.gov/2020/topicsobjectives 2020/overview.aspx?topicid=41

U.S. Department of Health and Human Services. (2010f). *2020 topics & objectives: Tobacco use: Objectives.* Retrieved from http://www.healthypeople.gov/2020/topics objectives2020/objectiveslist.aspx?topicid=41

U.S. Department of Health and Human Services. (2010g). *2020 topics & objectives: Tobacco use: Intervention and resources.* Retrieved from http://www.healthypeople. gov/2020/topicsobjectives2020/ebr.aspx? topicid=41

U.S. Department of Health and Human Services. (2010h). *Implementing Healthy People.* Retrieved from http://www .healthypeople.gov/2020/implementing/default.aspx

Williams, C., & Stanhope, M. (2008). Population-focused practice: The foundation of specialization in public health nursing. In M. Stanhope & J. Lancaster (Eds.), *Public health nursing: Population-centered health care in the community* (pp. 2–21). St. Louis, MO: Mosby Elsevier.

Winslow, C. E. A. (1920). The untilled fields of public health. *Science, New Series, 51*(1306), 22–33.

Wisconsin Department of Health Services. (2011). *Public health nursing: The public health intervention wheel.* Retrieved from http://www.dhs.wisconsin.gov/phnc/ InterventionWheel/index.htm

For a full suite of assignments and additional learning activities, use the access code located in the front of your book to visit this exclusive website: http://go.jblearning .com/londrigan. If you do not have an access code, you can obtain one at the site.

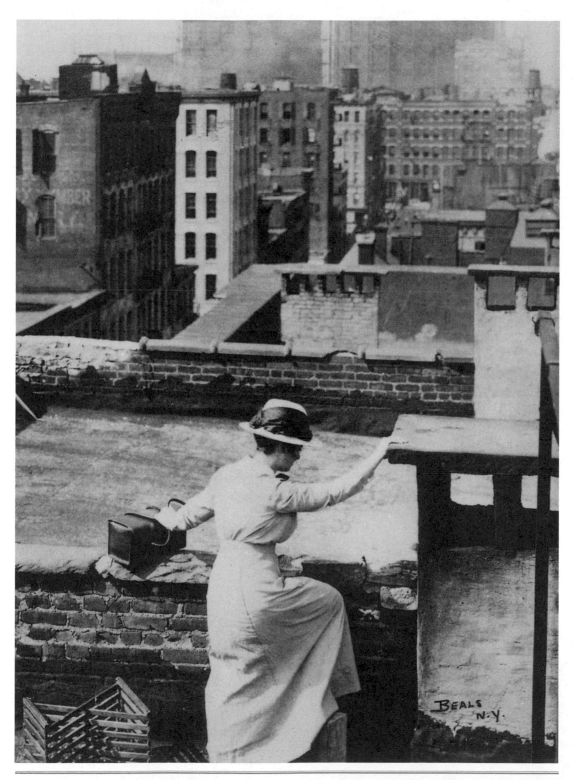

Source: Courtesy of the Visiting Nurse Service of New York.

Chapter 2

Public Health Nursing in the United States: A History

Sandra B. Lewenson

The history of public health nursing is continuous. What we are, we have become through those that have gone before, and the great leaders are of no country, but of the world (Gardner, 1933, p. 15).

LEARNING OBJECTIVES

www

At the completion of this chapter, the reader will be able to

- Define the various terms used to describe the work of nurses who have practiced in public health nursing over time.
- Describe the history of public health nursing.

- Explain the relevance of the history of nursing to current issues in public health nursing.

KEY TERMS

www

- ❏ Community health nurse
- ❏ District nurse
- ❏ Home care nurses

- ❏ Populations
- ❏ Public health nurse
- ❏ Visiting nurse

Hiestand (1982) called for the historian to reflect on "practice as it changed over time" because of its relevance to "understanding the nurses' experience" (p. 11). The purpose of this chapter is to reflect on the practice of public health nursing by examining the nurse's evolving experience in this role. This experience has been influenced by the type of agency where nurses worked, the community in which they served, the economic climate, the advances made in the sciences and technology, and other sociopolitical factors that shaped the kind of work being done (Bryant, 1968; Stewart & Vincent, 1968). The evolution of public health nursing reflects the response to these factors and the transformation that these nurses made in meeting the needs of individuals, families, **populations**, and communities (American Nurses Association [ANA], 2007). As the public health nursing role evolved, so did the nomenclature, leading some to question what a **public health nurse** is. This chapter examines public health nursing and the shift in roles as the names changed throughout the late 19th century until today. It also highlights the educational requirements for the public health nurse because as the titles and responsibilities changed to meet the needs of society, so did the educational requirements and expectations. Although this chapter seeks to explain the history of public health nursing and to address the question of what is a public health nurse, it raises more questions for the reader to consider than provides answers.

What Is a Public Health Nurse?

Early public health nursing leader Mary Gardner raised the question of what to call the nurse who provided care in the home in the preface of her 1933 book, *Public Health Nursing.* She decided on using the term "public health nurse" throughout her book instead of the other possible terms attributed to this role. Gardner (1933) explained as follows:

> *Certain questions of nomenclature have arisen, chief among them the name to be given to the nurse and to her work as described in these pages. In view of the present tendency toward more generalized methods of administration, and also because the functions of the various nurses are now so closely interwoven, the names "visiting nurse" and "visiting nursing associa-*

tion" have not been used in this book. "Public health nurse" and "public health nursing" have been substituted throughout to describe all types of nurses and organizations. (p. x)

Others questioned who was considered to be a public health nurse and the activities of this nurse. For example, Welsh (1936) wrote an article entitled, "What Is Public Health Nursing?," where she exclaimed that the very need for public health nursing to define itself after 50 years of organized activity was in itself an "indication of the lack of unity within the field itself" (p. 452). Confusion about who and what a public health nurse was stemmed from the increasing specializations that public health nurses were branching into other areas, such as tuberculosis nurses, maternity nurses, infant welfare nurses, and other specialty areas aside from **visiting nurses**.

The change in names used to describe the person who provided the care in the home has perpetually confused those in health care, as well as consumers of care (Geis, 1991; Humphrey & Milone-Nuzzo, 1996; Jones, Davis, & Davis, 1987; Levin et al., 2007; Roberts & Heinrich, 1985; Welsh, 1936). In schools of nursing, for example, students take courses in public health that are often labeled community health. Faculty members debate what they consider a "good" community clinical experience. This debate usually includes whether a visiting nurse experience ("carry the bag") or working in a health department or incorporating public health initiatives in a shopping mall or any number of combinations of experiences allow the student to understand the full dimension of public health nursing. This confusion stems from the faculty's orientation to this specialty and from the terminology used to describe the course: Is it public health or community health or both? Clark (2008) poignantly asks

Visiting nurse with a young boy.

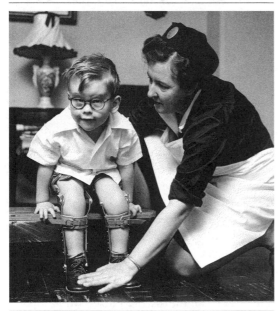

Source: Courtesy of the Visiting Nurse Service of New York.

what's in a name and tries to explicate the meaning of the various terms used to describe this specialty.

As the public health nursing role evolved, so did the names for this role. The changing names reflected the tensions between and among the stakeholders that shaped the work of public health nurses. The lack of cohesiveness of the various volunteer and public organizations and the separation of the preventive care from the curative aspects of the public health nurse's role led Buhler-Wilkerson (1993) to write, "it is little wonder, then that the question, 'What is a public health nurse' has been debated for more than 80 years" (p. 1783). The history of public health nursing provides the reader with the origins of the various names, the educational requirements for these roles, and insight into the debate that continues today as to what a public health nurse is.

Evolution of the Public Health Nurse

District Nurses

District nursing began in 1859 as part of an experiment where a hospital-based, trained nurse was sent to provide nursing care to the poor in "a small district" in Liverpool, England (Hughes, 1893/1949). From that early success the promoter of this experiment, William Rathbone, expanded this work, dividing Liverpool into 18 districts and supplying each district with its own **district nurse** (Hughes). The adoption of this successful form of nursing spread, and various agencies began to use district nurses throughout England.

English nursing leader Dacre Craven (1889/1984) wrote about the work of the district nurse in England and called Rathbone's experiment as the defining incident in identifying the distinct work of the district nurse. In Craven's description of the district nurse, she includes the care of the sick poor in their homes as the main focus of a district nurse. The responsibilities of the district nurse were carefully explained in Craven's work, *A Guide to District Nursing,* first published in 1889. Craven was considered one of the first superintendents of the central home where district nurses lived together. These nurses were drawn together from "the class of gentlewomen, with a view to bringing women of higher education and refinement to grapple with the special difficulties of the work" (Hughes, 1893/1949, p. 113).

District nurses addressed the health of the poor in the community and needed to have a "real love for the poor and a desire to lessen the misery" (Craven, 1889/1984, p. 1) that was found in the homes. Concern for the family and bringing cleanliness to the patient, the family, and the environment in which the family lived was part of the district nurse's role. The district nurse needed to know about the sanitary and charitable organizations in the district where the patients lived. In this way, when sanitary problems arose, such as a defective water supply, or "untrapped" cesspools or "unemptied dustbins," the nurse would notify the appropriate "sanitary committee of the district . . . who [would] take legal steps, if necessary, to compel the landlord to put the premises into a proper sanitary condition" (Craven, 1889/1984, p. 11). The daily work consisted of care of the sick poor and enabled the nurse to observe the sanitary conditions in the home that affected the health of the patient, the family, and the community (or district) in which the patient lived. Craven (1889/1984) gave the following examples of the sanitary work of the district nurse:

> Sometimes there is a plague of flies in the room, which can be traced to some foul or decaying animal or vegetable refuse. When the nurse carries down the dust and ashes to the dustbin she sees whether it ought to be emptied, and ascertains when this was last done. As she fetches water for the kettle she can find out whether it is from an impure and uncovered cistern, and as she empties the slops of her patient she ascertains whether the w.c. is in a good sanitary condition, and with a separate cistern from that used for drinking purposes (and she can herself occasionally flush the pan of the w.c.). (pp. 11–12)

Another important role of the district nurse was to educate patients, friends, and family about the need for a sanitary environment. The nurse taught about the need for personal cleanliness and hygiene, and she herself was expected to be a role model of both. The nurse's uniform, as Craven (1889/1984) described, reflected a clean and neat appearance. The district nurse was to be a paragon of excellence in the way she cared for the sick poor, managed the sanitation

of the environment, and educated others about cleanliness and sanitary principles. She also assumed the responsibility for the care of the dying patient and the dead. Craven (1893/1949) wrote that district nurses were instructed on the "best positions in which to place the dying, according to their ailment . . . so that they might breathe to the last without unnecessary effort or pain" (p. 133).

As the district nurses that Craven (1889/1984) wrote about carried on their work, they also were responsible for keeping records of what they did. Each district nurse spent time on paperwork documenting her caseload, the time she spent, and the care she provided in each home. The nurses shared this information with the superintendent of the district nurses, who collated their reports into a monthly report. The superintendent kept a log of all the cases the nurses managed. Based on the district nurses' work, reports included the number of new cases per month, the length of visits, and the number of visits required by the patients (Craven, 1889/1984, p. 131). Superintendents rated the work done and the data collected. For example, they would use ratings such as "excellent," "good," "moderate," "imperfect," or "nil" to rank such things as the patient's status; the cleanliness of the patient, the room, utensils, and beds; and the various kinds of treatments, like sponge baths, mouth care, precautions against bed sores, wound care, and other treatments. Records of various types of cases such as typhoid fever, diphtheria, puerperal disease, scarlet fever, obstetrical cases, and care of the newborn were also kept. In addition, the superintendent's report included an evaluation of the probationers, who acted as the district nurses, on their ability to observe the sick and manage the care of the sick (Craven, 1889/1984).

Knowledge about the work of these early district nurses in England spread to the United States. In 1893, Amy Hughes, Superintendent

Lillian Wald (left) and friends, 1915.

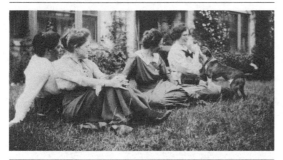

Source: Courtesy of the Visiting Nurse Service of New York.

of Nurses at the Metropolitan and National Nursing Association, one of the agencies to form in London, came to the United States to speak before the International Congress of Charities, Correction, and Philanthropy in Chicago. She explained to the American audience that "district nursing is the technical name for the work of nursing the sick poor in their own homes" (p. 111). Interest in district nursing spread as trained nurses from the early Nightingale-influenced training schools sought ways to improve the health of those who lived in the community. Miss C. E. Somerville, from Lawrence General Hospital in Massachusetts, said, "the last quarter of the century was well advanced when America caught the reflection of England's light, and the era of trained nursing for the poor began in this country" (Somerville, 1893/1949, p. 119).

Early district nursing associations, also called visiting nurse associations, organized in the United States. Some were established along religious missionary lines that expected the care of the sick to include a religious concern for the well-being of the patient. An early example of this was the Woman's Branch of the New York City Mission and Tract Society, which in 1877 used trained nurses to provide care to the sick in the home in New York City (Lewenson, 1993; Somerville, 1893/1949). Two years later the

Ethical Culture Society offered a nondenominational visiting nurse service that rendered care to the sick poor. Both associations began almost 20 years before the secular visiting nurse service was founded by Lillian Wald and Mary Brewster in 1893 at the Henry Street Settlement. Other early district and visiting nurse associations opened in Boston, Chicago, Philadelphia, and other cities across the United States, offering care to the sick poor and those of moderate means. They shared a common goal and assumed many of the same roles as their counterpart district nurses did in England (Somerville, 1893/1949).

Nightingale's paper "Sick Nursing and Health Nursing," presented at the Chicago World Fair in 1893, described the district nurse as providing care to the sick at home, as well as someone who assumed the work as a health missioner. A health missioner required additional training in how to teach healthy behaviors to mothers in the community and in the home. Nightingale outlined some of the content that was included in their additional training in areas such as sanitary conditions in the home, management of health of adults, women in childbearing years "before and after confinement," and infants and children (Nightingale, 1893/1949, p. 41).

Nightingale (1893/1949) believed that to improve the health of infants and babies, mothers needed to learn about healthier lifestyle behaviors. Nightingale used a population focus to explain why these health missioners needed to be concerned about the health of infants and babies. She wrote that,

The life duration of babies is the most 'delicate test' of health conditions. What is the proportion of the whole population of cities or country which dies before it is five years old? We have tons of printed knowledge on the subject of hygiene and sanitation. The causes of enormous child mortality are perfectly well known: they are chiefly, want of cleanliness, want of fresh air, careless dieting and clothing, want of white-washing . . . in one word, want of household care of health. (p. 29)

Nightingale's idea about health nursing extended to the community, and she summarized this in her paper by saying, "The health of the unity is the health of community. Unless you have the health of the unity there is no community health" (Nightingale, 1893/1949, p. 35).

The concept of health missioners or health nursing was embedded in the work of the visiting nurse in the United States as these nurses added to their work the ideas generated by the public health movement that was calling for ways to keep communities healthy. The public health movement was ongoing in the United States since the mid-1800s, when the Shattuck commission identified the need for the creation of local health boards that would collect statistical data on the population, including records of marriages, births, and deaths. States were called on to investigate "the cause of disease, abatement of the smoke nuisance, adoption of means for public health education, and other far-reaching measures" (Beard, 1922, p. 142). Scientific discoveries about the causes of the spread of certain diseases like yellow fever, malaria, tuberculosis, or poliomyelitis further advanced public health initiatives. Visiting nurses cared for the sick at home and provided the families they visited with information about how to keep their families and communities healthier.

Public health nursing leader Lillian Wald attended the Chicago exposition and was greatly influenced by Nightingale's paper describing health nursing (Haupt, 1953). Haupt wrote that Wald had "accepted Florence Nightingale's concept of 'health nursing' and put the word 'public' in front of it so that all the people would know that they could use it" (p. 81). The nurses

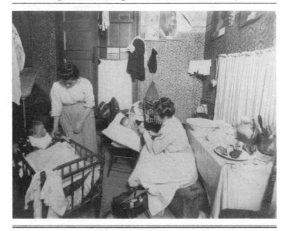

Philadelphia visiting nurse with a family.

Source: Courtesy of the Barbara Bates Center for the Study of Nursing History, University of Pennsylvania.

at the Henry Street Nurses Settlement, for example, cared for the sick at home and offered classes to mothers on how to keep their families healthier. Although the term "health missioner" is rarely seen in the literature describing public health nursing in the United States, the dimension of health promotion and disease prevention continued to be imbued in the work of public health nursing.

Visiting Nurse

Public health nursing leader Lavinia Dock addressed the issue of nomenclature in her text, *A Short History of Nursing* (Dock & Stewart, 1938). Dock wrote that the first evidence of the term "visiting nursing" was found in the early records of St. John's House, England, which began in 1848. During that period cholera and smallpox were rampant in England and the United States, and "Anglican and Catholic sisters spent their lives in visiting the poor and caring for the sick under the most terrible conditions" (Dock & Stewart, 1938, p. 305). By the

20th century, however, the role of the visiting nurse expanded into what was to become part of the larger "public health movement." Dock wrote, "In the twentieth century visiting nursing became one part of the broadening field of 'public health nursing,' as an ideal of the visiting nurse who was teacher, sanitarian, and public-spirited citizen as well as nurse, gradually took form" (Dock & Stewart, 1938, pp. 305–306). This new expanding field of public health nursing, Dock believed, was to become the "nursing of the future" (p. 306).

As mentioned earlier, public health nurses were closely aligned with the public health movement that flourished during the early 20th century. Fitzpatrick (1975a) described the noted public health expert Charles Winslow's identification of three phases of the public health movement: "the phase of empirical environmental sanitation, the bacteriological phase, and the educational phase" (p. 6). The fact that nurses were already engaged in providing both health care and health education within communities led Winslow and others to acknowledge the value public health nurses brought to the larger public health movement (Fitzpatrick, 1975a).

Modern Nursing Movement

The history of the modern nursing movement in the United States began in 1873 as Nightingale's work influenced the opening of schools for nurses in New York, Connecticut, and Massachusetts (Lewenson, 1993). It was a time of great change for women who sought a way to financially support themselves in some kind of labor outside of the home. Women read a description about one of the new training schools that had started at Bellevue Hospital in New York City in *The Century Magazine* (North, 1882), describing nursing as a "new profession for women" (p. 38). Once a nursing student completed the apprenticeship training at one of these hospital schools, however, she was sent out as a "trained nurse" into the community without the security of hospital employment. Instead of hiring their graduates, hospitals typically used their next class of nursing students to staff the hospital. A trained nurse consequently had to find employment elsewhere and usually worked as a private duty nurse, caring for one patient in the home setting, or as a public health nurse, working in public or privately-funded organizations with responsibilities for visiting patients in their homes and promoting health in the community.

By 1893, 20 years after the first few Nightingale-influenced training schools began, nursing superintendents of the schools that had already opened joined together with other women from around the world at the now famous Chicago World's Fair. It was at this international conference that professional nursing organizations in the United States began. The first organization to form was the American Society of Superintendents for Nurses, which was started by pioneering nursing superintendents who wanted to establish standards and control over the education and practice of nursing. These leaders banded together in 1893 and by 1912 became known as the National League of Nursing Education, which changed its name again in 1952 to the current title, the National League for Nursing (NLN). As this group formed, the leaders, Isabel Hampton Robb, Lavinia Dock, and others, saw the need to organize nurses working at the bedside. The need to control practice; lobby for state nursing registration laws, which were nonexistent at the time; and support those nurses in financial trouble led to the formation of the Nurses Associated Alumnae of the United States and Canada in 1896, which in 1911 became known as the American Nurses Association (ANA).

This need to control and standardize nursing education and practice extended to another group of nurses, marginalized because of racial bias.

Many African American nurses were excluded from joining the ANA as a result of a shift to statewide membership in the organization. Once that occurred in 1916, individual nurses no longer could join and relied on membership through their state nurses associations (Carnegie, 1991; Lewenson, 1993). Racist policies of many states, particularly in the South, prohibited African American nurses from membership and left them without the support of a professional organization. This meant issues such as control of education in their nursing schools and control of practice through state registration laws that often discriminated against them would be left unattended until 1908, when the National Association of Colored Graduate Nurses (NACGN) formed. Nursing leader Martha Franklin sought assistance from other African American nurses to establish this organization to support the needs of black nurses in the United States. This organization lasted from 1908 until 1952, when integration into the ANA was achieved (Carnegie, 1991).

Sophia Palmer, first editor of the *American Journal of Nursing,* wrote that, "Organization is the power of the age. Without it nothing great is accomplished" (Palmer, 1897/1991, p. 297). Organizations formed throughout the country, addressing many of the Progressive Era issues touching on the social, economic, and political welfare of the population. Nurses, by virtue of their education and practice, were aware of the connection between a healthy society and the right to vote (Lewenson, 1993). Concern for women's rights extended into the discussions of the NLN and the ANA, leading to organizational support of a woman's right to vote by 1912. The NACGN also supported women's rights initiatives, as evidenced by its support of the work of the International Council of Nurses in that area. The NACGN had sent a delega-

tion years ahead of both the NLN and the ANA to participate in discussions related to women's rights around the globe (Lewenson, 1993).

Public Health Nursing Emerges

Throughout the late 1800s and early 1900s, Lavinia Dock advocated suffrage for women and wrote extensively about this issue in the *American Journal of Nursing* and other journals of that period. Dock aligned the vote with health care and said that without it, nurses would not be able to effectively improve the health of society (Lewenson, 1993). Concern for the public's health was shared by others like Lillian Wald and Mary Brewster, who founded the Henry Street Settlement in New York City's Lower East Side in 1893 to address the health of the people who lived there. Graduates and friends from the New York Hospital training school, Wald and Brewster opened the nurses' settlement house in 1893 (2 years after they had graduated from the training school) to care for the population of immigrants who flooded into the United States during the late 19th and early 20th centuries. The spread of illness became a real threat to the many Americans who lived in the overcrowded cities and experienced firsthand the diversity of those who immigrated here (Fitzpatrick, 1975a; Lewenson, 1993).

Buhler-Wilkerson (1985) said the impetus of the wealthier parts of society to improve the health of the poor stemmed, in part, from an understanding of the germ theory along with the idea that infectious diseases could be spread easily to their own families and communities by those immigrants who "sewed clothes in their filthy tenement homes or who processed food" (p. 1155). Early visiting nurses were hired by philanthropic women who sought to provide the urban poor with assistance during times of illness. According to Buhler-Wilkerson (1985),

Henry Street nurses, 1903.

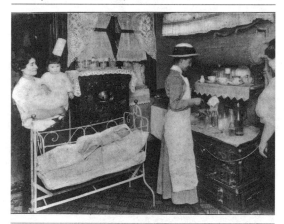

Source: Courtesy of the Visiting Nurse Service of New York.

the nurses hired by these lady philanthropists were to bring their shared vision of the "good society" by bringing "care, cleanliness, and character to the homes of the sick poor" (p. 1155). Nurses were to teach the families they visited about the ways of American life that would lead to the prevention of disease and promotion of health. Fear of the spread of illness prompted some of the concerns of those nurses and their benefactors in bringing health care to the homes of the sick poor (Buhler-Wilkerson, 1985).

Dock worked at the Henry Street Settlement alongside Wald and other colleagues, engaging in what we now call primary healthcare activities, including visiting homes of those who needed care related to an illness, participation in well-baby clinics, case finding, health-promoting activities, surveillance, and school nurse activities. They lived within the Henry Street settlement in the same community in which they provided nursing care. It was the comprehensive visiting nurse services like the ones delivered at Henry Street that proliferated throughout the country and offered another way for nurses to

support themselves while caring for individuals, families, populations, and communities. Nursing care included the care of the sick at home as well as well-baby classes and other health-promoting courses offered to the community.

Most nurses who graduated from the nursing schools in the late 1800s worked in private duty, providing nursing services to one patient in the home. This focus differed somewhat from that of the visiting nurse. Visiting nurses saw several patients in a day, and depending on the agency in which they worked, variable fees were attached to their visit based on the patients' ability to pay. While caring for the sick at home, they also provided much-needed health education. Often, the ability to care for the sick at home fostered a level of trust among the nurses and the families and community they served, which in turn provided them easier access to these same groups as they sought to provide health education. The work of the visiting nurse evolved into what became known as public health nursing and became a viable specialization for the graduate trained nurse. Having coined the term "public health nurses," Wald and other nursing leaders recognized a need to control the practice of this emerging specialization in nursing and founded the National Organization for Public Health Nursing (NOPHN) in 1912 (Buhler-Wilkerson, 2001).

National Organization for Public Health Nursing

The NOPHN grew out of a desire by public health nurses to control the practice and standards of the emerging field of public health nursing. By 1912, the number of public health nurses had grown to over 3,000 and their work was supported through private and public funding (Gardner, 1933). The work was accepted by the community and extended far beyond the care provided to the sick at home. The public health nurses' role had expanded to meet the needs of a growing American urban and rural population— public health nurses visited patients in the home and provided additional primary healthcare services. In 1933, Gardner described the increasingly expanded and valued role of the public health nurse as follows:

We find other agencies counting not only on her help in individual cases, but upon the knowledge which she has gained from her unique position. We see that she has had her effect on state and city legislation, and has influenced public opinion to effect non-legislative reform. We find her valued as a preventive agent and health instructor by municipalities and state bodies, and the usefulness of her statistics acknowledged by research workers. We find her acting as probation officer, tenement house and sanitary inspector, county bailiff, domestic educator, and hospital social workers. She is found in the juvenile courts and the public playgrounds, in the department stores and the big hotels, in the schools and factories, in the houses of small wage-earners and in the swarming tenements of the poor. We find her in the big cities, the small towns, the rural districts and the lonely mountain regions. We find her dealing with tuberculosis, babies, mental cases, industrial workers, expectant mothers, midwifery and housing conditions. (p. 25)

The expansion of the public health nurse's role in all facets of life grew in response to the needs of society. Visiting nurse associations proliferated throughout the early 20th century. Public health nurses worked for these newly forming visiting nurse associations throughout the country in both rural and urban settings. They provided care to the sick in their homes, educated the public on healthcare measures that would

Nurse teaching a nutrition class to a family, 1928.

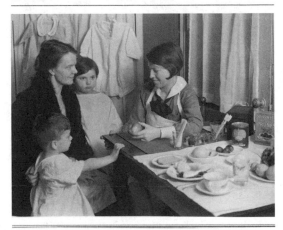

Source: Courtesy of the Visiting Nurse Service of New York.

prevent illnesses like tuberculosis and other communicable diseases, and promoted healthy behaviors. Each of these associations developed its own guidelines and was mostly organized by lay boards that did not have the same background as the public health nurses who founded some of the earlier visiting nurse associations, such as the Chicago Visiting Nurses Association or the Cleveland Visiting Nurse Association (Fitzpatrick, 1975a). Fitzpatrick (1975a) explained that, "Until the rapid extension of public health nursing associations took place, there had been some success in upholding higher ethical and professional practices as well as a certain degree of conformity among the largest associations. This was due, in part, to the exceptional leadership ability and ideals of the early pioneers in the movement" (pp. 18–19). Yet as public health nursing associations expanded in the early 1900s, the lack of appropriate supervision and the misplaced understanding by the lay boards that ran the newly organized visiting nurse associations caused many in nursing to be worried about a real "threat to sound nursing practice itself" (Fitzpatrick, 1975a, p. 19).

Without clarity about the nursing role in public health, without understanding what the educational requirement of this nurse should be, and without standards regarding the practice, public health nursing leaders believed it imperative to organize. Public health nursing educator Ella Crandall contacted several of her peers between 1910 and 1911, asking them for their thoughts on the need for another nursing organization that specifically focused on public health nurses. Crandall found support among her colleagues; however, support for the format of such an organization varied. Although all agreed that an organization was needed and all agreed to lay members being included, some favored becoming a committee of the already-existing ANA. Crandall's idea, however, was for a separate organization that focused on setting standards and guidelines for public health nursing practice and education (Fitzpatrick, 1975a).

In 1912 Crandall's idea for a separate organization prevailed and the NOPHN formed. Leaders in nursing, like Lillian Wald, Mary Beard, Mary Gardner, Edna Foley, Jane Delano, and Anna Kerr, participated in the organization of this newly formed group. They addressed the issues of standardizing public health nurse requirements, such as requiring them to be graduates of nurse training schools and registered nurses in states that required registration, and supported the idea of agency membership, which meant that non-nurses could be members of the organization, an idea that had not yet been practiced by the ANA or the National League of Nursing Education (forerunner of the NLN). The purpose of the NOPHN was to promote "sound public health nursing for the people of this country, who would be the recipients of the service" (Fitzpatrick, 1975a, p. 24).

A public health nurse weighing children, 1930.

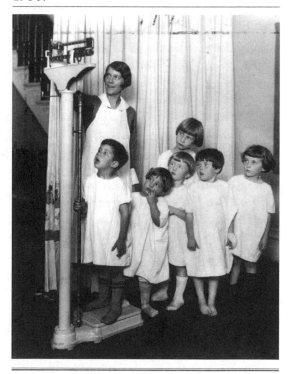

Source: Courtesy of the Visiting Nurse Service of New York.

The architects of this new organization struggled with what to name the group. Some wanted to reflect the name of the visiting nurse, whereas others, like Crandall, sought to use the term "public health nursing" in the title, because public health nursing was considered to be broader than the earlier term of visiting nurse. The leaders debated the name, and when they finally came up with the title, "National Association of Public Health Nurses," again Crandall argued that the name needed to reflect more than nurses. Edna Foley, another public health nursing leader, suggested the name, "National Organization for Public Health Nursing," which was unanimously agreed upon

(Fitzpatrick, 1975a). Wald was elected as the organization's first president.

One of the early NOPHN pamphlets (1914) described the public health nurse as follows:

A Public Health Nurse is a product of evolution. She has developed from the old-fashioned district or visiting nurse, who visits and nurses the sick, poor patient in his home. She is still that same visiting nurse and also, according to the demands of the community in which she serves, a public school nurse, an infant welfare nurse, a tuberculosis nurse, a hospital social service nurse, a sanitary inspector, a truant officer, a social worker, a visiting dietician, and even a midwife. Adequate preparation means special training and experience for each worker.

The idea that public health nursing evolved from the various terms to date—district nurse, visiting nurse—represented the full scope of practice that public health nurses were expected to provide. Public health nurses initially engaged in the wide range of practice, knowing that providing care in the home as visiting nurses afforded them access to where health-promoting behaviors could take place. Who paid for the care, whether the public or a privately-run voluntary or business association, often determined the types of services the nurse could provide. The earlier public health nurse found employment as school nurses, industrial nurses, visiting nurses, and in other settings where they could impact the health of a particular population; for example, they worked with mothers and babies or people with communicable diseases like tuberculosis. Providing preventive and health promotional education in the community was all part of the work of public health nurses regardless of particular setting or agency for whom they worked.

As public health nurses became more valuable to society, their numbers and the number of settings where they worked increased. Yet the tension between the privately-funded visiting nurse services, which offered more of the care of the sick at home, compared with publically-run health departments, which assumed more of the activities like surveillance of communicable diseases and health education, created a separation—perhaps a false one—of the work of the public health nurse. The frequently seen overlap of the public health nurse's role created confusion in both the public and the profession's understanding of that role (Buhler-Wilkerson, 1985).

The term "public health nurse" was continually being defined and refined. For example, in 1919, 5 years after the formation of the NOPHN, Executive Director Ella Crandall wrote to George Vincent at the Rockefeller Foundation, where she sent him a "corrected report" of a previously shared description of the term "public health nurse." Crandall (1919) wrote the following:

Term public health nurse considered for past five or six years by public health nurses and people administering visiting nurse associations as applicable to work of modern visiting nurse because (1) any nurse giving bedside care should realize opportunities for teaching health protection and hygiene; (2) individual illness not solely individual matter but lowers health standard for family, hence for community; consequently visiting nurse is a public health nurse; although usually supported by private funds, ultimate goal to have all public health nursing supported by public funds as are public school teachers, nurses employed by municipality not allowed time for bedside care; hence dependent on visiting nurse to round out her service; impossible to employ both kinds of workers in small and rural communities, therefore rural nurse must be trained in both.

There was a distinction in the work of the public health nurse based on the setting, the specialization, and the environment in which the public health nurse practiced. If the public health nurse worked in an urban setting, there were more resources in the community that addressed the various healthcare needs of the population. As a result, visiting nurses, in many instances, focused more on the care of the sick at home, whereas nurses who worked in public health departments focused more on the preventive and health-promoting kinds of education the public required. In rural settings where healthcare resources were more limited, the public health nurse would offer the full range of public health services, including the preventive and the curative.

In 1919 the NOPHN published a book presenting a description of the public health nurse that recognized that "public health nursing is a profession still in process of evolution" (Brainard, 1919, p. v). Anna Brainard (1919) wrote that although public health nurses worked in both publically and privately funded organizations, "It does not necessarily mean nursing done under the direction of a public department of health: it means nursing done for the health of the public. It does not mean merely bedside care; it means nursing care with an eye to the social as well as the medical aspects of the case" (p. 4). Her definition of a public health nurse included "any graduate nurse who is doing any form of social work in which the health of the public is concerned, and in which her training as a nurse comes into play or is recognized as a valuable part of her equipment" (p. 4).

The idea that public health nurses were found providing bedside care in the home as well as dispensing health information to the

A public health nurse with a child in Chinatown.

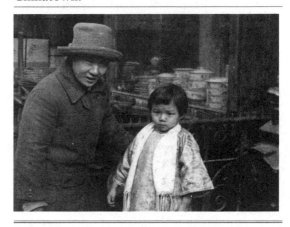

Source: Courtesy of the Visiting Nurse Service of New York.

public continued to create tension as to the role of the public health nurse. The public health nurse found herself dependent on the resources in the community. The division of the type of care the organization provided continued to be a source of concern for those in public health because it was viewed as necessary for the public health nurse to offer a full range of services to improve the health of the public.

Early Experiments in Public Health Nursing

METROPOLITAN LIFE INSURANCE COMPANY

In 1909, just before the founding of the NOPHN, the Metropolitan Life Insurance Company linked visiting nurses with home care services that were offered to millions of their policyholders. Wald was instrumental in setting the stage for the expanded role of public health nurses. Evidence of the efficacy of their care was collected by nurses through the statistics they kept of their work (Gardner, 1933). The public, as well as the company, valued the work of the visiting nurses who participated in this program, which lasted from 1909 until 1952. Almost 20 years before this successful experiment was to end, Gardner (1933) wrote, "the tendency of the Company towards an increase in the use of the nurse's time for instructive work in the home is an interesting comment on the value of such work in the actual conservation of life" (p. 24).

The visiting nurse brought health care and healthcare education into the homes of the families she visited. The number of visits to the homes of policyholders throughout the United States rose to one billion home visits, making Wald's experiment one of the "first national system[s] of insurance coverage for home-based care" (Buhler-Wilkerson, 1993, p. 1782). The demise of the Metropolitan Visiting Nurse experiment, however, came about because of many factors, one of which Hamilton (1988) related to tension created by two different approaches to care: an economic concern for cost containment, as espoused by the Metropolitan Life Insurance Company, and one embodying the concern to provide nursing services to those in need regardless of the need to contain costs. In addition, by 1952, the decline in policyholders coupled with the increasing cost of nursing service led the company to close this program (Buhler-Wilkerson, 1993). Although historians like Hamilton, Buhler-Wilkerson, and others critique the experiences of the past from a vantage point of time, Alma Haupt, who was the director of Nursing Bureau of Metropolitan Life Insurance Company from 1935 until it closed in 1952, expressed her more immediate and perhaps personal view of the program, highlighting its success. Haupt (1953) wrote the following:

> *"Metropolitan Nursing Service" has provided an example of how a profession and a business organization can work together for a common goal—better health, less sickness*

> *and death, and better business. It has shown that maintaining a high standard of nursing service depends on the availability and use of the cooperation, leadership, and standards of a profession. It has shown the advantages of having the prestige, leadership, and financial and organizational backing of the Metropolitan, a company whose contributions have had marked influence on the health of a nation. (p. 84)*

AMERICAN RED CROSS PUBLIC HEALTH NURSING SERVICE

Wald's insight into the needs of populations in both the urban and rural communities led to another important experiment in public health nursing. Buhler-Wilkerson (1993) describes this experiment as the founding of the American Red Cross Public Health Nursing Service (also known as Red Cross Town and Country Nursing Service) in 1912. Public health nurses were used to bring public health care to rural communities around the country. The Red Cross organized and standardized the work of these public health nurses to function in the community, providing an expanded role of public health nursing services that included home care and preventive care (Kernodle, 1949).

In keeping with the need to engage communities in the care of their health, the Red Cross published in 1913 a small text that accompanied a course that was given to mothers in the community. The purpose of this book was to promote healthy behaviors and prevent serious illness by involving the family, in most cases mothers, to support the work of public health nurses. In the preface of the book, Mabel Boardman, Chairman of the National Relief Board of the American Red Cross, wrote, "work as hard as they might, neither the medical nor nursing professions could alone accomplish much along sanitary lines until the people in general became aroused to the importance of such matters. Knowledge that personal health depends largely upon the health conditions of the community brings home to each individual a serious personal interest and sense of responsibility" (Delano & McIsaac, 1913, p. v). Nursing leaders Jane Delano and Isabel McIsaac, authors of this text, sought to educate the public about health as part of a broader public health initiative by the American Red Cross. This text was republished several times during the 1900s with different titles; in 1941, the title of the course offered to mothers was called "Red Cross Home Nursing," and a subsequent text was published in 1942 with that same title. The changing titles reflect the changes in public health nursing throughout the late 1900s through mid-twentieth century. In the preface of the 1942 version, Mary Beard, Director of Nursing Service at the American Red Cross, again made the strong connection between science and health and illness, stressing the need for healthcare professionals to be supported in their work by educating the homemaker about health. "The individual in the home—particularly the mother or homemaker—continues to hold a responsible place in relation to health. Her part is one of keeping herself and her family in good health, of assisting in giving proper care to members of her household when they are ill, and of supporting community action for the promotion of health" (Trott, 1942, p. v).

The American Red Cross National Nursing Service lasted until 1947, when fewer than 100 Red Cross services remained. The nurses who served in these rural areas provided both the nursing care at home and the health promotion and disease prevention activities that designated the ideal role of the public health nurse. This dichotomy of the two roles, although combined in most rural settings because of lack of services, was mostly reflected in urban settings where the split between the visiting nurse hired by voluntary agencies and the public health nurse hired in public agencies segmented the care that nursing could have more seamlessly provided (Roberts & Heinrich, 1985). Buhler-Wilkerson (1993) speaks in depth about the repercussions of this public health nursing experiment and the reasons for its demise. Although this discussion is beyond the scope of this chapter, the reader is encouraged to explore the reasons for this change because it relates to the lack of a cohesive plan of care that would translate Wald's vision of public health nursing to the American public. The division between the curative care provided to the sick at home and the activities of health promotion and disease prevention by competing healthcare agencies contributed to the end of this experiment and perhaps contributes to the continued confusion about the role of the public health nurse.

The Evolution Continues: Public Health Nursing in the 1930s

The 1930s saw the economic depression where unemployment in all communities permeated the well-being of those who lived during this period. Between 8,000 and 10,000 nurses were unemployed during this time (Abrams, 2007a). Nurses lost private duty positions and public health employment and found relatively few hospital jobs available (Ashmun, 1933; Fitzpatrick, 1975b). Public health nurses saw their salaries cut and their jobs lost (Abrams, 2007a). The New Deal, however, brought government-funded healthcare programs to American communities to improve economic conditions, hiring unemployed graduate nurses with or without public health experience in programs like the Children's Bureau. Both the public health movement and the need for communities to determine their healthcare needs faced the challenging economic downturn of the 1930s. Public health nurses, however, with help from various governmental programs, endured this economic crisis, continuing to find meaning in their work in both the public and private settings.

Toward the end of the depression, in 1938, a revised copy of the *Board Members' Manual for Board and Committee Members of Public Health Nursing Services* was published by the NOPHN. The purpose of such a manual was to offer guidance to the many local community advisory boards, comprised of lay and professional people, that formed in communities around the country to provide support "for public health activities of municipal and state governments" (NOPHN, 1938, p. vi). The preface of the manual reminded the reader that "at a time when some despairing folk would turn over all social activities to tax-supported agencies, it is well to remind ourselves that voluntary associations still have essential things to contribute: flexibility and willingness to experiment, standards of efficiency . . . creation of public opinion, discovery of community leaders" (NOPHN, 1938, p. vi.). Community boards undertook a variety of public health services in the community, including managing finances, determining public health policies, and deciding on the type of public health nursing programs that were needed in a community, such as "public health nursing associations, American Red Cross chapters, and tuberculosis associations" (NOPHN, 1938, p. ix). The *Board Members' Manual* supported these community advisory boards as both a guide and a reference because they served both public and private organizations engaged in public health activities.

The NOPHN (1938) *Board Members' Manual* also provided a definition of the term "public health nursing," stating that public health nursing includes "all nursing services organized by a community or an agency to assist in carrying out

any or all phases of the public health program. Services may be rendered on an individual, family, or community basis in home, school, clinic, business establishment, or office of the agency" (NOPHN, 1938, p. 4). The role of the public health nurse by the late 1930s still included both the care of the sick at home and the broader work of community education and health promotion activities. The idea of separating the services of the public health nurse, according to the *Board Members' Manual,* would fly in the face of "efficiency and economy" (NOPHN, 1938, p. 6). The range of functions that the public health nurse was responsible for were maternity health, infant and preschool health, school health, industrial nursing, adult health, communicable diseases, tuberculosis, syphilis and gonorrhea, noncommunicable diseases, orthopedic services, vital statistics, sanitation, mental hygiene, nutrition, reports and records, and medical standing orders (NOPHN, 1938). The care moved from the concern for individuals to concern for the health of the larger community. It was recommended that each community have public health agencies to engage in some, if not all, of the above activities as part of a planned approach to provide a comprehensive public health nursing program in the community.

C. E. A. Winslow (1938a), a professor of public health at the Yale School of Medicine, recognized the need for communities to organize all nursing care in the community to meet the health needs of the public. He spoke about the need for voluntary organizations to continue to be part of communities' planned public health resources. Winslow (1938a) wrote that

> *good public health nursing by its very nature is a generalized family service and the ideal toward which we are working is that of a single public health nurse in a given area providing both bedside care and health education to the families under her charge. Any administrative*

plan which tends to separate bedside care from health instruction, or nursing for the poor from nursing for the rich is undesirable. (p. 2)

Winslow saw public health nurses as providing a wide range of nursing services, all for the purpose of fostering health.

The need for more public health nurses in the community required financial support from both the public and private sector. Winslow (1938a) saw a need to coordinate all nursing services in the community, including those in the hospital, private duty, and public health:

Under an organized community plan it should be possible to develop effective coordination of all the nursing forces of the community. It is obvious that duplications of work by different agencies should be avoided, unfilled needs discovered and met, and the public informed as to the role of each agency . . . planning should make possible better service for the home and far more economical use of community resources. The respective fields of the hospital and public health nursing agency could be adequately defined and provision made for continuity of treatment upon discharge from the institution. (p. 4)

Simplistically, the coordination of community nursing services could ultimately enhance the health care of the public and could lead to such innovations as insuring the middle class with home healthcare service benefits, increasing the income of public health nurses, and ultimately supporting a "modern public health program" (Winslow, 1938a, p. 7). The need for public support of nursing education was also considered a part of the plan that Winslow saw as essential to improving and increasing the number of public health nurses.

Through the evolutionary development of community advisory boards and councils as well as the three nursing organizations (NLN, ANA, and NOPHN) and organizing the Joint Committee on Community Nursing Service (in 1934), coordination of public health nursing needs throughout the country was a goal that some believed could be established (Winslow, 1938a, 1938b). Winslow, along with others, looked toward these local and organizational councils to solve the concerns about providing for the health of the public. Winslow (1938a) wrote,

I am convinced that the development of a fully coordinated and truly effective system of community nursing, in home and in hospital, for rich and for poor, including health instruction and bedside care, is one of the most vital social problems of the present day . . . but the community councils of nursing can solve it if they have the courage and vision. (p. 8)

Nurses needed to organize and bring together the various stakeholders, hospitals, community agencies, and private duty nurses to coordinate and advance the public health nursing services in the community.

Public Health Nursing in the Second Half of the 20th Century

By the middle of the 1900s, the kinds of nursing services that communities would need as public health and public health nursing evolved in response to advances in science, new technologies, and social legislation. The advent of new drugs, like penicillin in the 1940s, created different challenges for public health nurses. Because people were living longer, nurses working in the community had to address the healthcare issues presented by an increasingly aging population, care for the chronically ill, and respond to cardiac diseases and cancer (Winslow, 1945, p. 989). The dramatic communicable illnesses at the beginning of the 20th century gave way to increased disabilities related to chronic illnesses later on. Even though the cost of care in

"She's something special in a very special service." A Visiting Nurse Service of New York flier, 1950.

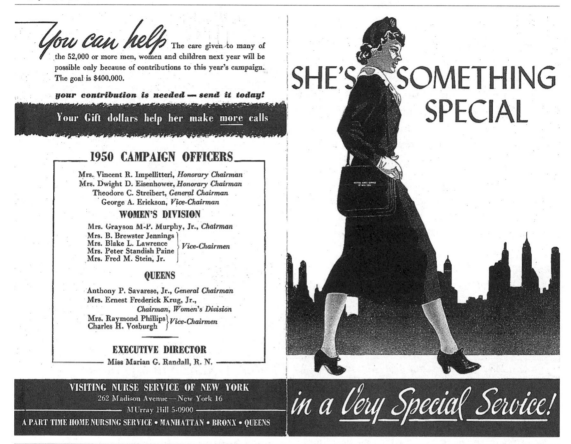

Source: Courtesy of the Visiting Nurse Service of New York.

the home was less than institutional-based care, the institution offered families some support from the daily responsibilities of providing care in the home (Buhler-Wilkerson, 2001).

In the 1950s the nursing profession underwent a transformation, as many of the earlier nursing organizations reorganized. The NOPHN, for example, was subsumed under the NLN, and public health nursing issues became one of many issues for the larger organization, which, in turn, may or may not have sufficiently addressed the needs of this important evolving nursing role. Nursing organizations sought to break down racial and gender bias in nursing, and the NACGN became extinct as it merged with the ANA in 1952. The profession also sought to move nursing education into institutions of higher learning and to encourage more men and women of diverse backgrounds into the profession (Brown, 1948). Esther Lucille

Brown, author of a noted study about nursing, also acknowledged that health care was changing and the existing barriers between healthcare institutions within the community and hospital were breaking down. Brown (1948) wrote that, "The hospital is moving out into the larger community; the community is moving into the hospital" (p. 30). The public health agencies that up to the 1940s had successfully focused on reducing morbidity and mortality rates were now poised to focus on diseases of middle age. Increasing amounts of federal funding in various statewide public health initiatives addressing the control of "venereal disease, tuberculosis, cancer, mental health, and maternal child health" (Brown, 1948, p. 31) added to a changing public health environment in which public health nurses worked. Nurses needed to meet different challenges that public health nursing afforded.

HOME HEALTH NURSING

The social upheaval of the 1960s, challenging women's rights, civil rights, as well as the U.S. military responsibility in Vietnam, also brought with it sweeping social reforms. Medicare legislation in 1965 included a home healthcare benefit to constituents that "increased the reach and visibility of home care and led to its significant growth" (ANA, 2008, p. 2). The 2008 ANA publication regarding the evolution of home health nursing refers the reader back to the founder of the modern nursing movement, Florence Nightingale, and to William Rathborn's district nursing. The evolution of the term "home health nursing" included similarly-expressed ties to the history of public health nursing in the ANA (2007) description of public health nursing. These two terms, home health nursing and public health nursing (and this may be too simplistic), diverged as more people were discharged earlier from hospitals by the 1970s as a result of a Medicare benefit

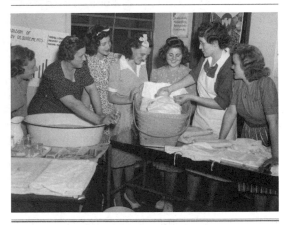

A public health nurse teaching a baby class, 1942.

Source: Courtesy of the Visiting Nurse Service of New York.

offering home care support. Acute care in the home, offered 24 hours a day, 7 days a week, was an outcome of the increased home care benefits reaped by this new social legislation.

By the 1980s, home care services became essential for those people being discharged earlier and earlier from hospitals as a result of the institution of diagnosis-related groups in hospitals across the United States. Home health nursing focused on acute care of individual patients in the home, similar to the focus of early district nurses on care of the sick in the home. Two national nursing organizations formed in the 1980s to address the needs of **home care nurses**, the Visiting Nurse Associations of America and the National Association for Home Care (ANA, 2008).

The ANA published the first standards in home care in 1986, which were subsequently revised in 1992, 1999, and more recently in 2008. Although the definition of home health nursing differs greatly from that of the more recent definition of public health nurse (ANA, 2007), they both share a similar history. However, this history diverged in the 1960s because of the social and political changes in healthcare benefits. The ANA (2008) definition of home health nursing describes it as providing nursing care to the "acutely ill, chronically ill, and well patients of all ages in their residences" (p. 3). The definition goes on to include that the home health nurse focuses on "health promotion and care of the sick while integrating environmental, psychosocial, economic, cultural, and personal health factors affecting an individual's and family's health status" (p. 3). This varies from the ANA (2007) definition of public health nursing, which states that "public health nursing is the practice of promoting and protecting the health of populations using knowledge from nursing, social and public health science" (p. 5). The ANA (2007) further delineates the practice of public health nursing as "population-focused with the goals of promoting health and preventing disease and disability for all people through the creation of conditions in which people can be healthy" (p. 5). According to the ANA (2008), home health nurses assume a greater responsibility in "managing the financial cost of care," and it is this aspect of their role that differentiates this specialty from other nursing specialties (p. 4). Because home health nurses work directly with both public and private payers of care, they must have knowledge of the financial systems that pay for this care to support the individuals and families within their care. The striking difference between the two nursing specialties seems to be the breadth in which they approach the care as well as the target of their care, and yet there seems to be overlap.

COMMUNITY HEALTH NURSE

A term of more recent origin was coined by the ANA to refer to all nurses who work outside of an institutional setting such as the hospital (Clark, 2008). The term **community health nurse** refers to nursing services in the community and

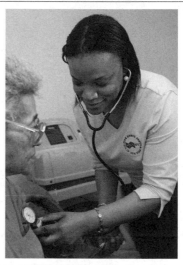

A public health nurse of today.

Source: Courtesy of the Visiting Nurse Service of New York.

encompasses the work of the public health nurse (Jones et al., 1987). In the 1980s, some viewed the terms "community health nurse" and "public health nurse" as interchangeable, whereas some interpreted public health nursing to be a specialty encompassed by the term "community health nurse" (Levin et al., 2007). In 1985 the term "community health nurse" meant that any nurse who worked in a community setting, whether or not he or she was educationally prepared for public health nursing, was considered a community health nurse (Levin et al., 2007). Public health nurses, however, needed advanced education at the master's or doctoral level that was based on public health science (Levin et al., 2007). A distinction between public health nursing and other community health nurses was made in 1992, calling for public health nurses to be "community-based and population focused" (Williams, as cited by Levin et al., 2007, p. 6). The noted nursing leader of the second half of the 20th century, Virginia Henderson, questioned how one could separate "home care from public health nursing . . . and [was] puzzled at the change that has come about in the public image of the community nurse" (Abrams, 2007b, p. 385).

Public Health Nurses in the 21st Century

The title of public health nurse has been used since Lillian Wald claimed the name for the work of the visiting nurse who provided both sick care in the home and the full range of health promotion and disease-preventing activities in the community in the early part of the 1900s. Wald collected statistical data on the work of the public health nurse of Henry Street, served as an advocate for healthcare policy reforms, refined the work of the public health nurse to include school nursing, and led the many early experiments in public health nursing as mentioned earlier in this chapter. As the 20th century progressed and public and private agencies divided the kinds of nursing services provided, the role of the public health nurse was often segmented into either the care of the sick or population-based health-promoting and disease-prevention activities. By the 1970s (and perhaps beginning earlier in the 1960s), community health nursing was the term that was frequently used instead of public health nursing, and in 1973 the ANA published for the first time standards of community health nursing practice (ANA, 2007). In 1986, the ANA defined the community health nursing practice as promoting and preserving the "health of populations by integrating the skills and knowledge relevant to both nursing and public health" (ANA, 2007, p. 56). The glossary of the 1986 document (that was reprinted in the 2007 edition of the *ANA Public Health Nursing: Scope and Standards of Practice*) stated that the terms "public health

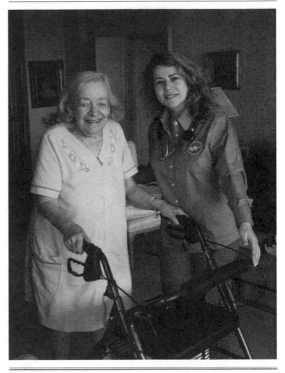

A public health nurse of today.

Source: Courtesy of the Visiting Nurse Service of New York.

nursing and community health nursing are synonymous" (ANA, 2007, p. 57).

The ANA (2007) described the distinguishing characteristic of public health nursing as population-focused with "goals of promoting health and preventing disease and disability as well as improving the quality of life" (p. 11). Public health nurses still cared for the sick at home as well as maintained an expanded role in the care of the public's health. Public health nurses were involved in eight content domains, including "informatics, genomics, communication, cultural competence, community-based participatory research, policy and law, global health, and ethics" (ANA, 2007, p. 2). The increasing complexity of the role was noted by the ANA (2007) as a result of societal and political events that signify challenges to the stability of a community, whether they are local, national, or global. The ANA (2007) identified the threats to the "health of populations as including a reemergence of communicable diseases, increasing incidence of drug-resistant organisms, overall concern about the structure of the health care system, environmental hazards, and the challenges imposed by the presence of modern public health epidemics such as obesity- and tobacco-related deaths" (p. 3). Public health nurses are now involved with "syndromic surveillance, mass casualty planning and the handling of biological and chemical agents" (ANA, 2007, p. 4). Partners in the community now include law enforcement officers, communication experts, postal workers, and others involved in the safety of the community-at-large. According to the ANA (2007), the public health nurse has a greater emphasis on population-based services than ever before. The level of understanding is greater and the demands for higher education more profound. Evidence-based practice guides public health nurses in their work with populations under duress. The current definition of the public health nurse described by the ANA (2007) has evolved into the following:

> *Public health nursing is the practice of promoting and protecting the health of populations using knowledge from nursing, social, and public health sciences (American Public Health Association, Public Health Nursing Section, 1996). The practice is population-focused with the goals of promoting health and preventing disease and disability for all people through the creation of conditions which people can be healthy. (p. 5)*

This text applies the Minnesota Department of Health Population-Based Public Health Nursing Practice Intervention Wheel as a model

Mothers and a public health nurse with babies.

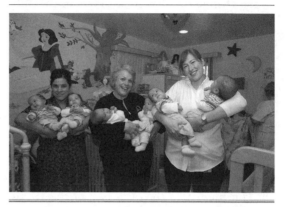

Source: Courtesy of the Visiting Nurse Service of New York.

to guide public health nursing practice. Public health nursing, according to the Minnesota Department of Health (2007), is defined as "the synthesis of the art and science of public health and nursing" (p. 2). This science and art focuses on the development of interventions to the population as opposed to the individual. This population may be defined as a population at risk or those with a common risk factor leading to the threat of a particular health issue. It also may be defined as a population of interest known as a healthy population who may in fact improve their health by making certain choices that will further promote health and/or protect against disease or injury—for example, an adolescent population that engages in alternative sports and chooses to wear protective gear avoids serious injury. Although public health nurses' primary focus is working with populations, their work often extends beyond this. Minnesota Department of Health (2001) noted the following:

> *Public health nurses work in schools, homes, clinics, jails, shelters, out of mobile vans and*

dog sleds. They work with communities, the individuals and families that compose communities and the systems that impact the health of those communities. Regardless of where public health nurses work or whom they work with, all public health nurses use a core set of interventions to accomplish their goals. (p. 1)

Public health nursing still maintains the need to provide care to those in the community, and the evolution of the term continues and seems to be the term that now describes the role of those nurses who work within the community.

A public health nurse weighs a baby.

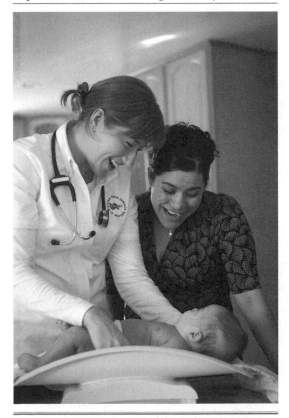

Source: Courtesy of the Visiting Nurse Service of New York.

Education of Public Health Nurses

Although the nomenclature of public health nurses changed over time, the one constant that can be found in the literature was the need for advanced education for those who worked in this specialization. From the inception of public health nursing in the United States, early nursing leaders recognized the need for public health nurses to have more education than the 3-year diploma training provided to support the work they did in this specialization. Programs such as the postgraduate course at the Instructive District Nursing Association of Boston in 1906 and the one started at Teachers College in 1910 were designed to better prepare nurses to take up the work of nursing in the community (Gardner, 1933; Haupt, 1939). By 1915 there were approximately four postgraduate programs in public health, which grew to over 15 in 1922. By 1952 there were over 28 programs set within colleges and universities approved by the NOPHN (NLN, 1952). The various studies that examined nursing in the early 1900s, like the Goldmark report, examined the kinds of advanced education required of public health nurses above and beyond the training they received in the 3-year programs (Crandall, 1922). Later studies, such as Brown's *Nursing for the Future* (1948), recognized that "as collegiate schools of nursing have developed . . . it has come to be believed that preparation designed for beginning positions in public health nursing can and should be built into the basic curriculum" (p. 96). Nurses entering the public health nursing field would be prepared at the baccalaureate level. The American Red Cross rural public health nursing service, known as the Town and Country, required its public health nurses to have additional education as a public health nurse before undertaking such a responsibility (Kernodle, 1949).

In 1952 a joint committee consisting of the NOPHN and the U.S. Public Health Service studied the curricular needs of the public health nurse. The number of public health nurses had increased to over 24,000 in 1952 from 3,000 in 1912 (Gardner, 1933; NLN, 1952). This increase in numbers constituted a "potent force in translating public health science into service" (NLN, 1952, p. iii). As before, public health nurses were responding to the changing concepts of public health that extended into all facets of life. The joint committee developed a public health nursing curriculum guide that reflected the current thinking of that period, which was that public health was "to provide, through community effort, those services for the saving of life, the prevention of disease, and the restoration to health which the individual or family is unable to provide, or to provide as well, by individual effort" (NLN, 1952, p. iii).

The joint committee noted that the profound changes in the science of medicine, public health, psychology, education, social organization, social sciences, and public health administration called for a new and more comprehensive curriculum guide than had previously existed. Recognizing the need for public health nurses to be responsive to future changes, the curriculum guide was designed to develop the professional skills of the individual to meet the needs for the "immediate future" as well as "be able to adjust to changing situations" (NLN, 1952, p. 2). The joint committee recognized the need for advanced content to be included in its guide; however, they seemed ambivalent about specifying the level in which the public health curriculum would be instituted (NLN, 1952):

While the Central Committee decided that an adequate basic nursing education in accor-

dance with generally accepted standards would be assumed in the preparation of the Guide, the Committee recognized that this raised certain practical questions. The actual curriculum content that is needed to produce the knowledge and skill required of the public health nurse today or tomorrow is of course conditioned by the students' previous educational and professional background. It has not been found possible nor deemed necessary to specify at each point in the Guide where the learning should take place—in the school of nursing, in the postgraduate program of study, or through a variety of other processes of education and professional experience. (p. 6)

Associate degree programs in nursing that originated in the early 1950s, with the intent of preparing the "technical" nurse, began to include community and home care in the curriculum in the 1990s (NLN, 1993). In 1993, the NLN published a booklet claiming a vision for nursing education that called for a population-based focus for all nursing programs. All nursing programs accredited by the organization, including baccalaureate, associate, diploma, and practical nursing programs, would ensure that all nurses "are prepared to function in a community-based, community-focused health care system" (NLN, 1993, p. 3). The idea that all types of entry into practice programs would include community content in their curriculum challenged the idea that this content had usually been reserved for baccalaureate and higher degree programs. Although the level of content may have varied, according to the ANA (2007) the "baccalaureate degree in nursing is the educational credential for entry into public health practice" and the master's level prepares a "nurse specialist level with specific expertise in population-focused care" (p. 10). The ANA (2007), however, acknowledges the roles that the associate degree and diploma graduate registered nurse, as well as the licensed practical nurse, have in a community setting. The graduates of these programs also practice in a community setting "where care is directed toward the health or illness of individuals or families, rather than populations" (ANA, 2007, p. 10).

The ANA (2007) describes the term "advanced practice public health nurse" as a master's-prepared public health nurse who functions as a clinical nurse specialist or a nurse practitioner using a population-focused care model. Doctoral education also affords additional opportunities for public health nurses to function in roles such as informatics, clinical practice, epidemiology, and education. Here too the coursework at the doctoral level would have a population focus that translates into the work of the public health nurse.

In 2006, Erie County, New York, advertised for a public health nursing position on the Internet. Anyone responding to this ad had to have a bachelor's or master's degree in nursing. Other states and counties may have different criteria for hiring, but for many agencies the bachelor's degree is the minimum requirement for public health nurses, just as it is in most literature about public health nurses. In a press release, the American Association of Colleges of Nursing again reiterated that one of the essentials of baccalaureate education is "health promotion and disease prevention at the individual and population levels" (2008, p. 2). Yet in keeping with the vast social and economic changes

that fostered a shift from hospital-based care to more home-based care, nursing care at all educational levels adjusted to accommodate to the care needed in the home.

Conclusion

The history of public health nursing tells the story of an extraordinary group of professionals who, over time, adapted to the healthcare needs of the public. Whether they cared for the sick poor or those who could pay, whether they worked in voluntary visiting nurses' organizations or in municipal health departments, whether they were educated in postgraduate programs or in baccalaureate degree programs, these nurses provided both curative and preventive services to the population living in the community. Changing names from district nurse to public health nurse to community nurse and back again to public health nurse only typified the efforts of nurses to adjust to changes that social, political, and economic factors required. The ability to continue to work in public health, regardless of the term applied to their work, shows the resiliency of public health nursing. The tradition whereby a need to redefine itself and reflect on the kinds of care they can provide in both the public and private sector continues with us today. As we read further in the text, it is important to remember the origins of the public health nurses' role as the intervention wheel is applied. Consider the many iterations of this role and how nursing continues to evolve, serve its present day populations, and learn from its past.

References

Abrams, S. E. (2007a). For the good of a common discipline. *Public Health Nursing, 24*(3), 293–297.

Abrams, S. E. (2007b). Nursing the community, a look back at the 1984 dialogue between Virginia

Henderson and Sherry L. Shamansky. *Public Health Nursing, 24*(4), 382–386.

American Association of Colleges of Nurses. (2008, October 30). *Press release: Nursing schools move to trans-*

form baccalaureate education in response to patient care needs and the changing nature of the registered nurse. Retrieved in a blast e-mail to Sandra Lewenson from the AACN; reader was directed to the following website for additional information: http://www.aacn.nche.edu/Education/pdf/BaccEssentials08.pdf

American Nurses Association (ANA). (2007). *Public health nursing: Scope and standards of practice.* Silver Spring, MD: Author.

American Nurses Association (ANA). (2008). *Home health nursing: Scope and standards of practice.* Silver Spring, MD: Author.

Ashmun, M. (1933). The cause and cure of unemployment in the nursing profession. *The American Journal of Nursing, 33*(7), 652–658.

Beard, J. H. (1922). Progress of public health work. *Scientific Monthly, 14*(2), 140–152.

Brainard, A. M. (1919). *Organization of public health nurses.* New York, NY: Macmillan.

Brown, E. L. (1948). *Nursing for the future: A report prepared for the National Nursing Council.* New York, NY: Russell Sage Foundation.

Bryant, Z. (1968). The public health nurses' expanding responsibilities. In D. M. Stewart & P. A. Vincent (Eds.), *Public health nursing* (pp. 3–9). Dubuque, IA: Wm. C. Brown Company.

Buhler-Wilkerson, K. (1985). Public health nursing: In sickness or in health? *American Journal of Public Health, 75*(10), 1155–1161.

Buhler-Wilkerson, K. (1993). Bringing care to the people: Lillian Wald's legacy to public health nursing. *American Journal of Public Health, 83*(12), 1778–1786.

Buhler-Wilkerson, K. (2001). *No place like home: A history of nursing and home care in the United States.* Baltimore, MD: Johns Hopkins University Press.

Carnegie, M. E. (1991). *The path we tread: Blacks in nursing 1854–1990.* New York, NY: National League for Nursing Press.

Clark, M. J. (2008). *Community health nursing* (5th ed.). Upper Saddle River, NY: Pearson-Prentice Hall.

Crandall, E. P. (1919). Letter dated January 9, 1919, from Ella Crandall, Executive Secretary, National Organization for Public Health Nursing, to Dr. George E. Vincent at the Rockefeller Foundation. Collect RC, Record Group 1.1, Series 200, Box 121, Folder 1494, Rockefeller Archives, Pocantico, NY.

Crandall, E. P. (1922). An historical sketch of public health nursing. *American Journal of Nursing, 22*(8), 641–645.

Craven, D. (1889/1984). *A guide to district nursing.* London, UK: Macmillan and Company. In S. Reverby (Series Ed.), *The history of American nursing, A Garland Series.* New York, NY: Garland Publishing.

Craven, D. (1893/1949). On district nursing. In I. A. Hampton and others, *Nursing of the sick 1893: Papers and discussions from the International Congress of Charities, Correction and Philanthropy, Chicago* (published in 1949 under the sponsorship of the National League of Nursing Education, pp. 127–133). New York, NY: McGraw-Hill.

Delano, J. A., & McIsaac, I. (1913). *American Red Cross textbook on elementary hygiene and home care of the sick.* Philadelphia, PA: P. Blakiston's Son & Co.

Dock, L. L., & Stewart, I. M. (1938). *A short history of nursing: From the earliest times to the present day* (4th ed. illustrated). New York, NY: G. P. Putnam's Sons.

Fitzpatrick, M. L. (1975a). *The National Organization for Public Health Nursing, 1912–1952: Development of a practice field.* New York, NY: National League for Nursing Press.

Fitzpatrick, M. L. (1975b). Nurses in American history: Nursing and the Great Depression. *American Journal of Nursing, 75*(12), 2188–2190.

Gardner, M. S. (1933). *Public health nursing* (2nd ed., completely rev.). New York, NY: Macmillan.

Geis, M. J. (1991). Differences in technology among subspecialties in community health nursing. *Journal of Community Health Nursing, 8*(3), 161–170.

Hamilton, D. (1988). Clinical excellence, but too high a cost: The Metropolitan Life Insurance Company Visiting Nurse Service (1909–1953). *Public Health Nursing, 5*(4), 235–240.

Haupt, A. C. (1939). Thirty years of pioneering: In public health nursing. *American Journal of Nursing, 9*(36), 619–626.

Haupt, A. C. (1953). Forty years of teamwork in public health nursing. *American Journal of Nursing, 53*(1), 81–84.

Hiestand, W. C. (1982). Nursing, the family, and the "new" social history. *Advances in Nursing Science,* April:1–12.

Hughes, A. (1893/1949). The origin and present work of Queen Victoria's Jubilee Institute for Nurses. In I. A. Hampton and others, *Nursing of the sick 1893: Papers and discussions from the International Congress of Charities, Correction and Philanthropy, Chicago* (published in 1949 under the sponsorship of the National League of Nursing Education, pp. 111–119). New York, NY: McGraw-Hill.

Humphrey, C. J., & Milone-Nuzzo, P. (1996). *Orientation to home care nursing.* Gaithersburg, MD: Aspen.

Jones, D. C., Davis, J. A., & Davis, M. C. (1987). *Public health nursing: Education and practice.* Springfield, VA: U.S. Department of Health and Human Services, Public Health Service, Health Resources and Services

Administration, Bureau of Health Professions, Division of Nursing.

Kernodle, P. B. (1949). *The Red Cross nurse in action 1882–1948.* New York, NY: Harper and Brothers.

Levin, P., Cary, A., Kulbok, P., Leffers, J., Molle, M., & Polivka, B. (2007). Graduate education for advanced practice public health nursing: At the crossroads. *Association of Community Health Nursing Educators,* 1–24.

Lewenson, S. B. (1993). *Taking charge: Nursing, suffrage, and feminism in America, 1873–1920.* New York, NY: Garland Publishing.

Minnesota Department of Health. (2001). *Public health interventions: Applications for public health nursing practice.* Retrieved from http://www.health.state.mn.us/divs/cfh/ophp/resources/docs/phinterventions_manual2001.pdf

Minnesota Department of Health. (2007). Cornerstone of public health nursing. Retrieved from http://www.health.state.mn.us/divs/cfh/ophp/resources/docs/cornerstones_definition_revised2007.pdf

National League for Nursing (NLN). (1952). *Public health nursing curriculum guide.* New York, NY: National League for Nursing Press.

National League for Nursing (NLN). (1993). *Vision for nursing education.* New York, NY: National League for Nursing Press.

National Organization for Public Health Nursing [NOPHN]. (1914). Pamphlet attached to a letter sent by Ella Crandall to John D. Rockefeller on October 13, 1914, requesting funding for the organization. Collect RC, Record Group 1.1, Series 200, Box 121, Folder 1498, Rockefeller Archives, Pocantico, NY.

National Organization for Public Health Nursing [NOPHN]. (1938). *Board members' manual for board and committee members of public health nursing services* (2nd ed., revised and reset). New York, NY: Macmillan.

Nightingale, F. (1893/1949). Sick nursing and health nursing: Addendum. District nursing. In I. A. Hampton and others, *Nursing of the sick 1893: Papers and discussions from the International Congress of Charities, Correction and Philanthropy, Chicago* (published in 1949 under the sponsorship of the National League of Nursing Education, pp. 24–43). New York, NY: McGraw-Hill.

North, F. N. (1882). A new profession for women. *The Century Magazine, 25*(1), 38–47.

Palmer, S. (1897/1991). Training school alumnae associations. In N. Birnbach & S. B. Lewenson (Eds.), *First words: Selected addresses from the National League for Nursing 1994–1933* (pp. 293–297). New York, NY: National League for Nursing Press.

Roberts, D. E., & Heinrich, J. (1985). Public health nursing comes of age. *American Journal of Public Health, 75*(10), 1162–1172.

Somerville, C. E. M. (1893/1949). District nursing. In I. A. Hampton and others, *Nursing of the sick 1893: Papers and discussions from the International Congress of Charities, Correction and Philanthropy, Chicago* (published in 1949 under the sponsorship of the National League of Nursing Education, pp. 119–127). New York, NY: McGraw-Hill.

Stewart, D. M., & Vincent, P. A. (1968). *Public health nursing.* Dubuque, IA: Wm. C. Brown Company.

Trott, L. L. (1942). *American Red Cross textbook on Red Cross home nursing. Prepared under the direction of nursing service, American Red Cross.* Philadelphia, PA: The Blakiston Company.

Welsh, M. S. (1936). What is public health nursing? *American Journal of Nursing, 36*(5), 452–456.

Winslow, C.-E. A. (1938a). Nursing and the community. *Public Health Nursing,* April. Reprint.

Winslow, C.-E. A. (1938b). Organizing for better community services. *American Journal of Nursing, 38*(7), 761–767.

Winslow, C.-E. A. (1945). Postwar trends in public health and nursing. *American Journal of Nursing, 45*(12), 989–992.

For a full suite of assignments and additional learning activities, use the access code located in the front of your book to visit this exclusive website: http://go.jblearning.com/londrigan. If you do not have an access code, you can obtain one at the site.

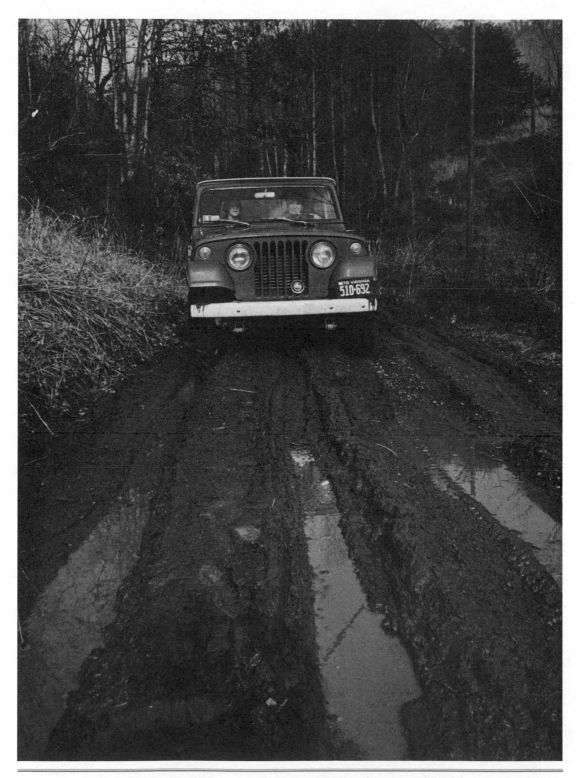

Chapter 3

Assessment: Using the Public Health Nursing Assessment Tool

Marie Truglio-Londrigan
Sandra B. Lewenson

The public health movement did not create the public health nurse, it found her at work in her district nursing the sick, watching over their families, and the neighborhood, and teaching in the homes those sanitary practices, those measures of personal and home hygiene, which do much to prevent disease and to promote health (Nutting, 1923/1991, p. 361).

LEARNING OBJECTIVES

www

At the completion of this chapter, the reader will be able to

- Identify the importance of a public health nursing assessment.
- Describe the components of the Public Health Nursing Assessment Tool.
- Apply the Public Health Nursing Assessment Tool.

KEY TERMS

www

❏ Assessment
❏ Determinants of health
❏ Disparities
❏ General health status
❏ Health-related quality of life and well-being

❏ Minnesota Department of Health Population-Based Public Health Nursing Practice Intervention Wheel Strategies

Assessment supports decision making in health care by providing information about the health of the individual, family, community, system, and population. Shuster and Goeppinger (2008) state that "community assessment is one of the three core functions of public health nursing and is the process of critically thinking about the community" (p. 351). Public health nurses recognize that communities in which the individual, family, system, or population reside influence the health and well-being of all stakeholders. Likewise, the individual, family, system, and population affect the health of the community and each other. An assessment tool guides the public health nurse through the process of discovery. This chapter presents the Public Health Nursing Assessment Tool (PHNAT), designed by Lewenson and Truglio-Londrigan, which uses the concepts found in *Healthy People 2020* (**Figure 3-1**) and the **Minnesota Department of Health Population-Based Public Health Nursing**

Figure 3-1 Graphic model of Healthy People 2020 determinants of health.

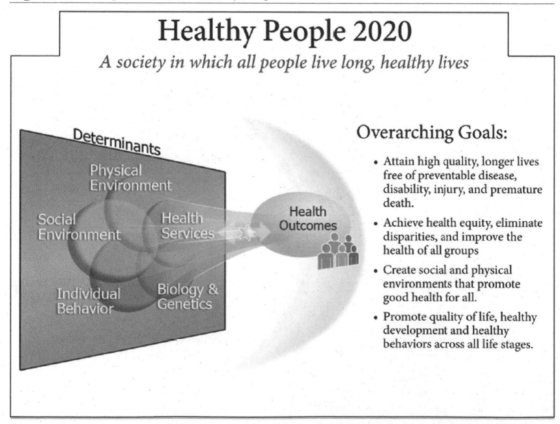

Source: U.S. Department of Health and Human Services [DHHS]. (2010a). *Healthy People 2020 framework.* Retrieved from www.healthypeople.gov/2020/consortium/HP2020Framework.pdf

Practice Intervention Wheel Strategies as its organizing framework. Specifically, the PHNAT uses the four foundation health measures that serve as indicators of progress toward achieving the goals of *Healthy People 2020*. These indicators include **general health status, health-related quality of life and well-being, determinants of health,** and **disparities** (U.S. Department of Health and Human Services [DHHS], 2010b, para. 4p). Using the four foundation health measures helps the public health nurse determine the priority needs of the community and then develop, implement, and evaluate a plan using the intervention wheel strategies as a guide. The PHNAT also asks the public health nurse to reflect on the experience of doing a public health nursing assessment. **Box 3-1** provides an outline of the organization of the PHNAT; it does not include all the detail that is found in the PHNAT, but rather provides a quick schematic.

Overview of the Unique Qualities of the PHNAT

The PHNAT offers a kaleidoscopic way to view the process of assessment. The authors see this kaleidoscopic capability as essential to public health nurses' practice as they work with a wide spectrum of clients. In the public health nurse's practice, clients include individuals, families, communities, systems, and populations. Therefore, a tool that permits the public health nurse to focus on each of these types of clients must be flexible. The PHNAT permits the public health nurse to assess the individual as well as simultaneously assess the community, population,

---

Box 3-1 Public Health Nursing Assessment Tool (PHNAT)

Schematic

Section I: Four Foundational Health Measures

Section I Part 1: Foundational Health Measures General Health Status (Certain aspects of this portion of the PHNAT may be directed toward the individual/family.)

A-1 Individual and Family	B-5 Population: Healthy Life Expectancy
B-1 Population: Vital Statistics	B-6 Population: Years of Potential Life Lost
B-2 Population: Mortality	(YPLL) (with international comparisons)
B-3 Population: Morbidity	B-7 Population: Physically and Mentally
B-4 Population: Life Expectancy (with international comparisons)	Unhealthy Days

Section I Part 2: Foundational Health Measures Health-Related Quality of Life and Well-Being (Individual/family assessment)

A-1 Individual and Family

Section I Part 3: Foundational Health Measures Determinants of Health

Part 3-1 Biology and Genetics

A-1 Individual and Family Assessment	B-3 Population: Race Distribution
B-1 Population Assessment	B-4 Population: Gender Distribution
B-2 Population: Age Distribution	

(continues)

Box 3-1 (continued)

Part 3-2 Social Factors

A-1 Social Determinants: Housing Conditions

A-2 Social Determinants: Transportation

A-3 Social Determinants: Workplace

A-4 Social Determinants: Recreational Facilities

A-5 Social Determinants: Educational Facilities

A-6 Social Determinants: Places of Worship

A-7 Social Determinants: Social Services

A-8 Social Determinants: Library Services

A-9 Social Determinants: Law Enforcement

A-10 Social Determinants: Fire Department

A-11 Social Determinants: Communication

A-12 Social Determinants: Employment Distribution

A-13 Social Determinants: Leading Industries in Community

A-14 Social Determinants: Educational Level of People Older Than 25 Years

A-15 Social Determinants: Family Income

Section I Part 3-2: Physical Determinants

B-1 Physical Determinants: History of the Community

B-2 Physical Determinants: Windshield Survey

B-3 Physical Determinants: The Built Environment

B-4 Physical Determinants: Natural Environment

B-5 Physical Determinants: Physical Barriers/ Boundaries

B-6 Physical Determinants: Environmental/ Sanitation/Toxic Substances

Section I Part 3-3: Health Services

A. Types of Services

A-1 Acute Care

A-2 Home Care

A-3 Primary Care

A-4 Long Term Care

A-5 Rehabilitative

A-6 Assistive Living

A-7 Mental Health Services

A-8 Occupational

A-9 School Health Programs

A-10 Dental

A-11 Palliative

Section I Part 3-3: Access to Care

B-1 Access to Care: Using the Seven A's

Section I Part 3-4: Policymaking

A-1 Local, State, and Federal Organizational Structure of Community

A-2 Political Issues in the Community

A-3 Health Policies

Section I Part 3-5: Behavior

A. Individual (choices for healthy living: exercise, stress reduction activities, sleep and rest, healthy diet, etc.)

B. Population (participation in town weight loss programs or exercise programs)

Section I Part 4: Foundational Health Care Disparities Assessment: Frequently takes place after the collection of data, during the analysis located in Part II of this document. The public health nurse, along with partners, may note disparities from their direct observations of the environment as well as noting disparities within data collected in all of the previous sections of this document. For example, 5-year cancer survival rate differences between races.

Box 3-1 (*continued*)

Section II: Analysis of Health Status

Section III: Prioritize Public Health Issues

Section IV: Plan and Implementation Using Minnesota Intervention Wheel Strategies

Section V: Tracking and Evaluation Section

Section VI: Reflection

Source: Public health nursing: Applying and doing. Sandra B. Lewenson and Marie Truglio-Londrigan. Adapted from U.S. Department of Health and Human Services. (2010a). *Healthy People 2020 framework.* Retrieved from www.healthypeople .gov/2020/about/default.aspx

and system, and this flexibility permits the public health nurse to shift his or her view back and forth depending on the area of focus and the priority needs at that moment in time. The authors developed the PHNAT using the Process Model for Healthy People 2020: Improving Health of Americans (Process Model) as a guide. It is located on the inside front cover of this text, and facilitates this shifting back and forth.

The PHNAT is embedded in and guides the user throughout the Mobilize, Assess, Plan, Implement, and Track (MAPIT) process discussed in Chapter 1, including the mobilization of partners who work together toward ensuring the health of the public. These partners participate in the assessment data gathering, analysis, planning, implementation, tracking of data, evaluation, and reflection. A visualization of the MAPIT process is also presented in the Process Model. Each part of the tool includes space for responses to questions, tables where data can be organized, and definitions for each of the foundational measures. The PHNAT prompts the user to analyze and reference the data collected. As the user becomes more familiar with the PHNAT, additional information and data may be sought, new tables formed, and original ones revised, depending on the needs of the user. For

example, if the user wants to compare the findings with national or global data, he or she can do so. An online version of the PHNAT further facilitates the use of this tool because it can be more easily manipulated and implemented. The comprehensiveness of the PHNAT also suggests that the completion of a public health nursing assessment would lend itself to group work in a course or in the practice setting.

The Internet provides a wealth of data that can be incorporated into the study. Information such as geography and history of a community, as well as census track boundaries and data, can also be found on the Internet and facilitates the assessment of the community. Online databases, such as those found in **Box 3-2**, are examples of important resources the public health nurse can use when completing the PHNAT. The data needed for many of the suggested tables on the PHNAT can be found through the Internet and the various electronic databases. The public health nurse should be sure to select reliable and valid sources on the Internet by taking the time to search sites to see what types of information they offer. When public health nurses come across other sites and resources, they can share them with their colleagues.

The various parts of the PHNAT can be completed in any sequence. This flexibility permits the group to work on this tool and collect the data simultaneously. Assessment is not a linear process and allows for the public health nurse to complete the process based on expediency, interest, time, and efficiency.

The PHNAT can be used by faculty to teach graduate and undergraduate nursing students. It is also meant to be used by public health nurses who work in all types of community settings such as home care, visiting nurse service, health departments, neighborhood health centers, schools, and industry. Because the PHNAT encourages mobilization and collaboration within a community, this tool can be shared and used by others in the community. The ethics of public health practice warrant that public health nurses who collect data be mindful and respectful of those they are assessing—for example, students assessing a community must schedule appointments with the various stakeholders rather than showing up unannounced. They also should carry identification and a letter of introduction from their school in some instances. Just as an assessment is never a static process, neither is the PHNAT a final product.

PHNAT Four Foundational Health Measures

General health status is one of the four foundational health measures. It refers to data that inform the public health nurse and partners in the health initiative about the health of the population and includes information located in Box 3-1 (U.S. DHHS, 2010c). It is important to note that some of this information is not population-focused, such as self-assessed health status; however, this is an example of how public health nurses serve individuals in the community as well as the general population.

Another foundational health measure is health-related quality of life. Health-related quality of life is a complex concept and focuses on "the impact health status has on quality of life" (U.S. DHHS, 2010d). This portion of the PHNAT also focuses on the individual and again sheds light on those public health nurses who do practice on a one-to-one basis with clients in the community. The particular areas included in this portion of the tool are (1) patient-reported outcomes measurement information system (PROMIS) tools to measure health outcomes from a patient perspective, (2) well-being measures, and (3) participation measures that also reflect an individual's perception of his or her health or ability to participate in and interact with the environment (U.S. DHHS, 2010d).

A major portion of the PHNAT includes the determinants of health. In this section the public health nurse collects information pertaining to those factors that determine the health of the individual, family, and the population living in a community. The health determinants that organize this section include biology and genetics, social factors, health services, policymaking, and individual behavior (U.S. DHHS, 2010e).

Biology and Genetics

The determinant of health under biology and genetics may include data that are individual/family-focused or population-focused. The public health nurse gathers the information on the individual and family with whatever health assessment tool he or she uses in the particular academic or clinical setting. Pertaining to the population, aggregate data such as age, race, and gender are important. Box 3-1 offers a comprehensive view of the type of information that needs to be collected. In addition, the databases listed in Box 3-2 help the public health nurse complete this section.

Examples of the types of questions the public health nurse may ask that are representative of this kaleidoscopic view include:

- Who is the client/family?
- What is the health of the client/family?
- What are the client's/family's health behavior and choices?
- Do these choices support health and a healthy lifestyle?
- What are the resources in the community that facilitate health?
- Does the client/family have access to these resources?
- What part of the population does the client/family represent?
- What is the status of health for this population?
- Who makes up this population?
- What do the aggregate data tell about this population?
- Is this family's particular issue reflected in the population as well?

Social Factors

Social factors, the next determinant of health to be considered, include social determinants of health and physical determinants or conditions in the environment (U.S. DHHS, 2010f). Social factors that the public health nurse assesses include the client's interactions and connections with family, friends, and others in the community. These interactions are important for positive health outcomes in individuals/families and a population. Social support is the type of supportive behavior offered to an individual/family or population by another person, family, or agency/organization. The support may be emotional, instrumental as in services provided, informational such as knowledge, and appraisal such as feedback (House, 1981). Social supports may be offered informally, as in the type of support offered to an individual by a family member or a friend, or they may be more formal, as in the support offered by an agency such as Meals On Wheels. The social assessment section of the PHNAT, as shown in Box 3-1, asks for information about formal and informal support systems in the community. Some of the areas that the public health nurse assesses include housing, transportation, work, recreation, education, places of worship, health care, social services, library services, law enforcement, fire protection, and communication services (U.S. DHHS, 2010f). As public health nurses assess these areas, they must pay careful attention to the Seven A's (Krout, 1986; Truglio-Londrigan & Gallagher, 2003; Williams, Ebrite, & Redford, 1991), which are discussed later in this chapter.

The second part of social factors includes physical determinants. The public health nurse must assess the physical environment of the community-at-large. The physical environmental factor informs the public health nurse about the health of the community and the population that resides in that community. Generally speaking, the physical environment is represented by that which can be seen, touched, heard, smelled, and tasted. However, the physical environment also contains less tangible elements, things such as radiation and ozone. The physical environment can harm individual and community health, especially when individuals and communities are exposed to toxic substances; irritants; infectious agents; and physical hazards in homes, schools, and work sites. The physical environment also can promote good health, for example, by providing clean and safe places for people to work, exercise, and play (U.S. DHHS, 2000, p. 19).

In *Healthy People 2020,* a limited definition is offered with an extensive list of physical environment examples that can be used throughout the PHNAT. Collecting assessment data on the physical environment includes what is often referred to as a "windshield survey" (Anderson & McFarlane, 1988; Stanhope & Lancaster, 2008). The windshield survey reflects what one can view from a car window as one drives through a community and contains observations of various components of the community such as housing, open spaces, transportation, race, ethnicity, restaurants, and stores. In urban areas where the use of cars is limited, walking through the community yields similar results. As public health nurses walk or drive through a community, they assess the physical environment using their five senses (Matteson, 1995). Are there trees, flowers, blue sky, trash, cracked asphalt, smokestacks, or garbage? Can birds, dogs, rain, car horns, screams, or traffic be heard? Can nurses smell flowers, grass, gas, or sewerage? And, finally, what tastes abound? In other words: Is the environment clean and safe for the people or are there hidden dangers such as radiation, ozone, carbon monoxide, and lead in their homes? The PHNAT asks the public health nurse to identify the boundaries of the community, the physical characteristics in relation to topography and terrain, the history of the community, sanitation services such as garbage pickup and recycling, and environmental programs that protect air, food, water, and provide animal and vector control. Here the public health nurse can obtain the data by using the Internet and electronic databases, by walking or driving through a community, or by interviewing members of the community.

HEALTH SERVICES

The determinant of health known as health services is more than a listing of the physical, social, and mental health programs offered to individuals/families or populations in a particular community (see Box 3-1). It also includes an assessment of access to these services. This access to quality care is an important part of the PHNAT. Most community- or population-based assessment tools request an assessment of health service organizations; however, the inclusion of access to care using the Seven A's is unique to the PHNAT. The Seven A's address more than the single concept of access. Whether or not there is access frequently depends on the additional factors of awareness, availability, affordability, acceptability, appropriateness, and adequacy of the service. It is essential for the public health nurse to assess and analyze each of these for whether individuals or populations can gain access to essential services that influence their health and well-being (Krout, 1986; Truglio-Londrigan & Gallagher, 2003; Williams et al., 1991).

The following Seven A's questions can assist the public health nurse in analyzing his or her findings:

- Is the population *aware* of its needs and the services of the community?
- Can the population gain *access* to the services that it needs?

- Is the service *available* and convenient to the population in terms of time, location, and place for use?
- How *affordable* is the service for the population in question?
- Is the service *acceptable* to the population in terms of choice, satisfaction, and cultural congruence?
- How *appropriate* is the service for the specific population, or is there a fit?
- Is the service *adequate* in terms of quantity or degree?

Policymaking

The public health nurse must also assess the policies that influence the health of the individual, family, community, system, and population under study. Examples include policies on seat belt use, helmet use, phone use and texting while driving, smoking, and child car seats. Each of these policies has had a positive influence on the health and well-being of individuals and the population at large, resulting in a decrease in disabilities and injuries. The public health nurse must be knowledgeable about how his or her community functions with regard to the political infrastructure, and as such must assess this infrastructure to be familiar with how it works: who are the formal and informal political leaders? How can they be reached? What initiatives have they supported in the past? What are the laws that affect the individual/family, population, and community with regard to the public's health? Are these laws upheld? Are there issues that have not been addressed, and, if so, what can be done to address these issues? The data collected in this section include the organizational structure of the community, a description of the political issues in the community, and an identification of some of the public health laws that affect the community and its mem-

bers' health. As the public health nurse conducts this portion of the assessment, it is important to explore what the local newspapers report, to meet with the local government, and to check out the school boards or any of the governing bodies in the area. Meet the candidates if it is an election year and listen to what the community is saying. Check websites, social networking sites, and local blogs. Using the Internet, here and throughout the PHNAT, assists the public health nurse in obtaining the necessary data and learning about the community.

Behavior (Individual and Population)

The data to be collected in this section of the PHNAT are the behaviors of individuals and families; however, population behavior may also be observed. The type of behavior an individual or population exhibits affects health—an individual who chooses to smoke cigarettes may have a different set of health outcomes compared to an individual who chooses not to smoke cigarettes. In recent years, there have also been examples of population-based behavior; for example, towns have gathered and participated in a collective great smoke-out or weight loss program. The public health nurse collects data on the individual and family that reflect their behavior and again turns the kaleidoscope to look outward to the community and population within that community. Some of the questions that provide insight into individual or population-based behavior are as follows:

- What does the assessment of the client tell about his or her behavior?
- What types of choices does he or she make with regard to diet, physical activity, alcohol, cigarette smoking or other drug use, and so forth?

- How does the family support health choices?
- How does the community support health choices?
- Have there been community-driven health promotion initiatives, like weight loss or physical activity programs such as a walk to school program?

Disparities is the fourth and final foundational health measure. According to *Healthy People 2020,* "If a health outcome is seen in a greater or lesser extent between populations, there is disparity. Race or ethnicity, sex, sexual identity, age, disability, socioeconomic status, and geographic location all contribute to an individual's ability to achieve good health" (U.S. DHHS, 2010g, para. 1). Frequently, the public health nurse will note disparities as he or she makes observations within the community and analyzes the data that are being gathered. Hence, for this foundational health measure much of the information needed is gathered throughout the PHNAT.

Analysis of Health

The public health nurse, along with other partnering members of a health initiative, analyzes the information gathered during the assessment process. Many times the public health nurse will examine past data to see whether trends and patterns have emerged over time. This process of analysis takes time and reflection. The key here is that the public health nurse does not do this alone but takes part in a partnership. This process identifies issues in a community and sets priorities.

Prioritize Public Health Issues

Once the public health nurse and partners conduct the assessment, an analysis of the data elucidates which priority public health issues exist in the community. In determining the priority health issues, the public health nurse, using a population-based focus, collaborates with other public health practitioners, key informants in the community, and any organization or agency that may have a voice with regard to the population and public health issue. In population-based care, partnerships form the necessary bonds to make sustainable changes necessary for health in the particular targeted population. Those involved in the partnership work together to form a common understanding of the issue. All involved, including the population of interest residing in the community, agree on the priority issue identified; this is essential for a positive outcome. Once the priority is noted, the partners confer with the *Healthy People 2020* topic areas and corresponding objectives for guidance in creating and implementing a plan to address the issue (U.S. DHHS, 2010h).

Plan and Implementation: Applying the Minnesota Intervention Wheel Strategies

In this section of the PHNAT, the public health nurse, along with any members of the partnership, develops a plan of action using the intervention wheel strategies. Again, working with members of the partnering organizations as well as other stakeholders is critical, because partnering is more likely to ensure a plan that is congruent with cultural ideas, values, and beliefs. It is also important to engage in reviews to determine a plan that is based in best practice. The PHNAT involves the application of the intervention wheel, which identifies 17 nursing interventions applied to three levels of practice: individual/family, community, and system. The intervention wheel began in the mid-1990s as part of a "grounded theory process carried out by the public health nurse consultants at the Minnesota Department of Health" (Keller, Strohschein, & Briske, 2008, p. 189). Questioning the contribution public health nurses made in population-based care, the consultants held a series of workshops that informed them of the work of public health nurses. Using a systematic, evidenced-based review of the literature, they analyzed the input of public health nurses who worked in a variety of community settings. This enabled the consultants to construct the wheel graph depicting the 17 intervention strategies applied to the three levels of practice (Stanhope & Lancaster, 2008). The intervention strategies visually depicted and color coded on the wheel are case finding, surveillance, disease and health event investigation, outreach, screening, referral and follow-up, case management, delegated functions, health teaching, counseling, consultation, collaboration, coalition building, community organizing, advocacy, social marketing, and policy development and enforcement. The intervention wheel was "conceived as a common language or catalog of general actions used by public health nurses across all practice settings" (Keller et al., 2008, p. 193).

For the purposes of this text, these intervention strategies have been separated out into five themes addressed in specific intervention chapters:

- *Hitting the pavement* includes the strategies of case finding, surveillance, disease and health event investigation, outreach, and screening.
- *Running the show* includes the strategies of referral and follow-up, case management, and delegated functions.
- *Working it out* includes the strategies of health teaching, counseling, and consultation.

- *Working together* includes the interventions of collaboration, coalition building, and community organizing.
- *Getting the word out* includes the interventions of advocacy, social marketing, and policy development and enforcement.

These intervention chapters focus on each of the themes noted above by using case study examples from public health nurses who use the intervention wheel strategies to address public health problems experienced by individuals, families, and populations within their communities. The reader can refer to these chapters when using the PHNAT.

Overall, when selecting the intervention strategy and developing a plan of action, the public health nurse works in concert with others in the community and considers the following:

- The population to be targeted for the plan
- Short-term goal(s), long-term goal(s)
- Community resources, including human, financial, time, technology, and educational resources
- Financing of the implementation and evaluation of the plan
- Evidence that supports the intervention for this population
- Evidence that the strategy is culturally appropriate
- Evidence that the Seven A's are accounted for
- Best place to implement the strategy
- Best person to implement the strategy
- How to evaluate whether or not the outcomes are met

Tracking and Evaluation

Tracking and evaluation are critical to the entire Process Model outlined on the inside front cover of this text and noted as the last part of the MAPIT process. While the partnership is determining what the plan will be and how the plan will be implemented, it is also important for them to determine what type of information will be collected, where it will be collected, who will collect it, where it will be stored, what kind of technology will be used, how it will be collected, and what type of resources will be needed. This is important for tracking so that the public health nurse and partners may determine if progress is being made in meeting objectives. If it is determined that there is progress, the public health nurse and partners will need to decide if the same plan and course of action will be sustained. If there are questions about the progress, changes may need to be initiated. This tracking of information and evaluation feed back to all levels of the Process Model. Over time, analysis of the data may inform the public health nurse and the members of the partnership that the vision or goals may need to change, or the partners may determine that the plan is not based in evidence or is not culturally congruent or that one or more of the Seven A's is not met and that these are the reasons for the weak outcomes. The tracking of data and evaluation, although at the bottom of the model, are important and inform every part of the Process Model. In 2010, the Institute of Medicine (IOM) published a report, *For the Public's Health: The Role of Measurement in Action and Accountability,* which speaks to some of the issues related to tracking and evaluation. Some of the interesting and complex questions raised include: How do we measure our progress as a nation in our movement toward a healthier America? What measurement approaches can we implement that will help us evaluate and critique agencies'/partnership's health initiatives with regard to population-based health outcomes? What are the best ways to gather and analyze data with a focus on all of the foundational health measures? So much time, energy, and resources are spent in partnership development, assessment, prioritizing of issues, planning, and in the implementation of health initiatives; tracking and evaluation are critical to all of these processes in that they bring us back to the three core functions of public health: assessment, policy development, and assurance.

Reflection

This final section of the PHNAT reminds the public health nurse to be reflective in his or her practice. Self-reflection aids in the decision-making process (Truglio-Londrigan & Lewenson, 2008) and causes the public health nurse to be vigilant during the assessment process and in the implementation of any plans. Questions that the public health nurse may ask include: What am I observing? What am I hearing? Am I seeing and hearing all that needs to be seen and heard? What am I missing? What feelings am I experiencing during this assessment process? Are these feelings facilitating this assessment or creating a barrier to the assessment? Are these feelings hindering the development of the partnership and the development of trust? Am I engaging in activities that help in mobilizing the community of interest?

The table in this reflection section asks the public health nurse to keep a record of the experience. The public health nurse can use this table to record when he or she worked on the assessment and how he or she responded to the various parts of the assessment, reflect on the group experience if the assessment was conducted in a group, or record any personal or professional reflection observed during the assessment process.

Conclusion

This chapter explains how to conduct a public health nursing assessment using the author-designed PHNAT. The unique qualities of the PHNAT include the use of the U.S. DHHS (2010a–h) foundational health measures including general health status, health-related quality of life and well-being, determinants of health, and disparities; application of the intervention wheel strategies; and self-reflection. The application of the PHNAT provides the public health nurse with the information that needs to be analyzed and ultimately determines the priority healthcare issues for a specific population within a community. To carry out the assessment, the public health nurse uses a variety of methods to obtain the data, including observation, interviews, Internet research, census tracks, government reports, newspaper accounts, and evidence of best practice. The public health nurse collaborates with other public health practitioners, key informants in the community, and other agencies to determine the priority. Once this priority is identified, the public health nurse works toward the development and implementation of a culturally congruent initiative based in evidence. The tracking evaluation of the initiative is part of the plan, as is the reflective piece by the public health nurse. Both the outcomes of the evaluation and the reflections provide rich feedback to the community and the public health nurse as he or she continues the ongoing assessment process.

References

Anderson, E. T., & McFarlane, J. (Eds.). (1988). *Community as client: Application of the nursing process.* Philadelphia, PA: Lippincott.

House, J. S. (1981). *Work stress and social support.* Reading, MA: Addison-Wesley.

Institute of Medicine (IOM). (2010). *For the public's health: The role of measurement in action and accountability.* Washington, DC: National Academies Press.

Keller, L. O., Strohschein, S., & Briske, L. (2008). Population-based public health nursing practice: The intervention wheel. In M. Stanhope & J. Lancaster (Eds.), *Public health nursing: Population-centered health care in the community* (7th ed., pp. 186–214). St. Louis, MO: Mosby Elsevier.

Krout, J. A. (1986). *The aged in rural America.* Westport, CT: Greenwood.

Matteson, P. S. (1995). *Teaching nursing in the neighborhoods: The Northeastern University Model.* New York, NY: Springer.

Nutting, A. (1923/1991). Thirty years of progress in nursing. In N. Birnbach & S. B. Lewenson (Eds.), *First words: Selected addresses from the National League for Nursing 1894–1933* (pp. 358–369). New York, NY: National League for Nursing Press.

Shuster, G. F., & Goeppinger, J. (2008). Community as client: Assessment and analysis. In M. Stanhope & J. Lancaster (Eds.), *Public health nursing: Population-centered health care in the community* (7th ed., pp. 339–372). St. Louis, MO: Mosby Elsevier.

Stanhope, M., & Lancaster, J. (Eds.). (2008). *Public health nursing: Population-centered health care in the community* (7th ed.). St. Louis, MO: Mosby Elsevier.

Truglio-Londrigan, M., & Gallagher, L. (2003). Using the Seven A's to determine older adults' community resource needs. *Home Healthcare Nurse, 21*(12), 827–831.

Truglio-Londrigan, M., & Lewenson, S. B. (2008). Know yourself: Reflective decisionmaking. In S. B. Lewenson & M. Truglio-Londrigan (Eds.), *Decision-making for nurses: Thoughtful approaches to practice* (pp. 1–11). Sudbury, MA: Jones and Bartlett.

U.S. Department of Health and Human Services. (2000). *Healthy people 2010* (Vol. 1). Washington, DC: U.S. Government Printing Office.

U.S. Department of Health and Human Services. (2010a). *Healthy people 2020 framework.* Retrieved from http://www.healthypeople.gov/2020/Consortium/HP2020Framework.pdf

U.S. Department of Health and Human Services. (2010b). *About healthy people.* Retrieved from http://www.healthypeople.gov/2020/about/default.aspx

U.S. Department of Health and Human Services. (2010c). *General health status.* Retrieved from http://www.healthypeople.gov/2020/about/GenHealthAbout.aspx

U.S. Department of Health and Human Services. (2010d). *Health-related quality of life.* Retrieved from http://www.healthypeople.gov/2020/about/QoLWBabout.aspx

U.S. Department of Health and Human Services. (2010e). *Determinants of health.* Retrieved from http://www.healthypeople.gov/2020/about/DOHAbout.aspx

U.S. Department of Health and Human Services. (2010f). *Determinants of health social factors.* Retrieved from http://www.healthypeople.gov/2020/about/DOHAbout.aspx#socialfactors.

U.S. Department of Health and Human Services. (2010g). *Disparities.* Retrieved from http://www.healthypeople.gov/2020/about/DisparitiesAbout.aspx

U.S. Department of Health and Human Services. (2010h). *Topics and objectives.* Retrieved from http://www.healthypeople.gov/2020/topicsobjectives2020/default.aspx

Williams, M., Ebrite, F., & Redford, L. (1991). *In-home services for elders in rural America.* Kansas City, MO: National Resource Center for Rural Elderly.

For a full suite of assignments and additional learning activities, use the access code located in the front of your book to visit this exclusive website: http://go.jblearning.com/londrigan. If you do not have an access code, you can obtain one at the site.

Public Health Nursing Assessment Tool

Designed by Sandra B. Lewenson and Marie Truglio-Londrigan

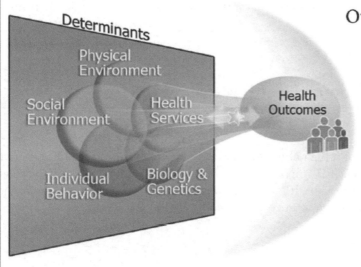

Healthy People 2020

A society in which all people live long, healthy lives

Determinants

Physical Environment

Social Environment

Health Services

Individual Behavior

Biology & Genetics

Health Outcomes

Overarching Goals:

- Attain high quality, longer lives free of preventable disease, disability, injury, and premature death.

- Achieve health equity, eliminate disparities, and improve the health of all groups

- Create social and physical environments that promote good health for all.

- Promote quality of life, healthy development and healthy behaviors across all life stages.

Suggestions for Table Use:

1. Read all horizontal and vertical columns. These will give clues about the key questions to ask.
2. Fill in the vertical column for each table that requests information on the Seven A's. When filling in these boxes, place the most pertinent information that you think informs the assessment.
3. When completing Section I *Part 3-3 (B-1)*: Access to Care, note that this is a summary of the work that you did in Part 1. Reflect on this information and arrive at your decisions pertaining to access to care.
4. In some instances, you need to consider collecting data on multiple years to identify trends. You can duplicate these tables and use them to collect the data on different years using census data.
5. Remember that this is a working document that you, the public health nurse, can adjust and revise to meet the needs of the community you are assessing. The collection of data is more than filling in the boxes. You may need to collect additional data in a particular area, depending on what you learn as you go. For example, you may fill in the boxes about the number of schools in a community, but you may also want to know the number of students per faculty member, if a community collaborator cited that as a concern.
6. In some instances, there will be overlap of data collection. Because information for this tool will usually be collected by a group, in qualitative research the overlap may be considered a saturation of data. In the analysis section, these data will provide a variety of perspectives.

Section I Part 1: Foundational Health Measures

General Health Status

Refers to information that will inform the public health nurse and partners in the health initiative about the health of the population. It is important to note that some of this information is not population focused such as self-assessed health status; however, this is an example of how public health nurses serve individuals in the community as well as the general population.

Section I Part 1

A-1 Individual and Family

When appropriate, the public health nurse will include self-assessed health status as well as history, physical, genogram, ecogram, and any other tools used by his or her organization. Summarize your finding in a narrative form below.

Source of Evidence: _____

Section I Part 1

B-1 Population: Vital Statistics

	Census Track		Community		County		State	
	#	%	#	%	#	%	#	%
Live births								
General deaths								

Source of Evidence: _____

Section I Part 1

B-2 Population: Mortality

Census Track	Community	County	State

Source of Evidence: _____

Section I Part 1

B-3 Population: Morbidity

Census Track	Community	County	State

Source of Evidence: _____

Section I Part 1

B-4 Population: Life Expectancy

Census Track	Community	County	State	National/International

Source of Evidence: _____

Section I Part 1

B-5 Population: Healthy Life Expectancy

Census Track	Community	County	State	National/International

Source of Evidence: _____

Section I Part 1

B-6 Population: Years of Potential Life Lost (YPLL)

Census Track	Community	County	State	National/International

Source of Evidence: _____

Section I Part 1

B-7 Population: Physically and Mentally Unhealthy Days

Census Track	Community	County	State	National/International

Source of Evidence: _____

Section I Part 2: Foundational Health Measures

Health-Related Quality of Life and Well-Being

Health-related quality of life is a complex concept and focuses on "the affect of health status on quality of life". This portion of the PHNAT also focuses on the individual and again sheds light on those public health nurses who do practice on a one-to-one basis with clients in the community.

Section I Part 2

A-1 Individual and Family*—Includes review of the following:

- Patient-Reported Outcomes Measurement Information System (PROMIS) (www.nihpromis .org/default.aspx) tools to measure health outcomes from a patient perspective
- Well-being measures
- Participation measures (activities of daily living, instrumental activities of daily living)

*There is no B in Section I Part 2.

Section I Part 3: Foundational Health Measures

Determinants of Health
Section I Part 3-1
Biology and Genetics

The determinants of health under biology and genetics include data that are individual/family focused or population focused. The public health nurse gathers the information on the individual and family as a client using whatever health assessment tool he or she uses in the particular academic or clinical setting. Pertaining to the population aggregate, data such as age, race, and gender would be considered important to gather.

Section I Part 3-1

A-1 Individual and Family Assessment

In this section, when appropriate, the public health nurse includes an assessment of the individual and family. Include the history, genogram, and ecogram. Special consideration is given to analysis of genetically defined diseases such as sickle cell anemia, cystic fibrosis, and BRCA1 or BRCA2.

Section I Part 3-1

B-1 Population Assessment

	Census Track	Community	County	State
Population at last census				
Population density				
Population changes in the last 10 years				

Source of Evidence: _____

Section I Part 3-1

B-3 Population: Race Distribution

	Census Track		Community		County		State	
	#	%	#	%	#	%	#	%
White								
Black/African American								
Hispanic								
Asian								
Native American								
Other								

Source of Evidence: _____

Section I Part 3-1

B-4 Population: Gender Distribution

	Census Track		Community		County		State	
	#	%	#	%	#	%	#	%
Female								
Male								

Source of Evidence: _____

Section I Part 3-2
Social Factors

Social factors, the next determinant of health to be considered, include social determinants of health and physical determinants or conditions in the environment. Social factors that the public health nurse assesses include the client's interactions and connections with family, friends, and others in their community. The second part includes physical determinants. The public health nurse must assess the physical environment of the community at large.

Section I Part 3-2
A-1 Social Determinants: Housing Conditions

Housing Characteristics	Total # of Units	Owner Occupied	Renter Occupied	Vacant	Housing Subsidies/Homeless Provisions

Source of Evidence: _____

Section I Part 3-2

A-2 Social Determinants: Transportation

	Description of Services: Cost, Destination of Service, Quality of Service, Condition of Services and/or Roads, Handicap Accessibility	Data Collection on Seven A's that will assist with determining adequacy or inadequacy
Train		
Bus		
Taxi including private services		
Major roads		
Minor roads		
Volunteers providing transportation		
School buses		

Source of Evidence: _____

Section I Part 3-2

A-3 Social Determinants: Workplace

List Places of Employment	Description of Workplace Professional, Industry, Factories, Schools, Town, City, County, Businesses	What Workplace Safety Measures Are in Place?	What Is the Estimated Yearly Salary Range of Employees?

Additional Questions to Ask:

- Do most people who reside in the community work in the community or do they commute?
- If they commute, what is their mode of transportation?
- What is the cost of that commute?
- What is the time of the commute?
- Does this commute impact quality of life?

Source of Evidence: _____

Section I Part 3-2

A-4 Social Determinants: Recreational Facilities

Recreational Facilities	Area Served/Services Provided, Cost, Population Served, Hours, Maintenance of Recreation Facilities (e.g., parks, playgrounds, athletic fields)	Data Collection on Seven A's that will assist with determining adequacy or inadequacy

Source of Evidence: _____

Section I Part 3-2

A-5 Social Determinants: Educational Facilities

	# of Public	# of Private (religious)	# of Private (secular)
Preschool			
Elementary			
Junior high			
Senior high			
Colleges/universities			
Early morning programs			
Recreational programs within school system			
After-school programs			

Source of Evidence: _____

Section I Part 3-2

A-6 Social Determinants: Places of Worship

Name/Address/Phone	Denomination	Services

Source of Evidence: _____

Section I Part 3-2

A-7 Social Determinants: Social Services

Agency Name/Address/Phone (food and clothing banks, homeless shelters, adult day care social services, child care)	Area Served/Services Provided/Cost of Services	Data Collection on Seven A's that will assist with determining adequacy or inadequacy

Source of Evidence: _____

Section I Part 3-2

A-8 Social Determinants: Library Services

Libraries Name/Address/Phone	Area Served/Services Provided	Data Collection on Seven A's that will assist with determining adequacy or inadequacy

Source of Evidence: _____

Section I Part 3-2

A-9 Social Determinants: Law Enforcement

Law Enforcement Services	Area Served/Services Provided, Size, Equipment, Response Time, Types of Calls Over Past 6 Months, Neighborhood Programs	Data Collection on Seven A's that will assist with determining adequacy or inadequacy
Police force		
Special services (SWAT, bomb squads, emergency response teams)		
Animal enforcement		
Senior watch patrols		
Private security		
Neighborhood watches		
Vigilante groups		

Source of Evidence: _____

Section I Part 3-2

A-10 Social Determinants: Fire Department

Fire Department Stations	Area Served/Services Provided, Number of Companies, Equipment, Response Time, Types of Calls Over Past 6 Months, Community Programs	Data Collection on Seven A's that will assist with determining adequacy or inadequacy
Fire fighters in company		
Special fire forces (emergency response teams)		

Source of Evidence: _____

Section I Part 3-2

A-11 Social Determinants: Communication

	Description of Services (include whether it is community based, state, or national)	Data Collection on Seven A's that will assist with determining adequacy or inadequacy
Television (e.g., educational, relaxation, emergency response)		
Radio (e.g., educational, relaxation, emergency response)		
Newsprint (e.g., educational, relaxation, emergency response)		
Internet/social networking/text messaging (e.g., educational, relaxation, emergency response)		
Newsletters		
Bulletin boards		
Telephone chains		

Source of Evidence: _____

Section I Part 3-2

A-12 Social Determinants: Employment Distribution

	# in Census Track	# in Community	# in County	# in State
Employed persons				
Unemployed persons				

Source of Evidence: _____

Section I Part 3-2

A-13 Social Determinants: Leading Industries in Community (name at least two)

Name	Address	Type	# of Employed

Source of Evidence: _____

Section I Part 3-2

A-14 Social Determinants: Educational Level of People Older Than 25 Years

	Census Track	Community	County	State
Ninth grade and lower				
High school graduate				
Some college				
College graduate (associ-ate's and baccalaureate)				
Median # of years of school completed				

Source of Evidence: _____

Section I Part 3-2

A-15 Social Determinants: Family Income

	Census Track	Community	County	State
$0–5,000				
$5,000–$9,999				
$10,000–$14,000				
$15,000–$24,999				
$25,000–$34,999				
$50,000–$64,000				
$65,000–$79,000				
$80,000 or more				
	100%	100%	100%	100%

Source of Evidence: _____

Section I Part 3-2

B-1 Physical Determinants: History of the Community

Write a narrative including information about the history of the community you are assessing. Include data that describe who started the community, any interesting stories that define the community.

Source of Evidence: _____

Section I Part 3-2

B-2 Physical Determinants: Windshield Survey

The windshield survey reflects what the public health nurse can view from a car window while driving through a community and contains observations of various components in the community such as housing, open spaces, transportation, race, ethnicity, restaurants, and stores.

Source of Evidence: _____

Section I Part 3-2

B-3 Physical Determinants: The Built Environment

The built environment describes the man-made structures in the community including the kinds of stores, buildings, and sidewalks that facilitate healthy behaviors (or not). Describe your observations about this built environment and how it may be a determinant of health.

Source of Evidence: _____

Section I Part 3-2

B-4 Physical Determinants: Natural Environment

Write a narrative that includes data on factors such as topography, climate, terrain, topographical features, and other factors in the community.

Source of Evidence: _____

Section I Part 3-2

B-5 Physical Determinants: Physical Barriers/Boundaries

Write a narrative that includes data such as geographical boundaries and man-made boundaries.

Source of Evidence: _____

Section I Part 3-2

B-6 Physical Determinants: Environmental/Sanitation/Toxic Substances

	Description of Services (include whether it is community based, state, or national)	Data Collection on Seven A's that will assist with determining adequacy or inadequacy
Water supply		
Sewerage supply		
Solid waste disposal		
Provisions or laws for recycling		
Air contaminants		
Vector control programs for deer, ticks, rabid animals, rodents		
Other		

Source of Evidence: _____

Section I Part 3-3

Health Services

The determinant of health known as health services is more than a listing of the physical, social, and mental health programs offered to an individual/family or a population in a particular community. It also includes an assessment of access to these services and uses the Seven A's. The Seven A's address more than the single concept of access. Whether or not there is access frequently depends on additional concepts of awareness, availability, affordability, acceptability, appropriateness, and adequacy of the service. Each of these is essential to assess and analyze for whether individuals or populations can access essential services that can influence their health and well-being.

Source of Evidence: _____

Section I Part 3-3

A-1 Acute Care

Agency Name/Address/Phone	Area Served/Services Provided, Cost, Hours, Population Served	Data Collection on Seven A's that will assist with determining adequacy or inadequacy

Source of Evidence: _____

Section I Part 3-3

A-2 Home Care

Agency Name/Address/Phone	Area Served/Services Provided, Cost, Hours, Population Served	Data Collection on Seven A's that will assist with determining adequacy or inadequacy

Source of Evidence: _____

Section I Part 3-3

A-3 Primary Care

Agency Name/Address/Phone	Area Served/Services Provided, Cost, Hours, Population Served	Data Collection on Seven A's that will assist with determining adequacy or inadequacy

Source of Evidence: _____

Section I Part 3-3
A-4 Long-Term Care

Agency Name/Address/Phone	Area Served/Services Provided, Cost, Hours, Population Served	Data Collection on Seven A's that will assist with determining adequacy or inadequacy

Source of Evidence: _____

Section I Part 3-3
A-5 Rehabilitative

Agency Name/Address/Phone	Area Served/Services Provided, Cost, Hours, Population Served	Data Collection on Seven A's that will assist with determining adequacy or inadequacy

Source of Evidence: _____

Section I Part 3-3
A-6 Assistive Living

Agency Name/Address/Phone	Area Served/Services Provided, Cost, Hours, Population Served	Data Collection on Seven A's that will assist with determining adequacy or inadequacy

Source of Evidence: _____

Section I Part 3-3
A-7 Mental Health Services

Agency Name/Address/Phone	Area Served/Services Provided, Cost, Hours, Population Served	Data Collection on Seven A's that will assist with determining adequacy or inadequacy

Source of Evidence: _____

Section I Part 3-3
A-8 Occupational

Agency Name/Address/Phone	Area Served/Services Provided, Cost, Hours, Population Served	Data Collection on Seven A's that will assist with determining adequacy or inadequacy

Source of Evidence: _____

Section I Part 3-3
A-9 School Health Programs

Agency Name/Address/Phone	Area Served/Services Provided, Cost, Hours, Population Served	Data Collection on Seven A's that will assist with determining adequacy or inadequacy

Source of Evidence: _____

Section I Part 3-3

A-10 Dental

Agency Name/Address/Phone	Area Served/Services Provided, Cost, Hours, Population Served	Data Collection on Seven A's that will assist with determining adequacy or inadequacy

Source of Evidence: _____

Section I Part 3-3

A-11 Palliative

Agency Name/Address/Phone	Area Served/Services Provided, Cost, Hours, Population Served	Data Collection on Seven A's that will assist with determining adequacy or inadequacy

Source of Evidence: _____

Section I Part 3-3

B-1 Access to Care

The following Seven A's questions can assist the public health nurse in analyzing his or her findings:

- Is the population aware of its needs and the services in the community?
- Can the population gain access to the services that it needs?
- Is the service available and convenient to the population in terms of time, location, and place for use?
- How affordable is the service for the population in question?
- Is the service acceptable to the population in terms of choice, satisfaction, and cultural congruence?
- How appropriate is the service for the specific population or is there a fit?
- Is there adequacy of service in terms of quantity or degree?

Section I Part 3-3

B-1 Access to Care: Using the Seven A's

	Adequate/ Inadequate	Identify as a Problem Statement
Is the individual/family or population aware of its needs and services in the community?		
Can the individual/family or population gain access to the services it needs?		
Is the service available and convenient for the individual/family or population in terms of time, location, and place for use?		
How affordable is the service for the individual/family or population?		
Is the service acceptable to the individual/family or population in terms of choice, satisfaction, and congruence with cultural values and beliefs?		
How appropriate is the service for the individual/family or population or is there a fit?		
Is there adequacy of service in terms of quantity or degree for the individual/family or population?		

Source of Evidence: _____

Section I Part 3-4
Policymaking

The public health nurse must also assess the policies that influence the health of the individual, family, community, system, and population under study. Examples include policies on seat belt use, helmet use, phone use and texting while driving, and child car seats. Each of these policies has had a positive influence on the health and well-being of individuals and the population at large, resulting in a decrease in disabilities and injuries. The public health nurse must be knowledgeable about how his or her community functions with regard to the political infrastructure and as such must assess this infrastructure to be familiar with how it works: who are the formal and informal political leaders? How can they be reached? What initiatives have they supported in the past? What are the laws that affect the individual/family, population, and community with regard to the public's health? Are these laws upheld? Are there issues that have not been addressed, and, if so, what can be done to address these issues? The data collected in this section include the organizational structure of the community, a description of the political issues in the community, and an identification of some of the public health laws that affect the community and its members' health. As the public health nurse conducts this portion of the assessment, it is important to explore what the local newspapers report, to meet with the local government, and to check out the school boards or any of the governing bodies in that area. Meet the candidates if it is an election year and listen to what the community is saying. Check websites, social networking sites, and local blogs. Using the Internet, here and throughout the PHNAT, assists the public health nurse in obtaining the necessary data and learning about the community.

Section I Part 3-4

A-1 Local, State, and Federal Organizational Structure of Community

In the following table, include the organizational structure of the community including political parties of leadership: governor, senators, assemblypersons, mayor, and boards.

Once you collect the data, include a narrative and an organizational chart that represents a visual model of the hierarchy.

- Titles
- Names
- Method of contact
- Initiatives supported in the past and presently
- Interview one of the officials or go to a town board meeting

Source of Evidence: _____

Section I Part 3-4

A-2 Political Issues in the Community

Political Issues	Action Taken/Policy

Source of Evidence: _____

Section I Part 3-4

A-3 Health Policies (e.g., seat belts, taxes on tobacco, smoking ordinances, cell phone and texting bans)

Health Policies	Action Taken/Policy

Source of Evidence: _____

Section I Part 3-5

Behavior

Collect data on the individual and family that reflect their behavior, and again turn the kaleido-scope to look outward to the community and population in that community.

The public health nurse gathers the information on the individual and family as a client using whatever health assessment tool he or she uses in the particular academic or clinical setting. Some of the questions that provide insight into individual or population-based behavior are as follows:

- What does your assessment of the client tell you about his or her behavior?
- What types of choices does he or she make with regard to diet, physical activity, alcohol, cigarette smoking or other drug use, and so forth?
- How does the family support health choices?
- How does the community support health choices?
- Have there been community-driven health promotion initiatives that support health such as weight loss or physical activity programs like a walk-to-school program?

Summarize your finding in a narrative form below.

Section I Part 4: Health Care Disparities

According to Healthy People 2020, "If a health outcome is seen in a greater or lesser extent between populations, there is disparity. Race or ethnicity, sex, sexual identity, age, disability, socioeconomic status, and geographic location all contribute to an individual's ability to achieve good health" (2010f, para. 1). Frequently, the public health nurse will note disparities as he or she observes within the community and analyzes the data gathered. Hence, for this foundational health measure much of the information needed is gathered throughout the PHNAT. Summarize your finding in a narrative form below.

Section II: Analysis of Health Status

The public health nurse, along with other partnering members of a health initiative, analyzes the information gathered during the assessment process. Many times, the public health nurse will examine past data to see whether trends and patterns have emerged over time. This process of analysis takes time and reflection. The key here is that the public health nurse does not do this alone. It is a process that takes shape and form in the partnership. From this process the issues in a community are identified and priorities are set. Summarize your findings below identifying community needs, topics, and objectives.

Section III: Prioritize Public Health Issues

In determining the priority health issues, the public health nurse, using a population-based focus, collaborates with other public health practitioners, key informants in the community, and any organization or agency that may have a voice with regard to the population and public health issue. In population-based care, partnerships form the necessary bonds that make sustainable change for health in particular targeted populations. Those involved in the partnership work together to form a common understanding of the issue. All involved, including the population of interest residing in the community, agree on the priority issue identified. This is essential for a positive outcome. Once the priority is noted, then the partnership will confer with the Healthy People 2020 topic areas and corresponding objectives (U.S. DHHS, 2010g).

Section III: Prioritize Public Health Issues in Order of Priority

Issues	Targeted Population	Short-Term Goal(s)	Long-Term Goal(s)

Section IV and Section V: Plan and Implementation Using Minnesota Intervention Wheel Strategies

Tracking and Evaluation

Minnesota Intervention Strategies and Levels of Practice

Interventions	Levels of Practice			
	Individual/ Family/ Population	Community	System	Track and Outcome Evaluation
Surveillance				
Disease and health threat investigation				
Outreach				
Screening				
Case-finding				
Referral/follow-up				
Case management				
Delegated functions				
Health teaching				
Counseling				

(continues)

Tracking and Evaluation (*continued*)

Minnesota Intervention Strategies and Levels of Practice

Interventions	Levels of Practice			
	Individual/ Family/ Population	Community	System	Track and Outcome Evaluation
Consultation				
Collaboration				
Coalition building				
Community organizing				
Advocacy				
Social marketing				
Policy development and enforcement				

Section VI: Reflection

This final section reminds the public health nurse to be reflective in his or her practice. This section can be completed throughout the PHNAT process. Some of the questions that the public health nurse may ask include the following:

- What am I observing?
- What am I hearing?
- Am I seeing and hearing all that needs to be seen and heard?
- What am I missing?
- What feelings am I experiencing during this assessment process?
- Are these feelings facilitating this assessment or creating a barrier to the assessment?
- Are these feelings hindering the development of the partnership and the development of trust?
- Am I engaging in activities that help in mobilizing the community of interest?

A. Reflection Gained During Public Health Nursing Assessment

Date	Reflection

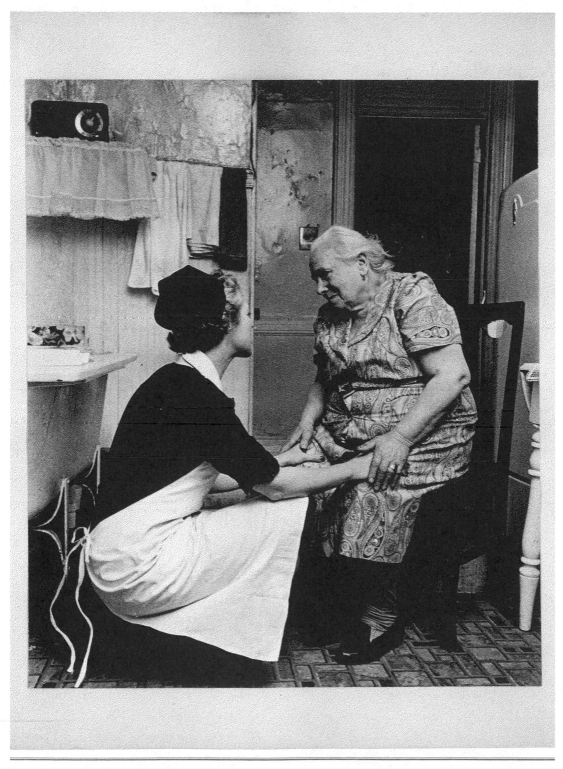

Source: Courtesy of the Visiting Nurse Service of New York.

Chapter 4

Fundamentals of Epidemiology and Social Epidemiology

Susan Moscou

Despite my experience in a large metropolitan hospital, and the subsequent knowledge gained through a year's residence in a reformatory and asylum for the waifs of New York, the exposure of that rear tenement in the lower East Side was a most terrible shock, a shock that was at first benumbing. A picture was presented of human creatures, moral, and, in so far as their opportunities allowed them, decent members of society, in rooms reached through a court that held open closets to be used by men and women, from some of which the doors had been torn away; up dirty steps into a sick-room where there was no window, the one opening leading into a small, crowded room where husband, children, and boarders were gathered together, impossible conditions under which to attempt to establish a home and bring up children (Wald, 1902, p. 567).

www

LEARNING OBJECTIVES

At the completion of this chapter, the reader will be able to

- Describe epidemiology and social epidemiology.
- Explain how the processes involved in epidemiology and social epidemiology are important within the context of providing for the public's health.

- Analyze the different perspectives of epidemiology and social epidemiology in the context of public health nursing.

KEY TERMS

Epidemiology Terms
- ❏ Age-specific rates
- ❏ Analytical epidemiology
- ❏ Attack rates
- ❏ Chain of infection
- ❏ Crude rates
- ❏ Descriptive epidemiology
- ❏ Epidemiological triad
  - ○ Agent
  - ○ Environment
  - ○ Host
- ❏ Incidence rates
- ❏ Prevalence rates
- ❏ Rate

Social Epidemiology Terms
- ❏ Developmental and life-course perspective
- ❏ Life course model
- ❏ Multilevel analysis
- ❏ Population perspective
- ❏ Social context
- ❏ Social determinants of health
  - ○ Discrimination
  - ○ Education
  - ○ Income
  - ○ Income inequality
  - ○ Occupation
  - ○ Socioeconomic position
  - ○ Socioeconomic status

This chapter discusses the concepts of epidemiology and social epidemiology and their use in public health nursing. Nursing students should use epidemiological tools when they want to understand how and why disease occurs within populations instead of individuals. Examples of populations are pregnant adolescents living in the South Bronx and college-aged students with sexually transmitted diseases. Nursing students use social epidemiological tools when they want to understand how the effects of poverty, **income inequality**, and **discrimination** contribute to how and why disease occurs within specific populations. The purpose of this chapter is to present the concepts of epidemiology and social epidemiology to the public health nurse for application in their practice.

Epidemiology

Epidemiology is the scientific discipline that studies the distribution and determinants of diseases and injuries in human populations

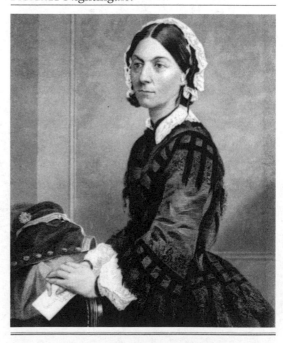

Florence Nightingale.

Source: Courtesy of the National Library of Medicine.

(Tarzian, 2005). The goal of epidemiology is to limit disease, injury, and death via specific interventions designed to prevent or limit outbreaks or epidemics (U.S. Department of Health and Human Services [DHHS] & Centers for Disease Control and Prevention [CDC], 1998, 2006). Epidemiology is concerned with the health of particular populations, whereas clinical nursing and medicine are concerned with individual health issues. The perspective of epidemiologists is to understand the source of the illness cause or exposure, ascertain who else has been exposed, if the exposure has spread beyond the initial point of contact, and to prevent additional cases or recurrences (U.S. DHHS & CDC, 1998, 2006). In comparison, the clinical perspective of medicine and nursing is to obtain information about the history of the present illness, conduct a physical, make a diagnosis, prescribe treatment—issues are considered on an individual basis and are treated as a single episode. Public health nurses are more in line with the epidemiology perspective because they are educated to integrate knowledge about the environment and the community with their understanding of health and illness as experienced by the individual, family, and population. The perspective in medicine tends to be focused on individual health, whereas the perspective in epidemiology tends to be focused on the population. **Box 4-1** illustrates the various ways these clinicians, practicing within these two frameworks, would

---

Box 4-1 Clinical vs. Epidemiology Perspective

Picnic Scenario: Fifty college students attend a picnic. The food is served at noon, and the students eat turkey, cornbread, tuna salad, and ice cream. The students return to campus. One student becomes sick and is taken to the student health center.

Clinical Perspective (Single Episode)
- History/physical finding of present illness
- Diagnosis
- Treatment

The clinician asks about the illness, diagnoses the ailment based on symptoms, and then treats.

Epidemiologist Perspective (Possible Multiple Episodes)
- History of present illness and observation for patterns
- How many students were at the picnic?
- Who else was sick?
- Timing
- What caused the illness?
  - Food
  - Heat
- Is this an epidemic?

The epidemiologist asks about the illness but also wants to know how many students attended the picnic and how many became sick. The epidemiologist also explores with the students what could have caused the illness: Was it the heat or the food? The epidemiologist would also analyze the food and ask if there was mayonnaise in the tuna salad, or how long had the tuna salad been sitting in the heat before it was served? Most importantly, after the epidemiologist gathers the information about the illness, the epidemiologist wants to make sure this is not an epidemic and learn how to prevent this illness in the future.

approach a situation in which a college student falls ill and is taken to the student health center.

Florence Nightingale applied this epidemiological framework when attending to soldiers in the Crimean War. Nightingale recognized that environmental problems such as poor nutrition, sanitation, and contaminated blankets contributed to infection and increases in mortality and morbidity. Nightingale's empirical observations of her surroundings enabled her to examine, methodically, the factors that contributed to disease (Pfettscher, 2002). This big picture allowed

Nightingale to deduce how illness occurred and what strategies reduced the spread of disease.

History

Epidemiological tenets have been used to describe and explain disease and the prevalence of these diseases since 400 B.C. A brief history of epidemiological events and well-known persons who used epidemiological thinking is found in **Table 4-1**.

This epidemiological history can be viewed within the context of two revolutions (**Table 4-2**). The first epidemiological revolution

---

Table 4-1 EPIDEMIOLOGICAL HISTORY AND EVENTS

400 BCE

Hippocrates (c. 400 BCE) provided an approach to those who wanted to investigate disease.

Hippocrates' treatise, *On Airs, Waters, and Places,* noted that these elements affected health.

Hippocrates believed that knowing how these elements were similar and different in specific areas would provide the basis to understand why a disease occurred and the probability of where the disease would occur.

17th Century

John Graunt (1620–1674) from London. Graunt published *Observations on the Bills of Mortality,* which quantified Britain's mortality data in 1662.

Graunt noted birth and death patterns, infant mortality, occurrences of disease, differences in disease by gender, differences in disease in urban and rural areas, and variations in disease by season.

18th Century

James Lind (1716–1794), studied scurvy (vitamin C deficiency) while sailing on a Navy ship in 1747.

In 1753, Lind published *A Treatise on Scurvy in Three Parts.*

This publication explained why scurvy occurred and the treatment for scurvy.

19th Century

William Farr (1807–1883) was responsible for the concept of surveillance data.

John Snow (1813–1858), an anesthesiologist, conducted investigations in London during the cholera outbreak.

20th Century

Joseph Goldberger (1874–1929) discovered why the disease pellagra (niacin deficiency) occurred.

The 1964 Surgeon General Report: *Smoking and Health: Report of the Advisory Committee to the Surgeon General* linked tobacco to lung cancer.

The Framingham Heart Study was initiated to identify factors contributing to heart disease in the United States.

The 1986 Surgeon General's Report: *The AIDS Epidemic.*

Sources: Adapted from Hippocrates (400 B.C.E.); The James Lind Library (n.d.); National Library of Medicine (n.d.a., n.d.b.); Office of History National Institute of Health (2005); Stephan (n.d.); UCLA Department of Epidemiology School of Public Health (n.d.).

Table 4-2 EPIDEMIOLOGICAL REVOLUTIONS

First Epidemiological Revolution (1870–1930)

The first epidemiological revolution was largely about infectious diseases. Scientists and public health practitioners discovered the causes of infectious diseases.

Immunizations discovered during this time period:
- Smallpox
- Polio
- Tetanus

Antibiotics discovered:
- Streptomycin: effective against tuberculosis (1947)
- Penicillin

Immunizations and antibiotics accounted for only a 5% drop in mortality rates.

Greatest advances of the first epidemiological revolution:
- Water purification
- Pasteurization
  - Decrease in diarrhea
  - Decrease in gastroenteritis

Second Epidemiological Revolution (1950–Present)

The second epidemiological revolution focused on chronic diseases such as asthma, cancer, and heart disease and on understanding levels of prevention.

Epidemiologists had little understanding of noninfectious diseases until 1950. During the second revolution, epidemiologists began to understand that 38% of deaths were a result of:
- Tobacco (lung cancer and heart disease)
- Diet and inactivity (heart disease, diabetes)
- Alcohol (heart disease, liver disease)

Understanding the factors that contribute to noninfectious diseases paved the way for interventions. Clinicians use the following levels of preventions with their clients:
- Primary (prevent from the outset)
  - Immunizations
  - Health education
- Secondary (early detection of disease)
  - Screening tests
    - PAP
    - Mammogram
    - Cholesterol
    - Colonoscopy
- Tertiary (reducing mortality and morbidity of the disease)
  - Cardiac rehabilitation

Source: Adapted from Bodenheimer and Grumbach, 2008.

focused on infectious diseases such as influenza, plague, and tuberculosis, which were largely responsible for illnesses and death in previous centuries. It was also during these times that scientists and public health practitioners discovered that the causes of infectious diseases were poverty, overcrowding, sanitation, and contaminated food and water supplies (Breslow, 2005). From 1870 to 1930, scientists and public health practitioners began to understand the cause(s) of infectious diseases. Once epidemiologists had an understanding of why infectious diseases occurred, public health interventions and some medical advances played a role in the reduction of those diseases.

The **rates** of morbidity and mortality of infectious diseases declined in the 18th and 19th centuries because of food production increases, leading to less malnutrition; improvements in nutrition leading to healthier adults and children; and improvements of overall living conditions as a result of improved sanitation and clean water, pasteurization of milk, and less overcrowding. It is important to note that this decrease in infectious disease rates occurred because of public health interventions.

The second epidemiological revolution began in 1950, when epidemiologists started to understand the causes of noninfectious diseases (e.g., heart disease, asthma, diabetes, violence). With this understanding public health practitioners could apply epidemiological principles to shed light on health promotion, disease prevention, and the role of risk factor identification and behavioral change in the promotion of health. Noninfectious diseases are discussed later in this chapter.

To summarize, during the first epidemiological revolution (1870–1930), scientists had little understanding about the causes of infectious diseases (e.g., tuberculosis and influenza). Reductions in infectious diseases were largely the result of public health interventions, whereas medical advances (immunizations and antibiotics) contributed about a 5% reduction in mortality rates. During the second epidemiological revolution (beginning in 1950), epidemiologists began to understand causes of noninfectious diseases such as heart disease, asthma, and diabetes, which paved the way for public health and clinical interventions (Bodenheimer & Grumbach, 2008).

Uses of Epidemiology

Why is it important to understand epidemiology and how it is used? In this section the reader will come to see how epidemiology is applied in public health nursing practice. This process includes the systematic collection of data and how the analysis of these data not only leads to a better understanding of a disease process, but the reduction of disease. The reader will also come to understand how the epidemiological process informs the public health nurse's decision making.

The collection and use of epidemiology data for decision making can be viewed in the following ways. Public health nurses engage in an assessment process that informs them about the health of the individual, family, population, and community. Chapter 3 is devoted to assessment. The process of assessment provides information so the public health nurse may engage in problem identification and/or potential problem identification, as well as information that may support program development and, at times, the development of public health policy. For example, the data collected by public health nurses may be presented to policymakers to shed light about the actual and potential problems seen in the population of their targeted home communities. Examples of this information may include data that highlight health, social, or environmental problems in a particular population in a policymaker's constituency; data on risks within their constituency; the history of health problems within a particular population, showing trends such as the increase or decrease of a particular disease; and the services available in a community. Knowing this information helps policymakers make decisions regarding the establishment of law and resource utilization and allocation.

Epidemiology plays a role in our day-to-day individual decisions pertaining to healthy behaviors such as smoking cessation, exercising, weight control, and eating healthy foods. These positive decisions are made because of epidemiological studies. Epidemiology has contributed to the fount of information about associations and causal relationships (we say causal relationships because research can never prove cause and effect) between obesity and diabetes, smoking and lung cancer, and risky sexual practices, such as engaging in unprotected sex, and sexually transmitted diseases. Without epidemiology we would not know how a disease is transmitted or the strategies to reduce our risks of contracting this disease. Public health nurses use this evidence daily in their practice as they develop educational programs for individuals, families, and populations in an effort to offer information that assists others to make healthy lifestyle choices.

The work of public health practitioners involves public health nurses, epidemiologists, health department officials, clinicians, physicians, scientists, media experts, educators, sanitation officials, and researchers. These individuals all provide particular worldviews that, when joined collectively, complete the clinical picture needed to understand the disease, the progression and trajectory of that disease, and interventions. Completing the clinical picture is identifying what the infectious agent is, why/how the disease is transmitted to the host, where the disease is most prevalent in terms of the place or location, when the disease most makes itself known with regard to time, and who the individual is that is affected by the disease. These are known

as the 5 W's of **descriptive epidemiology**, and are discussed below (U.S. DHHS & CDC, 2006, p. 31). Part of this clinical picture is an understanding of the determinants of health. One practitioner alone is unable to be a solo artist in this endeavor because effective public health strategies require collaborative and collective efforts between and among many different professions.

Human immunodeficiency virus (HIV) is an example of how epidemiologists were able to complete the clinical picture. In the early 1980s, a strange pneumonia affected five men who identified themselves as having sex with men. *Pneumocystis carinii* pneumonia was a relatively rare lung disease and appeared to be clustered only within this specific population (Sepkowitz, 2001). Additionally, clinicians were seeing Kaposi's sarcoma (KS), a relatively benign form of cancer, in their younger male patients who had sex with men. Kaposi's sarcoma was also relatively rare in the United States; the skin lesions associated with KS were usually localized to the lower extremities and affected older people in their 70s (Hymes et al., 1981).

Because these cases appeared to be clustered within a specific population and puzzled the medical community, the cases and laboratory results were reported to the CDC for further investigation. In 1981, the CDC provided information about the first cases of *P. carinii* pneumonia and KS among men who have sex with men (CDC referred to this group as homosexuals) to the medical community, and in 1982 the CDC named this disease "acquired immune deficiency syndrome" (known as AIDS). It was not until 1986 that the term "human immunodeficiency virus," or HIV, was adopted by the clinical community (Sepkowitz, 2008). Once a particular disease or health event is identified, healthcare professionals make the diagnosis in individual cases, whereas epidemiologists contribute to our understanding of the natural history of the disease. Since this time, the work pertaining to HIV has been carried on by a wide and varied group of healthcare professionals. Take a few minutes and just think. Who has contributed to the knowledge of this disease and the treatment of this disease? The list is rather overwhelming, yet at the same time it clearly presents for us the view that in order for the health of the public to be sustained there is a need for the collective wisdom of many working together. Public health nurses are a valued member of this collective group.

Finally, the search for causes is epidemiological research. This research is dedicated to the investigation of the causes and individual, societal, and environmental factors that contribute to a person's risk for contracting a disease and/or suffering injury. This research provides evidence for interventions that health professionals can use in their clinical practice, such as counseling about smoking, protective sexual practices, seat belts, car child seats, and immunizations. Public health nurses not only apply this research as evidence in their practice but raise questions for research and conduct research.

Epidemiological Approach

When we see a particular disease in our clinical practice or if we decide to explore a particular disease, we want to know who is affected by this disease, what factors contribute to this disease (environmental, social, or personal factors), if there are other cases, when this disease became known, why some individuals are more prone to this particular disease, and what common factors do diseased individuals have in common. Epidemiologists begin with case definition as the standard criteria to guide their practice.

A case definition is that which determines if a person has a particular disease. For example, an individual is diagnosed with diabetes if his or her blood sugar levels are above the cutoff point (126 mg/dL) on two separate occasions (U.S. Preventive Services Task Force, 2008). Case definitions standardize the diagnoses of a particular disease, thus ensuring that every case is similarly diagnosed. Additionally, case definitions consist of clinical criteria, including subjective data, which are client complaints, and objective data, which are the clinician's observations inclusive of physical, environmental, and laboratory findings.

Numbers and Rates

Epidemiologists are concerned about numbers and rates because it allows them to measure, describe, and compare the morbidity and mortality of a particular disease and/or injury in populations. Rates are "measures of frequency of health events that put raw numbers into a frame of reference to the size of a population. Rates are determined by statistical adjustments to the raw data, making them useful in making comparisons or examining trends" (Stotts, 2008, p. 91).

In epidemiology the numerator is the actual number of cases or events occurring during a given time period, and the denominator is the total population at risk during the same time period. The denominator is typically converted to a standard base denominator, such as 1,000, 10,000, or 100,000, so that comparisons can be made among at-risk populations, communities, and neighborhoods (Tarzian, 2005). Rates are useful to the public health nurse because they can help the nurse identify what populations in the community are at an increased risk for a particular disease and/or injury. For example, City A has a population of 130,000 nursing home residents. City A reported 100 cases of hepatitis A among nursing home residents to the Department of Health (DOH). City B has a population of 120,000 nursing home residents. City B reported 150 cases of hepatitis A among their nursing home residents to the DOH. The DOH determined that the specific rate for hepatitis A was 7.6 cases per 10,000 persons living in a nursing home in City A and was 12.5 cases per 10,000 persons in City B. The DOH specific rate calculations for these cities are found in **Box 4-2**. This type of data helps the public health nurse think about and develop initiatives that target nursing home residents who appear to be a high-risk population for contracting hepatitis A.

In addition to the above specific rates, there are many other rate definitions that measure morbidity (illness rates) or mortality (death rates) for populations at risk for contracting or dying from a particular disease, such as asthma, diabetes, or high blood pressure, or cause, such as a motor vehicle accident. Examples of these rates or statistical calculations are **incidence rates**, **prevalence rates**, **attack rates**, **crude rates**, and **age-specific rates** as listed in **Table 4-3**.

BOX 4-2 SPECIFIC RATE CALCULATIONS FOR HEPATITIS A FOUND IN CITY A AND CITY B

Numbers and rates permit the epidemiologist to measure, describe, and compare the morbidity and mortality of particular diseases. A rate is:

Number of cases or events occurring during a given time period
_____
          Population at risk during the same time period

In epidemiology, rates are changed to a common base such as 100,000 because it changes the result of the division into a quantity that permits a standardized comparison.

Example:

City A and City B saw an outbreak of hepatitis A in their nursing home residents. Each city reported these cases to the Department of Health. The Department of Health calculated the specific rates for each city using 10,000 as the standard base number. Hepatitis A specific rate for nursing home residents is calculated as follows:

City A specific rate:

    100 cases of reported Hep A cases
_____
130,000 City A nursing home residents

   City A specific rate: 7.6, which means that in nursing homes for City A, about seven to eight residents contracted hepatitis A.

   City B specific rate:

    150 cases of reported Hep A cases
_____
120,000 City B nursing home residents

City B specific rate = 12.5

By calculating the specific rate, the Department of Health can compare the hepatitis rates in City A and City B. Additionally, the Department of Health knows that nursing home residents are at risk for contracting hepatitis A.

_____
Source: Adapted from U.S. DHHS & CDC, 2006.

Table 4-3 Rate Definitions

Incidence Rate	Prevalence Rate	Attack Rate	Specific Rates	Crude Rate	Age-specific Rate
Applied in the study of acute diseases, a disease outbreak, or in the diagnosis of new cases. Incidence rates are the frequency with which a new condition or event occurs in a population over a period of time.	Applied in the study of chronic disease. Prevalence rate measures the number of people in a given population who have an already existing condition at a given point in time.	Important for the study of a single disease outbreak or epidemic during a short time period. The number is expressed as a percent.	These measure morbidity or mortality for a particular population: • Age specific • Gender specific • Income • Race/ethnicity • Infant mortality • Maternal mortality	A crude rate measures the experience of the entire population in a specific area with regard to the specific disease or condition being investigated. The crude mortality rate looks at the entire mortality rate from all causes of death for a population in a particular area during a specific time.	These rates provide age-specific information for a particular disease.
Example We want to know the number of new cases of flu. In the second week of November the student Health Services diagnosed 3 students with the flu. The total student population is 1,600.	*Example* We want to know the number of existing cases of flu. There were 3 new cases of the flu in the second week of November and 10 old cases of the flu in the first week of November.	*Example* 120 people flew from New York to Los Angeles. The meal served was meatloaf. Eighty people ate the meal and 40 people chose not to eat meatloaf. Twenty of those who ate meatloaf became ill.	*Example* Age-specific diabetes mortality in 45- to 55-year-olds	*Example* NYC death rate	*Example* Age-specific mortality rate is one limited to a particular age group. The numerator is the number of deaths in that age group and the denominator is the number of persons in that age group in the population. Examples include: Neonatal mortality rate Infant mortality rate
Calculation 3 new flu cases ÷ 1,600 (student population) × 1,000 (comparison denominator) Incidence rate is 1.8.	*Calculation* 3 + 10 cases ÷ 1,600 (student population) × 1,000 Prevalence rate is 8.1.	*Calculation* 20 (ill) ÷ 80 (meatloaf pop) × 100 Attack rate is 25%.	*Calculation* Number of diabetes deaths in 45–55-year-olds ÷ Population of individuals 45–55-year-olds × 1,000	*Calculation* The total number of NYC deaths reported during (1985) ÷ 5 million × 100,000	

Source: Adapted from U.S. DHHS & CDC, 2006.

DESCRIPTIVE EPIDEMIOLOGY

Descriptive epidemiology describes the extent of an outbreak in terms of who gets the disease, where the disease occurs, and when the disease occurred. These characteristics are described in **Table** 4-4. For example, Lyme disease was classified as a new disease when about 50 children were diagnosed with arthritis in Lyme, Connecticut. This cluster of arthritis in children caused an epidemiologist in Lyme, who was concerned because juvenile rheumatoid arthritis is relatively rare in children (France, 1999), to request that the CDC investigate this outbreak. The who in this outbreak were children, the where in this outbreak was a wooded hamlet at the mouth of the Connecticut River, and the when for this disease is typically the summer and fall when people tend to spend more time outdoors and thus are more at risk for a tick bite. The collection and analysis of this descriptive information form a critical first step in the epidemiological investigatory process.

This gathering and analyzing of data in descriptive epidemiology is also called the gathering of data on person, time, and place. This information allows the public health nurse to become knowledgeable about the public health problem being studied, thus enabling the public health nurse to provide a comprehensive picture of the health of the population under study and determine who is at risk for acquiring the particular disease. Another part of the epidemiological approach is known as **analytical epidemiology**, which facilitates the how and why of a particular disease.

ANALYTICAL EPIDEMIOLOGY

Analytical epidemiology illustrates the causal relationship between a risk factor and a specific disease or health condition. In other words, it seeks to answer questions about how and why disease occurs and the effects of a particular dis-

ease. Analytical studies use a comparison group to learn why one group has a disease and another does not. These groups are drawn from a healthy population living in the same community in which the disease has occurred. For example, a public health nurse was sent to a community where there was an outbreak of hepatitis A. The nurse interviewed the individuals who were diagnosed with hepatitis A and discovered that they had attended a graduation party at the local high school in the neighborhood. The public health nurse learned about the food that was served at this party and asked each person what he or she had eaten at the party. The public health nurse recognized the need for a comparison group for further investigation of this hepatitis A outbreak. The comparison group in this case would be those individuals at the same party who did not eat those same foods and who were not ill. "When . . . investigators find that persons with a particular characteristic are more likely than those without the characteristic to develop a certain disease, then the characteristic is said to be associated with the disease" (U.S. DHHS & CDC, 2006, p. 32). These characteristics include demographics such as age, race, or sex; constitutional characteristics such as immune state; behavioral characteristics such as smoking; or other characteristics, such as living next to a waste site (U.S. DHHS & CDC, 2006).

Analytical epidemiology attempts to search for the causes and effects of the disease under study. Further, epidemiologists discern how or why exposure to a particular agent results in the outcome of disease or no disease. Epidemiologists can study the occurrences of diseases in two ways: experimental studies and observational studies.

In an experimental study the researcher is the one who determines the exposure status of the individual or population. The researcher does not only observe, but also determines and

Table 4-4 DESCRIPTIVE EPIDEMIOLOGICAL VARIABLES

Person	Place	Time
Person variables are used to understand what makes a person susceptible to a disease or injury. Inherent characteristics include age, race, and sex. Acquired characteristics include marital status, education, occupation, living conditions, socioeconomic status, and access to health care.	Place variables describe the disease event by where the disease occurs, such as: • Place of residence • School district • Community • Country • State • Hospital unit	Time variables give information about how disease rates change over time. Time information can be reported in • Days • Weeks • Months • Years • Decades • Epidemic period: when the number of cases is greater than normal.
Inherent characteristics are considered fixed or unchangeable. A person's gender makes him or her at higher risk for some diseases, such as breast cancer. However, because age varies the person becomes more susceptible to illness as he or she ages.	Place information also provides insight into the geographical location and what factors in that environment facilitate the disease. For example, the temperature and climate may promote a place where a particular agent may grow and multiply.	Does the disease manifest itself during certain seasons? Is the presentation of the disease predictable? If so why? Can this information be used in the prevention of the disease?
Acquired characteristics may be modifiable via education.	Example Lyme disease was first characterized in Lyme, CT, because the lush wooded environment supported the agent, host, and environment cycle.	Example Seasonality may demonstrate disease occurrences by week or month over the course of a year. For example, flu season typically begins in November and ends in March.
Example A 50-year-old man develops lung cancer. He has smoked for 30 years. The smoking is considered an acquired characteristic because it is potentially modifiable with education. Behavioral changes (quitting or smoking fewer cigarettes) lead to a healthier life and prevention of lung cancer.		

Source: Adapted from U.S. DHHS & CDC, 2006.

actively initiates what the exposure is, where to deliver the exposure, how to deliver the exposure, when to deliver the exposure, and who will be the recipient of the exposure. The researcher determines recipient characteristics such as age, gender, and **socioeconomic status** (SES). The researcher then carries out the research design to determine the effects of the exposure on the experimental individual or population and compares these outcomes with those not having had the exposure. Those who have not been exposed are the comparison group. This type of study is sometimes referred to as prospective because the research moves forward in time to look at the effects of the exposure. It is also important to note that these studies rarely prove causation but often lead to more research. Experimental studies are generally used to determine the effectiveness of a treatment such as a vaccine or drug. These types of studies are considered the gold standard of clinical trials. Study participants in clinical trials are either given the medication or drug under study or given a placebo such as a sugar pill. Most of the major medications used to treat chronic diseases such as high blood pressure, diabetes, and asthma were subjected to trials in experimental studies.

Observational studies include cohort and case-control studies. In a cohort study, a cohort of healthy individuals that share similar experiences or characteristics are identified and classified by their exposures. For example, in a study that wishes to look at tobacco use and lung cancer, the cohort identified may be men 21 years of age who are actively engaged in smoking. This group is studied over a period of years, allowing researchers to compare the disease rates in the exposed group (those who smoked) with the unexposed group (those who did not smoke). In a case-control group the researcher identifies a group of people who have already been diagnosed with a disease (for example, women diagnosed with breast cancer) and a group without the disease. The researcher compares and contrasts the participants' past life experiences, characteristics, and exposures to determine patterns. Again, a comparison group is important in case-control studies. This type of research is sometimes referred to as retrospective because the researcher is looking at a situation in the present and linking it to situations or conditions in the past.

The Framingham Study is an example of a classic cohort study. Since 1949 the National Heart Institute of the U.S. Public Health Service observed men and women living in Framingham, Massachusetts, to identify factors related to developing coronary heart disease (Kannel, Schwartz, & McNamara, 1969). The Nurses' Health Study, another example of a cohort study, was started several decades ago to examine the relationship between oral contraception (birth control pills) and breast cancer (Colditz, Manson, & Hankinson, 1997).

Epidemiological Triad

The **epidemiological triad** (**Figure** 4-1) is the traditional model of infectious disease causation. The three components are agent, host, and environment.

Figure 4-1 Epidemiological triad.

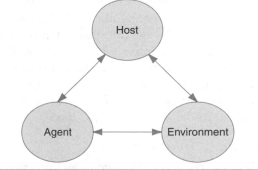

Source: Adapted from U.S. DHHS & CDC, 2006.

Agent factors refer to an infectious organism such as a virus, bacterium, parasite, or other microbe. **Host** factors that can mediate the effect of a particular agent are age, sex, **socioeconomic factors (SES) (education, income, occupation)** - behaviors (smoking, drinking, and exercise), and genetic factors. For example, a 95-year-old man with multiple chronic illnesses who does not get his yearly flu vaccine is more susceptible to influenza than a healthy 20-year-old college student. These host factors are also known as intrinsic factors. Environmental factors are known as extrinsic factors and include physical factors such as geography, climate, and physical surroundings (e.g., homeless shelters); biological factors such as insects that transmit the agent (e.g., mosquito transmits malaria); and socioeconomic factors such as sanitation and available health services that can determine the spread of a particular disease (e.g., tuberculosis increases with overcrowding) (U.S. DHHS & CDC, 2006).

Again, Lyme disease is an excellent example of the epidemiological triad. A particular deer tick infected with the bacterium *Borrelia burgdorferi* (the agent) infects a person (the host). The bacteria enter the skin at the bite site only after the infected tick has been in the host for 36 to 48 hours. The initial symptoms felt by the host are primarily the result of the body's response to this invasion. Specific factors such as exposure to heavily wooded areas (environment), the season (infection is most likely during the summer and fall), age (most common in children and young adults), and location (90% of cases occur in the coastal northeast as well as in Wisconsin, Minnesota, California, and Oregon) predispose the host to contracting Lyme disease (Depietropaolo, Powers, & Gill, 2005).

Chain of Infection

Diseases are classified as communicable or noncommunicable. Communicable diseases are considered infectious because they can be transmitted by an infected person to a noninfected person. The common cold, HIV, and tuberculosis are examples of communicable diseases. Diseases come about when the body (host) is exposed to an infectious agent (virus or microorganism) and the organism or virus grows within the body. If the organism or virus is able to grow within the host, the host at some point in time might become infectious and then can transmit the particular disease to another susceptible host. Noncommunicable diseases such as diabetes, asthma, and heart disease cannot be transmitted by the person who has that particular diagnosis. The contributing factors of noncommunicable diseases are genetics (e.g., Tay-Sachs disease), environmental factors (e.g., Love Canal), and behaviors such as overeating. These determinants of health are discussed in previous chapters and below.

The **chain of infection (Figure 4-2)** shows that infectious diseases result from their interaction with the agent, host, and environment. Transmission, direct or indirect, of an infectious agent takes place after the agent leaves its reservoir (host) by a portal of exit such as the mouth when coughing. The agent then enters the susceptible host via a portal of entry, such as a skin wound, to infect the susceptible host (U.S. DHHS & CDC, 2006).

Direct transmission modes are the immediate transfer of the disease agent between an infected person and susceptible person. Examples of direct transmission modes are direct contact via touching, kissing, and direct projection, which includes large short-range spray of droplets via sneezing or coughing. Indirect transmission takes place as an agent is carried from a reservoir to a host via air particles and gains access to the portal of entry via respiratory tract systems (e.g., mouth and nose). Vehicle-borne transmissions are contaminated materials or objects (fomites) in which communicable diseases are transferred (e.g., children's toys

Figure 4-2 The chain of infection.

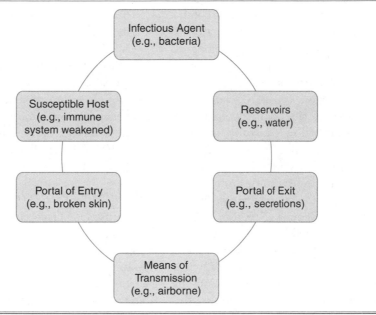

Source: Adapted from U.S. DHHS & CDC, 2006.

in a day care center) and vector-borne transmission methods transfer the disease by a living organism (e.g., mosquito) (U.S. DHHS & CDC, 2006).

Public Health Surveillance Data

Public health surveillance data are used by public health nurses and other health officials to understand disease prevalence and disease patterns. Surveillance data are critically analyzed and used by these individuals to make decisions about policy, funding, research, and program initiatives. Surveillance as an intervention strategy is discussed later in this text.

Social Epidemiology

Social epidemiology is the study of social conditions, such as poverty, socioeconomic status (SES), and discrimination, that play a role and influence the health of populations. Social epidemiology goes beyond the analysis of individual risk factors such as age and gender to include the study of the social context or societal implications in which the health–disease phenomenon occurs (Krieger, 2002). Social epidemiology measures the impact of the social environment on health outcomes, whereas epidemiology is more concerned with the impact of the physical environment on health outcomes (Berkman & Kawachi, 2000). Galea, Tracey, Hoggatt, DiMaggio, and Karpati (2011) examined the literature about social factors and health outcomes from 1980–2007. Galea et al. found that deaths attributed to low education numbered 245,000, racial segregation was 176,000, low social support was 162,000, impoverished individuals were 133,000, income inequality was 119,000, and area-level poverty accounted for 39,000.

Social epidemiology attempts to address social inequality's role in disease causation. Social epidemiologists investigate social conditions responsible for patterns of health, patterns of disease, and the well-being of populations, as well as examine how social inequality in the past and present has a role in the health or disease of populations (Krieger, 2001a). Social epidemiologists investigate the gradient of income on the health status of lower-income, middle-income, and upper-income classes in society. By looking at the health status at each income level, social epidemiologists can examine how income exerts an influence, either positive or negative, on health outcomes (Krieger, 2001b). For example, people growing up in poorer communities have worse health outcomes than those growing up in wealthier communities. Once a social epidemiologist teases out variations in health status by different income groups, the relationship between individual income, which is considered an individual factor, and income inequality, which is considered a contextual factor, can be explored (Subramanian, Kawachi, & Kennedy, 2001).

The concepts guiding social epidemiology are as follows:

- **Population perspective**, which means that because individuals are rooted in society, their risks for disease or staying healthy are situated with the population in which they belong.
- **Social context** of behavior, which means that certain behaviors such as smoking, drinking, and voter participation are shaped by social influences. For example, children who see their parents smoke are more likely to smoke when they get older, or communities with ample resources such as parks, grocery stores, and health clinics are more likely to shape healthier behavior.

- **Multilevel analysis**, which means that health outcomes are understood within the perspective of individual factors such as income and education, along with contextual factors that assess environmental exposures at the community, state, national, and global level.
- **Developmental and life-course perspective**, which means the early life experiences of an individual contribute to his or her susceptibility to disease later in life (**Table 4-5**).

Population Perspective

The population perspective is a guiding concept in social epidemiology. As discussed, the population perspective illustrates that an individual's risk for health problems cannot be isolated from the community in which he or she resides or from the population or society in which he or she belongs. Murray (2011) noted that "a population focus that addresses the social determinants of health is an essential component of primary health care" (p. 3); as such, an individual's risk for disease must be seen in the context of where he or she lives. For example, breast cancer survival rates in the population of Japanese women are higher than in the population of Japanese immigrants living in America and Japanese Americans. One explanation for the improved survival rate is the low dietary fat intake of Japanese women (Pineda, White, Kristal, & Taylor, 2001). This means that when a Japanese woman moves from Japan to the United States, her breast cancer survival rate would be less than if she lived in Japan.

Social Context of Behavior

The social context of behavior is a guiding concept of social epidemiology. As discussed, the social context of behavior addresses individual behavioral risk factors such as smoking and

Table 4-5 GUIDING PERSPECTIVES IN SOCIAL EPIDEMIOLOGY

Population	Social Context of Behavior	Multilevel Analysis	Developmental and Life Course
This perspective examines an individual's health in the context of the population where the person resides.	This perspective makes the case that risky behaviors such as smoking and drinking tend to be clustered in particular communities. The residents in these communities typically have less education, are more socially isolated, and have less access to health-promoting environments.	This perspective encourages a larger analysis of the problem by assessing all factors that contribute to disease.	This perspective examines the cumulative risk of health status based on early life exposures.
Example	This perspective recognizes that social environments have a large role in positive or negative health behaviors.	This analysis assesses the levels of exposures found at the community, state, national, and global level.	This perspective recognizes that disadvantages in one's early life may facilitate disease later in life.
Breast cancer survival rates for women in Japan are higher than for Japanese women who become U.S. immigrants.	Example	If we understand the relationship between the individual and the community level, we gain a larger understanding of health outcomes for the individual.	Example
	Communities with higher rates of smoking live in areas where smoking is heavily advertised.	Example	A child grew up in a poor neighborhood next to a medical incinerator. Additionally, several family members smoked cigarettes. The family did not have health insurance until the child was 10 years old. The child, however, was healthy and did not need medical attention. The child went to college and became quite wealthy. The early life experience of deprivation for this child, however, may contribute to developing asthma when older even though the new environment is less conducive to developing asthma.
		A person lives in a community that does not have grocery stores with fresh food, but there are several fast food restaurants on every block. Eating fast food almost every day might contribute to becoming overweight and might lead to diabetes in the future.	

Source: Adapted from Berkman and Kawachi, 2000.

drinking and examines these behaviors in a larger social context or by the social influences or conditions that contribute to specific behaviors. For example, the number of green spaces, such as parks, and supermarkets in a neighborhood often determine how an individual will behave and the choices the person has to make to maintain health and reduce his or her susceptibility to disease. Public health nurses working in the South Bronx, where many of the adults are overweight and at risk for diabetes or high blood pressure, recommend a diet and exercise regimens for these individuals. But, because there are few green space areas, no access to walking paths, no gym facilities, and the neighborhood feels less safe in the evening, many of these individuals do not adhere to the diet and exercise recommendations.

Social conditions often determine behavior and play a role in how susceptible a person is to disease. Growing up in poverty or wealth determines the type of neighborhoods where people can live (e.g., unsafe vs. safe), the environmental exposures in certain neighborhoods (e.g., lead), how people in these neighborhoods access health care (e.g., emergency room vs. private healthcare office), and the levels of educational attainment (e.g., high-school degree vs. college degree). For example, people living in poorer communities face increased risks of environmental exposures such as living near a medical incinerator, which might cause more asthma; lack of adequate housing that might lead to overcrowding, which can increase the prevalence of tuberculosis; reduced availability of medical resources that might lead to the increased use of the emergency room versus seeing a primary care clinician; and lower educational attainment that creates the context for detrimental behaviors such as smoking and drinking, which contribute to disease later in life such as lung cancer, cirrhosis of the liver, or emphysema.

Social conditions do not create disease but generate a susceptibility to disease. Social epidemiology takes into account that the continued exposure to adverse social conditions has a role in how well the host can resist disease and that these exposures often lay the groundwork for poorer health in the future (Berkman & Kawachi, 2000).

In summary, the whole notion of social context of behavior may also be viewed from a positive perspective in which the population's strengths are identified and engaged. In other words, how healthcare practitioners work with the population in shaping the social context of where they live can enhance health. Carthon (2011) engaged in a historical inquiry focusing on two civic associations that functioned in Philadelphia during the 1900s. The population of individuals consisted of primarily Black Americans who lived in economically and medically under-resourced communities, which accounted for poorer health rates. The utilization of community and social networks provided the population with resources needed to effect change.

The above is also an exemplar of social capital at work. Social capital structures are systems of networks, norms, and trust relationships that allow communities to address common problems (Pronyk et al., 2008). Putnam (1995) has defined social capital as social relationships (interpersonal trust norms of reciprocity and civic responsibilities) within communities that act as resources for individuals and facilitate collective action for a mutual benefit. Residents of a community with high social capital may provide one another with greater instrumental and psychosocial support than residents of a community with low social capital. Further, the community's level of interconnectedness and trust may reduce or increase barriers to care (Perry, Williams, Wallestein, & Waitzkin, 2008).

Multilevel Analysis

Multilevel analysis is a guiding concept of social epidemiology. As discussed, multilevel analysis is necessary to understand all factors that contribute to disease at the group and individual levels. It is an approach that permits simultaneous examination of group and individual level variables on individual level outcomes (Diez-Roux, 2000). It has already been noted that individuals are influenced by their social context. Therefore using a multilevel analysis will assist those in public health to look at independent and interacting effects of individual level factors as well as group-level factors on health outcomes. An example of this is noted by Diez-Roux (2000):

> *Within this field, one of the main research areas in which multilevel models have been applied is the investigation of the effects of neighborhood social environments on health outcomes. . . . A key issue in investigating neighborhood effects on health is separating out the effects of neighborhood characteristics (context) from the effects of individual-level attributes that persons living in certain types of areas may share (composition). Because neighborhoods can be thought of as groups or contexts with individuals nested within them, multilevel models have been used to investigate how neighborhood factors, individual-level factors, and their interactions influence health. (p. 181)*

Life Course Model or Perspective

The life course perspective is a guiding concept in social epidemiology. The **life course model** puts forward that the **socioeconomic position** of the family during childhood affects the child's health status, educational choices, and occupation choices in the future. Children growing up in families with less economic means or a lower socioeconomic position might have more health problems than children growing up in families with more economic means or a higher socioeconomic position. For example, children growing up in poverty might have more health problems

such as asthma, which then might contribute to a lower level of education because frequent asthma episodes result in more school absences, which in turn leads to less occupational choices because they did not do well enough in school to attend college, and less education results in lower income levels that can precipitate downward mobility (Dike van de Mheen, Stronks, & Mackenbach, 1998). Children, however, growing up in more prosperous neighborhoods tend to have better health outcomes than children in economically disadvantaged communities because they attend better schools, have access to health care, and their parents are better educated and therefore have better jobs (Acevedo-Garcia, Lochner, Osypuk, & Subramanian, 2003). Economic disadvantages in early life can set in motion negative consequences that build up over time to produce disease after 20, 30, 40, or 50 years of being disadvantaged (Berkman & Kawachi, 2000).

Multilevel Approaches to Understanding Social Determinants of Health

Social determinants of health refer to the interaction of environmental and social processes that can affect an individual's biological processes that make him or her susceptible to a disease. For example, a child is exposed to secondhand smoke and develops asthma when he or she is 6 years old. Additionally, this child might even develop lung cancer later in life because of the continued exposure to secondhand smoke and the early development of lung disease. We know that early life experiences can contribute to subsequent health outcomes, good or bad. Solving the direct effects of material conditions such as pollution, malnutrition, and housing are important, but the person might still be at risk for health problems depending on how long he or she was exposed to the offending agent or experienced economic or social deprivation.

Socioeconomic factors such as income, education, occupation, medical care, healthcare barriers, language, environmental exposures, discrimination, and so forth are all correlated with health outcomes in one context or another. The public health nurse considers the above variables to bring about a better understanding of health disparities noted in individuals, families, populations, and communities. Additionally, analyzing the interaction between socioeconomic factors, health, and discrimination gives the public health nurse a framework to develop interventions for specific individuals, families, or populations in specific areas. What follows is a discrete and detailed discussion of these social determinants of health.

SOCIOECONOMIC STATUS AND SOCIOECONOMIC POSITION

The relationship of SES and health status has been documented for centuries (Lynch & Kaplan, 2000; Mirowsky, Ross, & Reynolds, 2000). Socioeconomic status consists of family income, educational level, and occupation. Additionally, SES determines an individual's socioeconomic position within society. How much money, level of educational attainment, and the occupation a person has have a bearing on and reflect his or her socioeconomic position or standing in society. Additionally, populations have a socioeconomic position, and this is based on the economic resources available to the community. Like SES, the relationship between the socioeconomic position of a person or population and health status has been well established (Lynch & Kaplan, 2000). The effects of SES and socioeconomic position on health have been consistent with regard to health outcome disparities across different time periods, different geographical areas, and in nearly all measurements used to assess health and disease (Lantz et al., 2001).

An individual's SES and socioeconomic position in society are based on his or her educational level, annual income, occupation, and level of assets such as stocks, bonds, and home ownership. A person's SES and socioeconomic position matter to health status because living in a relatively poor community can be bad for one's health, whereas living in a relatively affluent community can be good for one's health. The SES or socioeconomic position of an individual or population contributes to positive or negative health behaviors (Stringhini et al., 2010). For example, individuals growing up in lower socioeconomic circumstances are more likely to live in an area where there may be health-damaging exposures, such as living near a sewage treatment plant, as opposed to individuals in upper socioeconomic circumstances who are more likely to grow up in communities with health-enhancing resources, such as supermarkets containing fresh fruits and vegetables (Lynch & Kaplan, 2000). The SES and socioeconomic position of an individual or group reflect the social and economic risks (e.g., living in unsafe neighborhoods) or rewards (e.g., living in safe neighborhoods) of that particular class in society (Mirowsky et al., 2000).

INCOME

One of the most significant determinants of good health is income; therefore, many have suggested that economic policy is a powerful form of health policy. By increasing a person's income, you increase the health status for everyone in society (Kaplan, 2001). Income matters in society because income gives a person access to resources that are necessary to maintain health (Kawachi, 2000; Wilkinson, 1999). For example, stress has been shown to have a negative impact on one's health, so being able to relieve stress is an important resource. A 55-year-old executive is able to relieve stress during the day because she has access to a gym in her office, whereas a 55-year-old bus driver does not have that resource available. The bus driver's inability to relieve stress makes him more susceptible to health problems.

Public health nurses work with individuals, families, and populations who experience stressors daily. How one responds to a particular stressor sets in motion physiological, behavioral, and psychological responses in the person. Additionally, how one handles a particular stressor depends on his or her coping mechanisms, support systems, and personality (Marmot, 2000). Sister Callista Roy, although not a social epidemiologist but a nursing theorist, recognized that adaptation to a particular stimuli is shaped by perceptions of the event and interpretation of the event. How the person interprets an event brings about a particular adaptive response. This response could have been formed by earlier life experiences. The Roy Adaptation Model puts forth that adaptation mechanisms used by a person have health consequences in the present and possibly in the future (Phillips, 2002). This example is presented for the reader in an attempt to demonstrate that public health nurses must also bring into their practice nursing's own unique body of knowledge.

INCOME INEQUALITY

Income inequality describes where wealth is concentrated and who controls the wealth in society. Income inequality measures the degree of income variation in a population, and income inequality on a community level contributes to the loss of social capital. Social capital refers to social resources such as parks, medical facilities, schools, and economic investments that are needed to ensure that communities have the resources to maintain health (Kawachi, 1999). Hence, communities with higher income are more likely to have higher social capital or resources—such as parks for their population to enjoy and enhance health—as opposed to communities with lower income and lower social capital. Income inequality also influences the average life expectancy for citizens in society.

Income inequality is either relative or absolute. Relative income inequality (growing up poor in a rich society vs. growing up poor where everybody is poor) has health consequences because individuals' perceptions of the social and material world can trigger biological processes (e.g., stress), which can lead to a current illness such as a headache or a future illness such as heart disease. For example, a child whose family is lower-income attends an expensive preparatory school on scholarship. This child is surrounded by students who have money and privilege. Further, the child's classmates vacation in Europe, wear the latest fashions, and see a movie every weekend. The child often feels sad because he or she does not have the money to buy new clothes, go to the movies, or travel. Had this child, however, gone to the local school with children of similar economic means, he or she might have better health outcomes in the present and the future. This model posits that socioeconomic inequalities as experienced by this child may activate psychosocial factors that contribute to health and illness (Wilkinson, 1999).

EDUCATION

Education is positively associated with employment and an important variable in understanding the social determinants of health. For example, an individual with a college degree is more likely to have employment that is more secure, higher paying, with health benefits, and has limited environmental exposures to hazards than an individual with a high-school diploma. The *New York Times* reported that staying in school for a long period of time and not smoking resulted in the best outcomes; thus, extreme education has a role in longevity (Kolata, 2007).

Adults with more years of education are less likely to engage in risky health behaviors such as smoking and drinking. Additionally, more education leads to a greater sense of personal efficacy. Of note, educational attainment and income returns vary over time and often differ by gender, race, and ethnicity. For example, what this means is even though women may have the same educational degree and same occupation, they make less than men because they are paid less for the same work.

Occupation

Occupation is studied less by researchers in the United States but is still an important indicator in health outcomes; Great Britain uses occupation in its analysis of health outcomes. A person's occupation tells us about his or her educational opportunities, economic independence, environmental exposures, and likely health stressors. For example, a coal miner in West Virginia has limited educational opportunities and less economic independence because he or she has skills that are unique to coal mining. These same individuals are exposed to coal dust, which affects their lungs and can lead to illnesses such as asthma, emphysema, and chronic respiratory infections. Further, coal miners experience a multitude of on-the-job stressors. Existing health problems may be worsened by stress because coal miners have less autonomy in their job and are unable to control or relieve their stress levels. A white-collar worker or executive has more education; thus his or her job is considered more prestigious. The more prestigious jobs are more likely to be held by individuals who are healthier, wealthier, and have more autonomy, which contributes to feelings of control. Further, autonomy or how well one controls his or her life can improve social status and social supports and lead to better health status (Marmot & Wilkinson, 2006).

Discrimination, Disparity, and Health

Studies of racial and ethnic disparities find that being a member of a minority group is a risk factor for less intensive and lower quality of healthcare services (Institute of Medicine, 2002). Racial and ethnic disparities have been consistently noted in cardiovascular procedures (LaVeist, Arthur, Plantholt, & Rubinstein, 2003), cancer diagnosis and treatment (Shavers & Brown, 2002), and colorectal cancer (Cooper, Yuan, & Rimm, 1997). Thinking about how discrimination harms health requires the public health nurse to consider the different experiences of those considered a dominant group, such as white men, and those considered a subordinate group, such as women. Social epidemiology considers that discrimination has an adverse effect on health, and some social epidemiologists hypothesize that discrimination actually creates a biological pathway for disease to occur in the body.

Social epidemiologists posit "inequality hurts and discrimination harms health" (Krieger, 2000, p. 36). How discrimination affects one's health status necessitates a conceptual framework that provides measurements and methods that permit an analysis of how discrimination can affect health in the present and in the future. Discrimination is the process by which people are treated differently because they are members in a particular group. Particular "isms" such as racism (bias against racial and ethnic groups), sexism (bias against women), ageism (bias against elders), heterosexism (bias against gays and lesbians), ableism (bias against disabled), and classism (bias against lower incomes) are forms of discrimination. How these "isms" become pathways for poor health is called the ecosocial theory of disease distribution. Ecosocial theory seeks to integrate the biological and social mechanisms of discrimination within a historical and multilayered analytical perspective. Ecosocial theory leads social epidemiologists to develop knowledge about (1) how a person embodies disease or how disease grows within the body, (2) the social and biological pathways that contribute to this embodiment, and (3) the cumulative interaction between exposure, susceptibility, and resistance to disease (Krieger, 2001c). Additionally, ecosocial theory examines the biological and social mechanisms of discrimination and how they become expressions for disease or poor health.

The public health nurse assesses discrimination on an individual level and a population level. The individual level examines indirect or unobserved forms of discrimination (how clinicians treat their clients differently based on race or gender) and direct forms of discrimination as reported by the client, then links these to an observable outcome measure such as uncontrolled high blood pressure, as noted in **Figure 4-3**.

Figure 4-3 Conceptual model to understanding discrimination.

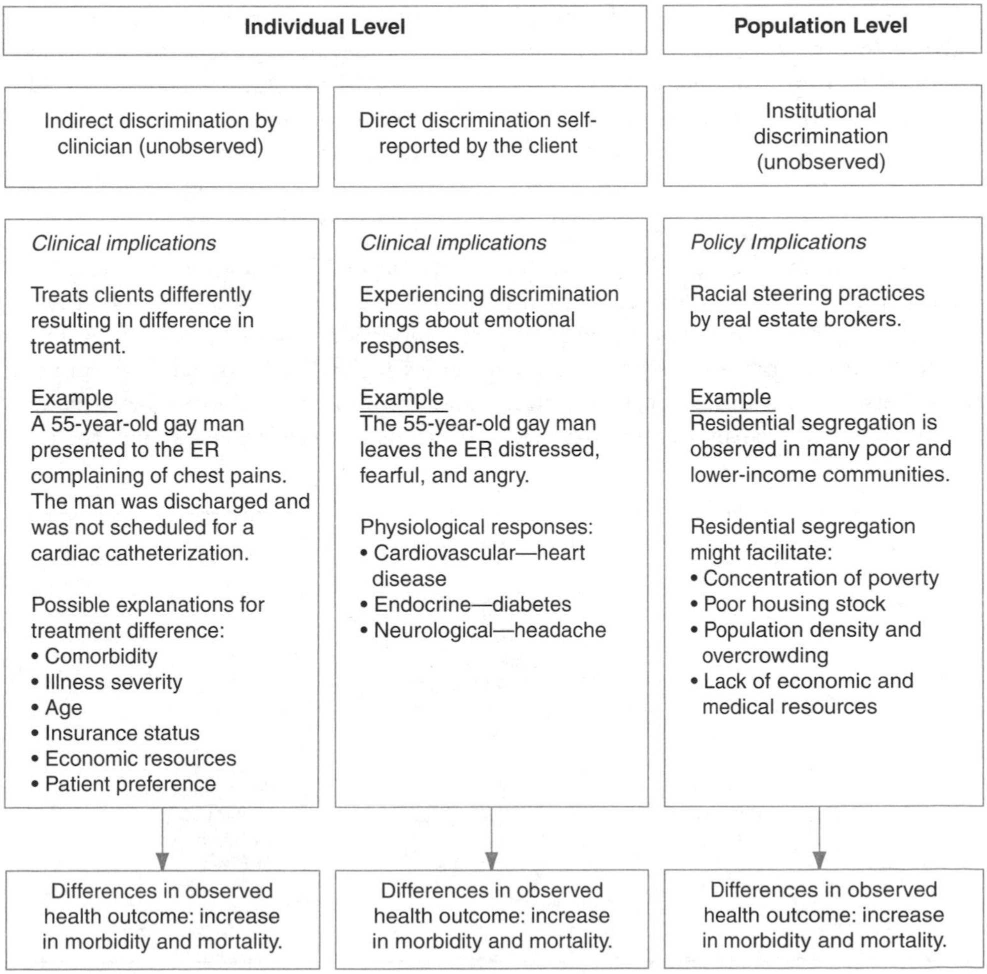

Individual Level		**Population Level**
Indirect discrimination by clinician (unobserved)	Direct discrimination self-reported by the client	Institutional discrimination (unobserved)
Clinical implications Treats clients differently resulting in difference in treatment. Example A 55-year-old gay man presented to the ER complaining of chest pains. The man was discharged and was not scheduled for a cardiac catheterization. Possible explanations for treatment difference: • Comorbidity • Illness severity • Age • Insurance status • Economic resources • Patient preference	*Clinical implications* Experiencing discrimination brings about emotional responses. Example The 55-year-old gay man leaves the ER distressed, fearful, and angry. Physiological responses: • Cardiovascular—heart disease • Endocrine—diabetes • Neurological—headache	*Policy Implications* Racial steering practices by real estate brokers. Example Residential segregation is observed in many poor and lower-income communities. Residential segregation might facilitate: • Concentration of poverty • Poor housing stock • Population density and overcrowding • Lack of economic and medical resources
Differences in observed health outcome: increase in morbidity and mortality.	Differences in observed health outcome: increase in morbidity and mortality.	Differences in observed health outcome: increase in morbidity and mortality.

Source: Adapted from Krieger, 2000.

On the population level, institutional discrimination is examined. Institutional discrimination refers to policies that are part of the standard working relationships of institutions. An example is corporate policies that often make it difficult for women or people of color to advance into upper management even though they are qualified. The public health nurse should always consider how the individual level and population level of discrimination contribute to poorer health outcomes as evidenced by increases in morbidity and mortality rates.

Discrimination can tell the public health nurse how groups are treated differently. Racism is a subset of discrimination. Jones (2001) developed a framework for understanding racism on three levels: institutionalized, personally mediated, and internalized.

- Institutionalized racism describes resources that are available to certain groups in society and their ability to access them. For example, the wait times in the emergency room in a private hospital are less than the wait times in a public hospital. Additionally, a wealthy community will

have more grocery stores with fresh food than a poorer community.
- Personally mediated racism describes prejudice and discrimination as experienced by particular groups of people because of their race. This type of racism can be intentional or unintentional. For example, a black student attending Yale might experience feelings of racism when a classmate asks if he or she was accepted into Yale because of the affirmative action program.
- Internalized racism describes how members of a stigmatized race accept or internalize the negative messages about their abilities. Manifestations of internalized racism might be hopelessness, self-devaluation, and other behaviors that reflect loss of self-esteem. For example, a child of color may play only with a white doll.

Understanding how racism exemplifies itself on all three levels gives the public health nurse an understanding of the resulting health outcomes for individuals, families, populations, and communities. **Figure 4-4** illustrates the relationship between and among the three.

Figure 4-4 Impact of racism on health outcomes.

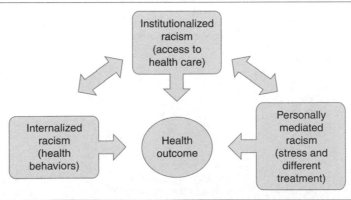

Source: Adapted from Jones, 2001.

Conclusion

A historical review of epidemiology looked at special events in history that facilitated the need for epidemiological practices. Further, epidemiological practices evolved after each significant revolution (infectious disease control vs. noninfectious disease control). Today, public health nurses and other public health practitioners apply epidemiological principles and tools to systematically collect health-related data, analyze these data, interpret these data, and recommend public health actions in terms of policy initiatives that address preventing and controlling disease(s) in particular populations and communities. Descriptive and analytical epidemiology was described and explored as well as the epidemiological triad and the chain of infection. Examples were offered throughout the reading to bring this material to life for the readers.

Social epidemiology makes the case that social determinants of health, which consists of SES (income, occupation, and education), socioeconomic position, and discrimination can influence health outcomes in the future. Additionally, it is the economic and educational advantages of an individual that facilitate better health outcomes. Social epidemiologists study how social equality and inequalities contribute to the biological expression of disease and positive or negative health outcomes.

References

Acevedo-Garcia, D., Lochner, K. A., Osypuk, T. L., & Subramanian, S. V. (2003). Future directions in residential segregation and health research: A multilevel approach. *American Journal of Public Health, 93*(2), 215–221.

Berkman, L. F., & Kawachi, I. (2000). A historical framework for social epidemiology. In L. F. Berkman & I. Kawachi (Eds.), *Social epidemiology* (pp. 3–12). New York, NY: Oxford University Press.

Bodenheimer, T. S., & Grumbach, K. (2008). *Understanding health policy: A clinical approach* (5th ed.). New York, NY: McGraw-Hill Lange Medical Books.

Breslow, L. (2005). Origins and development of the International Epidemiological Association. *International Journal of Epidemiology, 34,* 725–729.

Carthon, M. B. (2011). Making ends meet: Community networks and health promotion among blacks in the city of brotherly love. *The American Journal of Public Health, 101*(8), 1392–1401.

Colditz, G. A., Manson, J. E., & Hankinson, S. E. (1997). The Nurses' Health Study: 20-year contribution to the understanding of health among women. *Journal of Women's Health, 6*(1), 49–62.

Cooper, G. S., Yuan, Z., & Rimm, A. A. (1997). Racial disparity in the incidence and case-fatality of colorectal cancer: Analysis of 329 United States counties. *Cancer, Epidemiology, Biomarkers, & Prevention, 6,* 283–285.

Depietropaolo, D. L., Powers, J. H., & Gill, J. M. (2005). Diagnosis of Lyme disease. *American Family Physician, 72*(2), 297–303.

Diez-Roux, A. V. (2000). Multilevel analysis in public health research. *Annual Review of Public Health, 21,* 171–192.

Dike van de Mheen, H., Stronks, K., & Mackenbach, J. P. (1998). A lifecourse perspective on socioeconomic inequalities: The influences of childhood socioeconomic conditions and selection processes. In M. Bartley, D. Blane, & G. D. Smith (Eds.), *The sociology of health inequalities* (pp. 193–216). Oxford, UK: Blackwell.

France, D. (1999, May 4). Scientists at work: Allen C. Steere; Lyme disease expert developed the big picture of tiny tick. *The New York Times.* Retrieved from http://query.nytimes.com/gst/fullpage.html?sec=health&res=9C00EED8173CF937A35756C0A96F958260

Galea, S., Tracy, M., Hoggatt, K. J., DiMaggio, C., & Karpati, A. (2011). Estimated deaths attributable to social factors in the United States. *American Journal of Public Health, 101*(8), 1456–1465.

Hippocrates. (400 B.C.E.). Translated by Francis Adams. *On airs, waters, and places.* Retrieved from http://classics.mit.edu//Hippocrates/airwatpl.html

Hymes, K. B., Cheung, T., Greene, J. B., Prose, N. S., Marcus, A., Ballard, H., . . . Laubenstein, L. J. (1981).

Kaposi's sarcoma in homosexual men—A report of eight cases. *Lancet, 318*(8247), 598–600.

Institute of Medicine. (2002). *Unequal treatment: Confronting racial and ethnic disparities in health care.* Washington, DC: Author.

The James Lind Library. (n.d.). *Treatise of scurvy.* Retrieved from http://www.jameslindlibrary.org/trial_records/17th_18th_Century/lind/lind_tp.html

Jones, C. P. (2001). Race, racism, and the practice of epidemiology. *American Journal of Epidemiology, 154*(4), 299–304.

Kannel, W. B., Schwartz, M. J., & McNamara, P. M. (1969). Blood pressure and risk of coronary heart disease: A Framingham study. *Chest, 56*(1), 43–52.

Kaplan, G. A. (2001). Economic policy is health policy: Findings from the study of income, socioeconomic status, and health. In J. A. Auerbach & B. K. Krimgold (Eds.), *Income, socioeconomic status, and health: Exploring the relationships* (pp. 137–149). Washington, DC: National Policy Association.

Kawachi, I. (1999). Social capital and community effects on population and individual health. *Annals of New York Academy of Sciences, 896,* 120–130.

Kawachi, I. (2000). Income inequality and health. In L. F. Berkman & I. Kawachi (Eds.), *Social epidemiology* (pp. 76–94). New York, NY: Oxford University Press.

Kolata, G. (2007, January 3). A surprising secret to long life: Stay in school. *The New York Times.* Retrieved from http://www.nytimes.com/2007/01/03/health/03aging.html

Krieger, N. (2000). Discrimination and health. In L. F. Berkman & I. Kawachi (Eds.), *Social epidemiology* (pp. 36–75). New York, NY: Oxford University Press.

Krieger, N. (2001a). Theories for social epidemiology in the 21st century: An ecosocial perspective. *International Journal of Epidemiology, 30,* 668–677.

Krieger, N. (2001b). Historical roots of social epidemiology: Socioeconomic gradients in health and contextual analysis. *International Journal of Epidemiology, 30,* 899–900.

Krieger, N. (2001c). A glossary for social epidemiology. *Journal of Epidemiology and Community Health, 55,* 693–700.

Krieger, N. (2002). A glossary for social epidemiology. *Epidemiological Bulletin, 23*(1). Retrieved from http://www.paho.org/English/SHA/be_v23nl-glossary.htm

Lantz, P. M., Lynch, J. W., House, J. S., Lepkowski, J. M., Mero, R. P., Musick, M. A., & Williams, D. R. (2001). Socioeconomic disparities in health change in a longitudinal study of US adults: The role of health-risk behaviors. *Social Science and Medicine, 53,* 29–40.

LaVeist, T. A., Arthur, M., Plantholt, S., & Rubinstein, M. (2003). Explaining racial differences in receipt of coronary angiography: The role of physician referral and physician specialty. *Medical Care Research and Review, 60*(4), 453–467.

Lynch, J., & Kaplan, G. (2000). Socioeconomic position. In L. F. Berkman & I. Kawachi (Eds.), *Social epidemiology* (pp. 13–35). New York, NY: Oxford University Press.

Marmot, M. (2000). Multilevel approaches to understanding social determinants. In L. F. Berkman & I. Kawachi (Eds.), *Social epidemiology* (pp. 349–367). New York, NY: Oxford University Press.

Marmot, M., & Wilkinson, R. (2006). *Social determinants of health* (2nd ed.). Oxford, UK: Oxford University Press.

Mirowsky, J., Ross, C. E., & Reynolds, J. (2000). Links between social status and health. In C. E. Bird, P. Conrad, & A. M. Fremont (Eds.), *Handbook of medical sociology* (pp. 47–78). Upper Saddle River, NJ: Prentice Hall.

Murray, L. R. (2011). Public health and primary care: Transforming the U.S. health system. *The Nation's Health, 41*(5), 3.

National Library of Medicine (n.d.a). *The reports of the surgeon general: The AIDS epidemic.* Retrieved from http://profiles.nlm.nih.gov/NN/Views/Exhibit/narrative/aids.html

National Library of Medicine. (n.d.b). *The reports of the surgeon general: The 1964 report on smoking and health.* Retrieved from http://profiles.nlm.nih.gov/NN/Views/Exhibit/narrative/smoking.html

Office of History National Institute of Health. (2005). *Dr. Joseph Goldberger & the war on pellagra.* Retrieved from http://history.nih.gov/exhibits/goldberger/index.html

Perry, M., Williams, R. L., Wallerstein, N., & Waitzkin, H. (2008). Social capital and health care experiences among low-income individuals. *American Journal of Public Health, 98*(2), 330–336.

Pfettscher, S. A. (2002). Florence Nightingale: Modern nursing. In A. M. Tomey & M. R. Alligood (Eds.), *Nursing theorists and their work* (5th ed., pp. 65–83). Philadelphia, PA: Mosby.

Phillips, K. D. (2002). Sister Callista Roy: Adaptation model. In A. M. Tomey & M. R. Alligood (Eds.), *Nursing theorists and their work* (5th ed., pp. 269–298). Philadelphia, PA: Mosby.

Pineda, M. D., White, E., Kristal, A. R., & Taylor, V. (2001). Asian breast cancer survival in the US: A comparison between Asian immigrants, US-born Asian Americans, and Caucasians. *International Journal of Epidemiology, 30,* 976–982.

Pronyk, P. M., Harpham, T., Morison, L. A., Hargreaves, J. R., Kim, J. C., Phetla, G.,. . . Porter, J. D. (2008).

Is social capital associated with HIV risk in rural South Africa? *Social Science and Medicine, 66*(9), 1999–2010.

Putnam, R. D. (1995). Bowling alone: America's declining social capital. *Journal of Democracy, 6,* 65–78.

Sepkowitz, K. A. (2001). AIDS—The first 20 years. *New England Journal of Medicine, 344*(23), 1764–1772.

Sepkowitz, K. A. (2008). One disease, two epidemics—AIDS at 25. *New England Journal of Medicine, 354*(23), 2411–2414.

Shavers, V. L., & Brown, M. L. (2002). Racial and ethnic disparities in the receipt of cancer treatment. *Journal of the National Cancer Institute, 94*(5), 334–357.

Stephan, E. (n.d.). John Graunt. Retrieved from http://www.edstephan.org/Graunt/graunt.html

Stotts, R. C. (2008). *Epidemiology and public health nursing.* Clifton Park, NJ: Delmar Cengage Learning.

Stringhini, S., Sabia, S., Shipley, M., Bruner, E., Nabi, H., Kivimaki, M., & Singh-Manoux, A. (2010). Association of socioeconomic position with health behaviors and mortality. The Whitehall II study. *Journal of American Medical Association, 303*(12), 1159–1166.

Subramanian, S. V., Kawachi, I., & Kennedy, B. P. (2001). Does the state you live in make a difference? Multilevel analysis of self-rated health in the US. *Social Science & Medicine, 53,* 9–19.

Tarzian, A. J. (2005). Epidemiology: Unraveling the mysteries of disease and health. In F. A. Maurer & C. M. Smith (Eds.), *Community/public health nursing practice: Health for families and populations* (3rd ed., pp. 150–174). St. Louis, MO: Elsevier Saunders.

UCLA Department of Epidemiology School of Public Health. (n.d.). *John Snow.* Retrieved from http://www.ph.ucla.edu/epi/snow.html

U.S. Department of Health and Human Services (DHHS) & Centers for Disease Control and Prevention (CDC). (1998). *Principles of epidemiology: An introduction to applied epidemiology and biostatistics* (2nd ed.). Atlanta, GA: Author.

U.S. Department of Health and Human Services (DHHS) & Centers for Disease Control and Prevention (CDC). (2006). *Principles of epidemiology: An introduction to applied epidemiology and biostatistics* (3rd ed.). Atlanta, GA: Author.

U.S. Preventive Services Task Force. (2008). *Guide to clinical preventive services: Recommendations of the U.S. Preventive Services Task Force.* Rockville, MD: Agency for Healthcare and Research Quality.

Wald, L. (1902). The nurses' settlement in New York. *American Journal of Nursing, 2*(8), 567–575.

Wilkinson, R. (1999). Income distribution and life expectancy. In I. Kawachi, B. Kennedy, & R. Wilkinson (Eds.), *The society and population health reader: Income inequality and health* (pp. 28–35). New York, NY: The New Press.

For a full suite of assignments and additional learning activities, use the access code located in the front of your book to visit this exclusive website: http://go.jblearning.com/londrigan. If you do not have an access code, you can obtain one at the site.

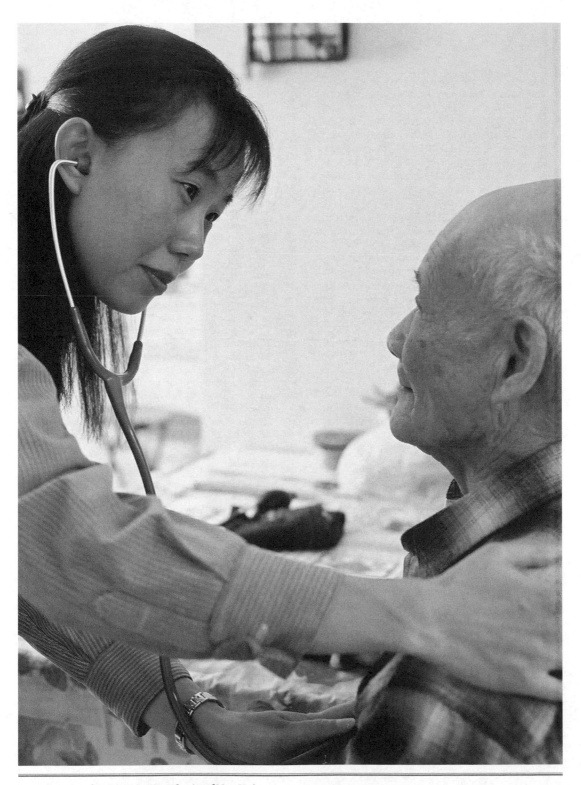

Source: Courtesy of the Visiting Nurse Service of New York.

Chapter 5

Evidence-Based Practice From a Public Health Perspective

Joanne K. Singleton
Renee McLeod-Sordjan

No system can endure that does not march (Nightingale, 1893/2004, p. 216).

www

LEARNING OBJECTIVES

At the completion of this chapter, the reader will be able to

- Define evidence-based practice.
- Describe the systematic approach to finding best available evidence.

- Explore the application of evidence-based practice to public health issues of health literacy and tobacco use.

www

KEY TERMS

- ❏ Evidence-based medicine
- ❏ Evidence-based practice

- ❏ Health literacy
- ❏ Tobacco use

Introduction to Evidence-Based Practice and Public Health

"In a world where public health threats range from AIDS and bioterrorism to an epidemic of obesity, the need for an effective public health system is as urgent as it has ever been" (Gebbie, Rosenstock, & Hernandez, 2003, p. 1). This quotation comes from an Institute of Medicine (IOM) report, *Who Will Keep the Public Healthy?*

Educating Public Health Professionals for the 21st Century. Although this report is aimed primarily at schools of public health, it includes recommendations for schools of nursing and medicine as well. For schools of nursing, the recommendations address the inclusion of an ecological perspective of health in nursing curricula, collaboration among all public health professionals from a variety of disciplines, and the provision of clinical experiences in the public health arena.

The 2011 IOM report, *The Future of Nursing: Leading Change, Advancing Health* considers key messages and recommendations that pertain to nursing. One of the key messages specifically addresses the improvement of nursing education to ensure the delivery of "safe, quality, patient-centered care across all settings, especially in such areas as primary care and community and public health" (p. 6).

An important aspect of these recommendations is the acknowledgment of **evidence-based practice (EBP)**. The IOM published *Health Professions Education: A Bridge to Quality* (Griener & Knebel, 2003), which included the following new vision for all health professions education: "All health professionals should be educated to deliver patient centered care as members of an interdisciplinary team, emphasizing evidence-based practice, quality improvement approaches, and informatics" (p. 3). This challenge was answered in 2006 with the Quality and Safety Education for Nurses (QSEN) initiative funded by the Robert Wood Johnson Foundation (QSEN, 2007). This initiative sought to identify the knowledge, competencies, and attitudes that nurses need to know to practice with quality and safety in mind. The six major areas of practice include: patient-centered care, teamwork and collaboration, evidence-based practice, quality improvement, safety, and informatics (Cronenwett et al., 2007).

What Is an Evidence-Based Practice Lens for Viewing Population-Based Health Issues?

The term "evidence based" was first used by medicine in 1992 by Gordon Guyatt, a Canadian physician from McMaster University, and the Evidence-Based Medicine Working Group. Although the term **evidence-based medicine** originated within the medical profession as a new paradigm for medical practice (Oxman, Sackett, & Guyatt, 1992), the essence of this paradigm—using research evidence as the best evidence to guide professional decision making—has recently spread to other professions both within and outside the healthcare arena. Singleton, Levin, and Keefer (2007) discussed several examples from the disciplines of law, education, and management. In addition, Cullum, Ciliska, Haynes, and Marks (2008) cite the use of the term "evidence based" in professions such as physiotherapy and police science.

Regardless of the field or discipline in which this paradigm or model is applied, EBP has several conceptual and process components that cross disciplinary boundaries. Evidence-based practice is a framework for decision making that uses the best available evidence in conjunction with the professional's expertise and the client's, customer's, or consumer's values and preferences to guide problem solving and judgments about how to best approach a situation to achieve desired outcomes (Melnyk & Fineout-Overholt, 2011; Straus, Richardson, Glasziou, & Haynes, 2005). The key to the EBP model is the systematic approach to finding the best available evidence to answer a focused question and to implement the answer in practice as follows:

1. Ask and frame a clinical question.
2. Find the evidence to answer the question.
3. Appraise the evidence for validity, source reliability, and applicability to practice.
4. Select and synthesize the best evidence for use.
5. Implement the evidence-based intervention in practice.
6. Evaluate the intervention and results.

The search for and retrieval of this evidence are not always approached in the systematic way

---

---

advocated in the EBP paradigm, which is to try to find the highest level of evidence first and then proceed methodically through the hierarchy of evidence that exists to answer the focused question. Some types of evidence carry more weight than other types of evidence. For example, a single study carries less weight than a systematic review, because a systematic review combines the results of several studies on the same clinical question or questions. We always want to use the highest level of evidence available to guide our clinical practice. Health professionals, therefore, have developed schemata that rank evidence according to levels. The higher the level of evidence, the more confidence we are able to have in a study's validity. There are

many different schemata for ranking the level of a piece of evidence. Based on the work of others, Melnyk & Overholt (2011) pre-sent seven levels in the hierarchy of evidence (see **Box 5-1**).

Although it is important to determine the levels of evidence upon which a recommendation for practice is based, it is also important to assess the quality of that evidence, whether it is a study or expert opinion. The quality of evidence depends on the critical appraisal of the study or the background of and resources used by an expert panel. The schema shown in **Box 5-2** provides one approach for assigning a quality rating to a piece of evidence. Using this approach, a rating for any level of evidence may range from A to D and reflects the basic

---

Box 5-2 Quality Ratings

A: A very well-designed study/project (Stetler et al., 1998)
B: A well-designed meta-analysis with at least 5 studies but less than 12; well-designed meta-analysis with large sample but some flawed studies*; individual studies in level IV, which may have a large sample size, but are secondary analyses of previously conducted randomized clinical trials (Singleton et al., 2005)
C: Well-designed individual studies with small sample sizes (Singleton et al., 2005)
D: Study/project has a major flaw that raises serious questions about the validity of the findings (Stetler et al., 1998)

*For example, use of nonrandomized trials in a meta-analysis seeking to answer questions of treatment effectiveness.

Source: From Singleton, Levin, Feldman, & Truglio-Londrigan (2005); Stetler et al. (1998).

scientific credibility of the overall study/project or other type of evidence.

Leveling schemes and quality ratings may differ according to the agency or organization or author. Under any circumstances, however, the leveling and determination of the quality of evidence are essential components of this model. Some evidence-based guidelines, such as the tobacco-dependence guidelines introduced later in this chapter, identify and define "strength" of evidence for the specific guideline. When reading EBP guidelines, therefore, it is important to identify the criteria used to assess the level, quality, or strength of evidence. This is the approach we have taken in providing readers with the best available evidence on two very important public health challenges: helping people to stop smoking and increasing the health literacy of our population.

Healthy People 2020—Public Health Conditions: An Evidence-Based Perspective

Healthy People 2020 is a federal government initiative that contains health objectives for the citizens of our nation (U.S. Department of Health and Human Services [U.S. DHHS], 2010a). This document is built on past government initiatives intended to guide action that would improve the nation's health. *Healthy People 2020* addresses many objectives. This chapter focuses on two health conditions from a public health perspective: health literacy and tobacco addiction. We discuss the national incidence and prevalence and morbidity and mortality of these health conditions, the evidence to guide or develop population-focused interventions for these conditions, and specific public health interventions in action for health literacy and tobacco addiction.

The first topic that will be highlighted in this chapter is Health Communication and Health Communication Technology. This topic, along with its specific objectives, may be viewed in its entirety under *Healthy People* tab, *2020 Topics and Objectives* (U.S. DHHS, 2010b). Under this topic area there are 13 objectives. One of the specific objectives for this topic area is:

HC/HIT-1: (Developmental) Improve the health literacy of the population

The second issue to be highlighted is under the topic area of Tobacco Use. This topic, along with specific objectives, may be viewed in its entirety under the *Healthy People* tab *2020 Topics and Objectives* (U.S. DHHS, 2010b). There are a total of 20 objectives under the topic area of **Tobacco Use**. Two of the specific objectives for tobacco use are:

TU-1: Reduce tobacco use by adults.
TU-2: Reduce tobacco use by adolescents.

The focus of this chapter is on an evidence-based approach to these two very important public health topics: health literacy and tobacco use. Before discussing these two public health topics and introducing the EBP approach to understanding them, an overview of population-based concepts will help you to put the subsequent discussions about specific public health issues in context.

Health Literacy as a Public Health Condition: Overview and Definition

Before the 1990s, the impact of literacy on population health in the United States was either unappreciated by health professionals or was generally thought of as a problem of an individual; literacy was not considered to be a public health condition. Today, it is known that literacy and its healthcare counterpart, health literacy, have far-reaching effects on both the individual with low health literacy and the U.S. population as a whole (Shohet & Renaud, 2006). *Healthy People 2020* has formally included health literacy as one of the defined objectives for study and intervention for 2010–2020 (U.S. DHHS, 2010b).

The definition of **health literacy** is continually being refined. The most widely-accepted definition states that health literacy is "the degree to which individuals have the capacity to obtain, process, and understand basic health information and services needed to make appropriate health decisions" (Nielsen-Bohlman, Panzer, & Kindig, 2004, p. 32). This definition has been expanded more recently to reflect the even broader impact that health literacy has on individual lives. "Literacy facilitates access to information, and enables individuals to make informed health decisions, to influence events, and to exert greater control over their lives" (Shohet & Renaud, 2006, p. 10). In more concrete terms, health literacy impacts an individual's ability to access health care, to make choices in obtaining appropriate health insurance coverage, and to seek out high-quality facilities to obtain evidence-based health screening and illness care as well as comprehend health information about disease prevention or self-care of chronic disease. Nine out of ten English speaking patients lack proficiency to comprehend everyday health communication (Nielsen-Bohlman et al., 2004). In addition, if an individual is the caregiver of children or elderly family members, the individual needs to advocate and make decisions for those in his or her care. Clearly, health literacy has far-reaching effects on individuals, families, communities, and the U.S. population as a whole.

INCIDENCE, PREVALENCE, MORBIDITY, AND MORTALITY

Incidence and Prevalence. Although low health literacy is now widely recognized to have a significant negative impact on both the individual and public health, tools to measure health literacy and strategies to improve care of the low literacy population have been developed only recently. For the third time in as many decades, the National Center for Education Statistics (2006) measured the English literacy of the U.S. population in the 2003 National Assessment of Adult Literacy. This survey was the first to include measurement of health literacy in addition to overall U.S. English literacy. The National Assessment of Adult Literacy surveyed a representative sample of 18,000 U.S. households as well as 1,200 persons in prisons. For the purpose of this study, health literacy was defined using the previously quoted IOM definition (National Center for Education Statistics, 2006).

Health literacy was measured using the three literacy measures used in the overall English literacy assessments by the 2003 National Assessment of Adult Literacy survey: prose, document, and quantitative measures. Prose literacy is defined as the ability to search, comprehend, and use information from continuous text. Document literacy is defined as the ability to search, comprehend, and use information from noncontinuous text (e.g., application forms or maps). Quantitative literacy is defined as the ability to identify and perform computation using numbers embedded in print materials (e.g., balancing a checkbook). In addition, three domains specific to health literacy were identified and measured: clinical, prevention, and navigation of the health system. The clinical domain was defined as the activities involved in the provider–patient interaction, such as completing forms and understanding medication dosages. The prevention domain was defined as activities related to disease prevention and self-management of illness. Navigation of the health system included activities such as understanding health insurance plans and consent forms.

Results of the 2003 adult health literacy survey showed that 36% of the U.S. population, or approximately 87 million adults, had either below basic (14%) or basic (22%) health literacy levels, defined as

- Below basic: No more than the most basic and concrete literacy skills
- Basic: Skills necessary to perform simple and basic everyday activities

Disparities among particular subpopulations were also noted. Hispanic populations had the lowest percentage of health literacy among ethnic groups. More men (16%) than women (12%) had below basic health literacy levels. Persons who did not speak English before attending primary school had lower health literacy than those who spoke English at early ages, and adults over age 65 had lower health literacy than other age groups. Educational attainment was significantly associated with below basic health literacy: 49% of individuals who did not complete either high school or a General Educational Development program had below basic health literacy scores. Adults living in poverty had lower health literacy levels than other socioeconomic groups, as did persons who had self-perceived overall health at lower ratings. Persons who had no health insurance or had Medicaid/Medicare had lower health literacy levels. Those who obtained their basic health information from television or radio had lower health literacy than those who obtained information from print media (National Center for Education Statistics, 2006).

Low health literacy may contribute significantly to the notable health disparities across specific populations in the United States. One of the overarching goals of *Healthy People 2020* (U.S. DHHS, 2010c) is to reduce these health disparities, which lead to increased morbidity and mortality as well as inefficient and ineffective use of public resources. Estimates of the cost of low health literacy to U.S. society range from $106 to $236 billion annually (Vernon, Trujillo, Rosenbaum, & DeBuono, 2007). When future and indirect costs are accounted for, this estimate increases to a range from $1.6 to $3.6 trillion annually (Vernon et al., 2007). Clearly, low health literacy is a public health condition of great consequence.

Morbidity and Mortality and Level of Evidence. Many studies have documented how low health literacy impacts a person's ability to obtain preventive screening services and to manage one's chronic diseases. Based on the level of evidence ratings in Box 5-1, the following evidence is reported. In a systematic review of the literature, Berkman, Sheridan, Donahue, Halpern, and Crotty (2011) found that patients with low health literacy used health resources less frequently than their higher literacy counterparts (level I). Maniaci, Heckman, and Dawson (2008) found that patients with lower levels of health literacy were found to have less medication knowledge after hospital discharge (level IV). In addition, patients with type 2 diabetes mellitus and low health literacy were found to have higher HgA_{1C} levels and higher rates of retinopathy than those with higher health literacy levels (Schillinger et al., 2002) (level IV). Patients with low health literacy were less likely to use preventive services (IOM, 2004) (level V). Also, higher mortality rates were associated with lower health literacy scores (Baker et al., 2007) (level IV). Patients with low health literacy have higher rates of hospitalizations and complications and higher emergency room use (Baker, Parker, Williams, & Clark, 1998; Baker et al., 2002) (level IV). Among elderly patients 65 and older, low health literacy was associated with increased hospitalizations, higher emergency room utilization, poor medication adherence, and impaired ability to interpret health messages (Berkman, Sheridan, Donahue, Halpern, Viera, et al., 2011) (level I). Moreover, patients with low health literacy were two to three times more likely to experience poor outcomes (DeWalt, Berkman, Sheridan, Lohr & Pignone, 2004) (level I).

EVIDENCE TO GUIDE POPULATION-FOCUSED INTERVENTIONS

Evidence on the morbidity and mortality related to health literacy provides guidance on population-focused interventions. The burden of low health literacy on the health of society mandates action to improve the problem. Population-focused interventions occur within the national, state, and local arenas.

In 2010, President Obama signed the Plain Writing Act of 2010, which was designed to promote communication that the public can understand. In response, the U.S. DHHS released a National Action Plan to Improve Health Literacy. The National Action Plan aims to eliminate complex medical jargon in health communication. The National Action Plan suggests a "universal precautions" approach to health literacy and communication. By adopting universal precautions, health professionals use clear communication that is culturally appropriate regardless of the perceived health literacy skills of the client. Health information comes from various sources across multiple disciplines (e.g., websites and social media; health professionals, caregivers, and public health officials; schools; television and radio). As a result of multiple health messages, national evidence-based strategies must be adopted to improve clear communication.

An exemplar health literacy intervention that addresses communication is the three-pronged strategy adopted by The Joint Commission (Murphy-Knoll, 2007). The first strategy makes clear communication an organizational priority.

The second strategy mandates that clear communication needs to be addressed across the continuum of care, from the acute care to the primary care setting. The third strategy states that policy changes must be pursued to improve provider–patient communication. *Health Literacy Innovations* is a computer-based software system used by the National Institutes of Health to improve the readability of health information by translating technical information into simpler terms.

Another national intervention involves increasing access to healthcare coverage for the entire population. During 2010, 50.7 million persons in the United States under the age of 65 were uninsured (DeNavas-Walt, Proctor, & Smith, 2011). In 2014, an estimated 32 million Americans will be newly insured by the Affordable Health Care for America Act (ACA), H.R. 3962. The law includes provisions to communicate healthcare information clearly, promote prevention, promote patient-centered interventions and create healthy homes, ensure equity and cultural competence, and deliver high-quality care. The ACA provides that language within state programs must be readable for those with low health literacy as well as culturally and linguistically appropriate.

The ACA also establishes workforce training opportunities to improve the patient–provider interaction. This interaction could be improved by increasing basic health literacy education of primary care providers. The ACA pushes for curriculum changes to teach health professionals skills for communicating with persons of low health literacy. Methods such as "teach back" (Pfizer Clear Health Communication Initiative, 2008) and "ask me three" (National Patient Safety Foundation, 2008) have been shown to improve patient comprehension and ability for self-care. Healthcare providers need to be educated that health education materials should be written in easy-to-use formats, with large font, short sentences, and action-oriented content to improve readability and patient comprehension (Doak, Doak, & Root, 1998). Curriculums in health-related professions need to reflect training in culturally diverse education techniques. In a study by Volandes and colleagues (2008), specific teaching techniques were shown to enhance decision-making ability regarding end-of-life care preferences.

Statewide initiatives in health literacy are overseen by the U.S. DHHS Office of Disease and Health Promotion. State and local collaborations between academic, government, and nonprofit organizations with a health literacy focus are funded across five priorities:

1. Incorporate health literacy improvement in mission, planning, and evaluation.
2. Support health literacy research, evaluation, training, and practice.
3. Conduct formative, process, and outcome evaluations to design and assess materials, messages, and resources.
4. Enhance dissemination of timely, accurate, and appropriate health information to health professionals and the public.
5. Design health literacy improvements to healthcare and public health systems that enhance access to health services.

For example, The Institute for Healthcare Advancement (2011) is a not-for-profit, privately operating California initiative that provides translation of patient education materials, delivers primary care in a community health setting, and also provides outreach services within the community.

Within communities, impaired health literacy negatively impacts the self-esteem of individual clients. The literature suggests that individuals do not access health care because of the "shame" related to their literacy problems. Organizations and healthcare providers can make changes to reduce this negative impact by creating "shame-free environments." Providing written materials at low literacy levels and offering assistance for those completing intake forms are suggested methods to remove barriers to care for those with low health literacy. It is important at a local level to assess the learning needs of disparate communities in a culturally competent manner. Multiple instruments (e.g., Newest Vital Sign, Test of Functional Health Literacy in Adults) exist to assess the health literacy of disparate communities and should be incorporated into daily practice to tailor individualized learning plans (Hanchate, Ash, Gasmararian, Wolf, & Paasche-Orlow, 2008; McLeod-Sordjan, 2011; Weiss et al., 2005).

Health Literacy and Tobacco Use: Specific Public Health Interventions (Case Study)

An organization reviews the current tobacco use health education materials it provides to nonsmoking adolescent clients (e.g., Did you know that tobacco addiction is one of the hardest habits to break?). These education materials could be evaluated for both reading level, using the Simplified Measure of Gobbledygook (McLaughlin, 2008), or Fry formula (Doak et al., 1998), and readability, using the Suitability of Assessment Materials, or SAM, tool (Doak et al., 1998). When designing materials for adolescents, in particular, it is important that patients "see themselves" in the illustrations on the material. The SAM tool gives very valuable guidelines that improve design for health education materials that are targeted to a specific audience. Revision of an organization's existing tobacco use materials to reduce reading level, improve readability, and clearly target a specific population is one example of a low cost and effective means to begin a system-wide movement toward clear communication.

FUTURE PROJECTIONS

Unfortunately, the problem of low health literacy may worsen in the United States across racial and generational groups. Kutner et al. (2007) reports 66% of adults aged 65 and older were classified with low health literacy. It is projected that Hispanics aged 65 and older are estimated to increase to 19.8% of the U.S. population by the year 2050 (Heron & Smith, 2007). If healthcare systems and individual providers do not make health literacy and clear communication a priority, public health outcomes can be expected to decline over future decades.

Tobacco Dependence as a Public Health Condition: Overview and Definition

Tobacco, a green leafy plant that grows in warm climates, has a long history in America. Dating back to the first American settlers in 1621 in Jamestown, Virginia, tobacco was the first crop grown for money in North America. Tobacco is dried and can be smoked or chewed. There are over 4,800 chemicals in tobacco and its smoke; nicotine is the chemical that makes tobacco addictive. Although the first settlers used tobacco in small amounts, the invention of the cigarette-making machine in 1881 resulted in widespread cigarette smoking. Nevertheless, it was not until 1964 that the Surgeon General of the United States reported on the dangers of cigarette smoking, identifying that the nicotine and tar in cigarettes may cause lung cancer. The U.S. Congress in 1965 passed the Cigarette Labeling and Advertising Act that required every cigarette pack to carry on its side the warning "Cigarettes may be hazardous to your health." This was followed by later legislation in 1971 banning radio and television advertising

of cigarettes. Cigarette companies responded to the government warnings about the hazards of smoking related to tar: By the 1980s, cigarette companies made, sold, and promoted low and ultra-low tar cigarettes. Congress passed another law in 1984, the Comprehensive Smoking Education Act, which created four different warning labels (**Figure 5-1**) and required cigarette companies to rotate among these warnings every 3 months.

Federal, state, and local governments, as well as private companies, have been taking action since the 1980s to restrict and ban smoking in public places. The American Lung Association tracks and reports tobacco control trends in the United States (see http://stateoftobacco control.org). As of 2010, the American Lung Association's smoke-free map reveals that only 27 states plus the District of Columbia have enacted comprehensive smoke-free laws

Figure 5-1 Cigarette health warnings.

SURGEON GENERAL'S WARNING: Smoking Causes Lung Cancer, Heart Disease, Emphysema, and May Complicate Pregnancy.

SURGEON GENERAL'S WARNING: Quitting Smoking Now Greatly Reduces Serious Risks to Your Health.

SURGEON GENERAL'S WARNING: Smoking by Pregnant Women May Result in Fetal Injury, Premature Birth, and Low Birth Weight.

SURGEON GENERAL'S WARNING: Cigarette Smoke Contains Carbon Monoxide.

Source: Public Law 98-474, Comprehensive Smoking Education Act, 1984. Smoking Tobacco & Health, Centers for Disease Control and Prevention.

to protect their citizens. One hundred million Americans remain unprotected by a lack of comprehensive smoke-free laws. On June 12, 2009, President Obama signed the Family Smoking Prevention and Tobacco Control Act (H.R. 1256) into law. The U.S. Food and Drug Administration (FDA) was granted the authority to regulate the sales, advertising, and ingredient content of all tobacco products marketed in the United States. The law also limits advertising to youth and requires graphic cigarette warning labels to cover 50% of the front and rear of the cigarette pack. (As of the writing of this chapter, there are issues surrounding graphic warning labels that are being challenged in the courts.)

Incidence, Prevalence, Morbidity, and Mortality

In the United States, cigarette smoking continues to be identified as the most avoidable cause of death and disability (Centers for Disease Control and Prevention [CDC], 2007a). Tobacco use begins in adolescence, with first use almost always occurring before 18 years of age. Cigarette smoking carries a significant disease burden for the primary smoker that may result in respiratory diseases, lung cancer, and/or cardiovascular disease; may have harmful reproductive effects; and results in more than 438,000 deaths per year in the United States (CDC, 2007b). Exposure to secondhand smoke for the nonsmoker creates a significant health risk, especially for individuals with respiratory or cardiac conditions, and can result in premature death and disease. In addition, 8.6 million Americans live with a significant tobacco-related illness (CDC, 2007b). According to a CDC (2008) report, direct medical costs in the United States from tobacco dependence are more than $96 billion per year and an additional $97 billion resulting from lost productivity.

Although most smokers report a desire to quit, most quit attempts fail. New smokers from adults to children are continually recruited. Not only are interventions critical to help those who already smoke to quit, interventions to prevent people, especially children, from starting to smoke are essential to eliminating smoking-related illnesses.

About 45 million adults (21%) in the United States smoke (CDC, 2007a), and each day about 4,000 children ages 12 to 17 smoke their first cigarette, with about 1,200 becoming addicted to tobacco (CDC, 2006; Substance Abuse and Mental Health Services Administration [SAMHSA], 2005, 2007, 2008). In 2006, it was reported that 3.3 million adolescents aged 12 to 17 years were tobacco users, with 2.6 million of this population cigarette smokers (SAMHSA, 2008). About 82% of adolescent smokers are interested in quitting, but only about 4% of the 77% who attempt to quit are successful (Engels, Knibbe, de Vries, & Drop, 1998; Zhu, Sun, Billings, Choi, & Malarcher, 1999). Quit attempts in adolescents are usually unassisted and unplanned, yet those who enroll in quit programs are twice as likely to succeed as those who are not enrolled (McCuller, Sussman, Wapner, Dent, & Weiss, 2006).

An estimated 6 million youths will die prematurely from cigarette-related deaths. (U.S. DHHS, 2010d). Over the past 50 years, the prevalence of smoking in the United States has decreased by about 50%, to about one fifth of the population. Men smoke more than women (23% vs. 19%). Native American/Native Alaskans smoke more (33%) than blacks and whites (both at 21%), Hispanics (15%), and Asians/Pacific Islanders (11.3%). In 2005, 19 million adults attempted to quit, but only 4 to 7% are estimated to have been successful (Hughes, 2003). In 2009, the rates of teen smoking declined to 20%, yet monitoring teen smoking is important because 80% of adult smokers began before the age of 18 (CDC, 2010b). Although there is now "a robust evidence base about effective interventions. . .the United States has not yet achieved the goal of making tobacco use a rare behavior" (CDC, 2008, p. 7).

EVIDENCE TO GUIDE POPULATION-FOCUSED INTERVENTIONS

Enormous health-related disparities exist in second-hand smoke exposure. Among the highest exposed are children aged 4–11 and low-income individuals at 61% and 63%, respectively (CDC, 2008b). Decreasing smoking in public places not only protects nonsmokers from the effects of secondhand smoke, but it may also promote smoking cessation by restricting smoking behavior. Comprehensive multicomponent strategies to enforce no-smoking policies within organizations were found to be the most effective strategies to decrease smoking in public places. The ACA of 2009 granted the FDA authority to regulate tobacco products to prevent illness within the population. The law creates a Prevention and Public Health Fund that provides states with financial incentives to encourage healthy behaviors among Medicaid recipients (U.S. DHHS, 2010d).

The evidence for tobacco cessation is reviewed in *Ending the Tobacco Problem: A Blueprint for the Nation* (IOM, 2007). This publication endorses innovative social policies that translate the scientific evidence into action. Sample interventions include:

- counter-marketing youth-targeted smoking cessation mass advertising,
- adopting comprehensive smoke free laws,
- increasing healthcare access to smoking cessation programs,
- restricting smoking-related advertisements, and
- increasing the federal excise tax on cigarettes.

A moderate effect was found with the use of educational material and posted warnings to enforce no-smoking policies (Serra, Bonfill, Pladevall, & Cabezas Pena, 2008). From 2002 to 2004, smoking prevalence in New York City decreased from 21.5 to 17.5%. This has been attributed to increased taxes that raised the price of cigarettes as well as the law that made all indoor workplaces smoke free. This percentage decrease equates with approximately 240,000 fewer smokers (CDC, 2007a). The rate of teen smoking in New York City is half of the national rate. Increasing the federal excise tax has shown national benefits as well. As of December 2010, the following five states had set excise tax rates of $3 or more per pack: New York ($4.35), Rhode Island ($3.46), Washington ($3.025), Connecticut ($3), and Hawaii ($3). For every 10% increase in the price of tobacco products, consumption falls by approximately 4% overall, with a greater reduction among youth. In 2009, the ACA enactment of the 62-cent federal cigarette excise tax increase is projected to prevent initiation of smoking by nearly two million children, cause more than one million adult smokers to quit, and prevent nearly 900,000 smoking-attributed deaths (U.S. DHHS, 2010). The long-term healthcare savings by reducing tobacco-related healthcare costs is estimated to be $44 billion.

Mass media interventions are used as part of a comprehensive tobacco cessation program, and they can be effective strategies for adults (Bala, Strzeszynski, & Cahill, 2008). Mass media interventions, such as those delivered by leaflets, booklets, posters, billboards, newspapers, radio, and television, are used to promote smoking cessation. One example of this type of intervention is the media campaign initiated by the New York City Department of Mental Health and Hygiene. In 2006, the Department launched a television advertising blitz with disturbing images and graphic descriptions of the health consequences of smoking. One vignette showed a man speaking with a robotic voice after a laryngectomy made necessary by throat cancer. This campaign reduced smoking rates overall among men and Hispanic New Yorkers (CDC, 2007a). A prominent national campaign resulted in approximately 450,000 fewer adolescents initiating smoking (Farrelly, Nonnemaker, Davis, and Hussin, 2009). A cost-utility analysis found that the campaign recouped the $234 million in media-related costs and just under $1.9 billion in medical expenses averted for society over the lifetimes of the youth who did not become smokers (Holtgrave, Wunderink, Vallone, & Healton, 2009).

In May 2008, the U.S. Public Health Service released the updated guidelines on tobacco use, treatment, and dependence (Fiore et al., 2008). These evidence-based guidelines recommend treatment for individuals who are tobacco dependent. Recommendations from the guidelines represent strength of evidence with A through C ratings. The strongest recommendations, A, are based on multiple, well-designed, randomized trials that are directly relevant to the recommendation. Level B ratings indicate that some evidence from randomized clinical trials supported the recommendation but the scientific support was not optimal. Level C ratings are "reserved for important clinical situations in which the Panel achieved consensus on the recommendation in the absence of relevant randomized controlled trials" (Fiore et al., 2008, p. 15). According to the guidelines, "It is difficult to identify any other condition [than tobacco dependence] that presents such a mix of lethality, prevalence, and neglect, despite effective and readily available interventions" (Fiore et al., 2008, p. 2).

The guidelines strongly recommend that clinicians screen and document patients' tobacco use status and deliver evidence-based tobacco dependence treatment (strength of evidence A) (Fiore et al., 2008). Simple reminders, like chart stickers or electronic prompts, can be instituted within an organization to remind clinicians to ask about smoking status. For smokers who are not currently interested in quitting, motivational techniques can be used to encourage a future quit attempt (strength of evidence B). Clinicians and clinicians-in-training should be taught effective smoking cessation strategies to assist individuals who want to make a quit attempt and those who are not yet motivated to do so (strength of evidence B). Further, because the tobacco dependence treatments identified in the guidelines are cost effective, they should be offered to all smokers (strength of evidence A). Counseling for tobacco-dependent adolescents has been found to be effective and therefore is recommended (strength of evidence B). Web-based interventions may be useful in assisting tobacco cessation (strength of evidence B). Cessation counseling has been found to be effective with parents to help protect children from secondhand smoke (strength of evidence B).

What Does Additional Evidence Tell Us About Adolescents?

The evidence indicates that tobacco advertising and promotion increase the likelihood that nonsmoking adolescents will become smokers at a later time (Lovato, Linn, Stead, & Best, 2003). The three most heavily branded cigarette companies accounted for 80% of adolescent cigarette brands (SAMHSA, 2007). "Joe the Camel" was an example of an advertising strategy that was specifically directed to promote adolescent smoking.

The National Cancer Institute (2010) concluded that there is a causal relationship between smoking initiation in teens and exposure to media depictions of smoking. In a 2010 meta-analysis of four studies, Millett and Glantz found that viewing tobacco use in movies contributed to a 44% rate of smoking initiation among pediatric populations. Overall, there is weak evidence that mass media can be effective in preventing young adults from starting to smoke. Mass media campaigns that developed and focused their message based on their target audience were more effective than those that did not use this strategy. Campaigns of greater intensity and duration were more successful than those that were not (Sowden, 1998).

Media communications has played a key role in branding cigarettes and creating an image for adolescents. Adolescents experience tremendous social marketing and peer pressures that can promote risky behaviors like smoking. In 2005, tobacco industries spent $13.5 billion in advertisements (National Cancer Institute, 2008). Tobacco advertisers targeted adolescents by aiming their message at the emotional developmental needs of this age group, such as popularity, peer acceptance, and positive self-image. Tobacco print and media ads create the perception that smoking will satisfy these needs.

Many population studies have documented decreases in teen smoking when social media interventions are combined with public health initiatives. In 2000, the American Legacy Foundation began the largest social media effort to prevent teen smoking, entitled "truth" (National Institute for Health Care Management [NIHCM], 2009). Farrelly et al. (2009) concluded that the truth campaign accounted for approximately a 22% decline in adolescent smoking. An example of a media campaign targeting young adults was the billboard advertising in New York City featuring star athletes from various local sports teams. The slogan, "I don't smoke, do you?" was prominently displayed along major highways throughout the city.

Other interventions are directed toward the selling of tobacco. It is believed that if young people are unable to purchase cigarettes, this may reduce the number who start to smoke. Although warnings and fines levied against retailers to discourage the illegal sale of cigarettes were shown to be effective in decreasing sales, the outcome of this intervention has not shown a clear effect (Stead & Lancaster, 2005). Further, it is believed that the behavior of a child's/adolescent's family may influence the likelihood of the child/adolescent starting to smoke. Although there is evidence that family interventions may prevent adolescents from smoking, other evidence showed neutral or negative outcomes (Thomas, Baker, & Lorenzetti, 2007).

Do school-based programs prevent children who are nonsmokers from becoming smokers? Thomas and Perera (2006) reviewed 23 high-quality, randomized controlled trials. The interventions in these studies included information giving, social influence approaches, social skills training, and community interventions. Information giving alone was not supported by the evidence as an effective intervention, and there was limited evidence for the effects of the other interventions. Peterson et al. (2009) demonstrated the effect of motivational interviewing on teen smoking cessation. In a randomized control trial of 50 high schools in Washington, abstinence from smoking increased 4% in teenagers who received personalized telephone calls and motivational interviews.

Through increased implementation of evidence-based interventions, tobacco dependence in adolescents declined 40% from 1997 to 2003. Prior to 2009, progress stalled, possibly because of decreased state funding for tobacco dependence prevention programs, increased tobacco industry marketing, and decreased effectiveness of mass media campaigns (CDC, 2007a).

In 2009, the National Youth Tobacco Survey still revealed a decline in smoking among middle school and high school students. The prevalence of current tobacco use among middle school students declined (15.1 to 8.2%), as did current cigarette use (11.0 to 5.2%) and cigarette smoking experimentation (29.8 to 15.0%). Similar trends were observed for high school students (current tobacco use: 34.5 to 23.9%; current cigarette use: 28.0 to 17.2%; cigarette smoking experimentation: 39.4% to 30.1%). The CDC (2010b) reports that despite the decline in teenage smoking by interventions, state programs remain underfunded. The tobacco epidemic in the United States is an example of how utilizing EBP public health measures at a national level can stop this epidemic and accelerate declines in the related morbidity and mortality associated with tobacco dependence.

PUTTING EVIDENCE INTO PRACTICE

Traditional smoking cessation counter-marketing strategies employed a wide range of efforts, including paid television, radio, billboard, print, and web-based advertising at the state and local levels; media advocacy through public relations efforts, such as press releases; and local events, media literacy, and health promotion activities (Fiore et al., 2008). In today's technologically-dependent society, social media has emerged as a popular source of health information. Innovations in tobacco cessation health communication should include targeting smoking audiences through personal communication devices (e.g., text messaging) and online networking environments, as well as fostering dissemination of health messages through innovative channels (such as weblogs or "blogs").

Approximately 62% of the U.S. population report that they use the Internet, with greater than 50% of adults reporting health-related information searches (CDC, 2010a).

Internet-based interventions provide an excellent public health opportunity to impact tobacco use at a population level. There is a positive association between web-assisted tobacco interventions and successfully quitting (An et al., 2008). A systematic review of web-based interventions demonstrated a 17% increase in 6-month tobacco abstinence (Shabab & McEwen, 2009).

An exemplar of a web-assisted, EBP smoking social networking site is QuitNet. QuitNet is an Internet-based intervention that provides telephone intervention, 24-hour social networking, and smoking cessation medication and email support. QuitNet first launched on the World Wide Web in 1995. Dr. Nathan Cobb created the concept, which was later adopted by Join Together, a project of Boston University School of Public Health. With the University's help, QuitNet.com, Inc. was formed in 2000 to take on the role of expanding QuitNet into a self-supporting service operating worldwide. QuitNet is utilized in several statewide smoking initiatives including Utah and North Dakota. Utah has the lowest smoking rate in the country at 8.8% (Utah Department of Health, 2010). In 2011, 860 Utahans per month were served with free tailored interventions by QuitNet and telephone-based quit interventions. Structured interventions that reach the entire community have shown to improve smoking cessation in Utah: 93% of Utahans have implemented rules against smoking in their homes, and 98% of Utah children are without secondhand exposure in their homes (Utah Department of Health, 2010). Clearly, more research needs to be done to explore outcomes with Internet-based smoking programs. Yet, web-based interventions are important in population-based strategies for tobacco cessation. The Internet programs can be self-tailored and are an inexpensive way to deliver to large populations, because they require low personnel costs.

TOBACCO DEPENDENCE: FUTURE DIRECTIONS THROUGH BEST PRACTICES

According to the U.S. DHHS (2010), the most effective evidence-based, population-based approaches result from the synergistic effect produced by putting into place the following program components: state and community interventions, health communication interventions, cessation interventions, surveillance and evaluation, and administration and management. The IOM (2007) put forth the goal of reducing smoking so that it is no longer a significant health problem for our nation. The IOM believes, based on substantial evidence, that this can be achieved through state tobacco control programs that are comprehensive, integrated, and maintained over time. The U.S. DHHS strategic plan, *Ending the Tobacco Epidemic,* focuses on improving American health by strengthening existing EBPs as well as stimulating new tobacco cessation research. Putting into practice national evidence-based interventions is an example of how to curtail a public health condition such as the tobacco epidemic in the United States.

References

An, L. C., Schillo, B. A., Saul, J. E., Wendling, A. H., Klatt, C. M., Berg, C. J.,... Luxenberg, M. G. (2008). Utilization of smoking cessation informational, interactive, and online community resources as predictors of abstinence: Cohort study. *Journal of Medical Internet Research, 10*(5), e55.

Baker, D. W., Gamarazian, J. A., Williams, M. V., Scott, T., Parker, R. M., Green, D.,... Peel, J. (2002). Functional health literacy and the risk of hospital admission among Medicare managed care enrollees. *American Journal of Public Health, 92*(8), 1278–1283.

Baker, D. W., Parker, R. M., Williams, M. V., & Clark, W. S. (1998). Health literacy and the risk of hospital admission. *Journal of General Internal Medicine, 13*(12), 791–798.

Baker, D. W., Wolf, M., Feinglass, J., Thompson, J. A., Gasmaranian, J. A., & Huang, J. (2007). Health literacy and mortality among elderly persons. *Archives of Internal Medicine, 167*(14), 1503–1509.

Bala, M., Strzeszynski, L., & Cahill, K., (2008). Mass media interventions for smoking cessation in adults. *Cochrane Database of Systematic Reviews* (Issue 1), Art. No.: CD004704. doi: 10.1002/14651858. CD004704.pub2

Berkman, N., Sheridan, S., Donahue, K., Halpern, D., & Crotty, K. (2011). Low health literacy and health outcomes: An updated systematic review. *Annals of Internal Medicine, 155*(2), 97–107.

Berkman, N., Sheridan, S., Donahue, K., Halpern, D., Viera, A., Crotty, K., ... (2011). *Health Literacy Interventions and Outcomes: An Updated Systematic Review. Evidence Report/Technology Assessment No. 199.* (Prepared by RTI International–University of North Carolina Evidence-based Practice Center under contract No. 290-2007-10056-I.) AHRQ Publication Number 11-E006. Rockville, MD: Agency for Healthcare Research and Quality.

Centers for Disease Control and Prevention (CDC). Office on Smoking and Health. (2006). Sustaining State Programs for Tobacco Control: State Data Highlights. Retrieved from http://www.cdc.gov/tobacco/data_statistics/state_data/data_highlights/2006/pdfs/dataHighlights06rev.pdf

Centers for Disease Control and Prevention (CDC). (2007a). *Best practices for comprehensive tobacco control programs—2007.* Atlanta, GA: U.S. Department of Health and Human Services, Centers for Disease Control and Prevention, National Center for Chronic Disease Prevention and Health Promotion, Office on Smoking and Health.

Centers for Disease Control and Prevention (CDC). (2007b). Cigarette smoking among adults—United States, 2006. *Morbidity and Mortality Weekly Report, 56,* 1157–1161.

Centers for Disease Control and Prevention (CDC). (2008a). Smoking-attributable mortality, years of potential life lost, and productivity losses—United States, 2000–2004. *Morbidity and Mortality Weekly Report, 57*(45), 1226–1228.

Centers for Disease Control and Prevention (CDC). (2008b). Disparities in secondhand smoke exposure—United States, 1988–1994 and 1994–2004. *Morbidity and Mortality Weekly Report, 57*(27), 744–747.

Centers for Disease Control and Prevention (CDC). (2010a). *Vital Signs.* Retrieved from http://www.cdc.gov/vitalsigns/tobaccouse/smoking/latestfindings.html

Centers for Disease Control and Prevention (CDC). (2010b). Tobacco use among middle and high school students—United States, 2000–2009. *Morbidity and Mortality Weekly Report, 59*(33), 1063–1068.

Cronenwett, L., Sherwood, G., Barnsteiner, J., Disch, J., Johnson, J., Mitchell, P., . . . Warren, J. (2007). Quality and safety education for nurses. *Nursing Outlook, 55*(3), 122–131.

Cullum, N., Ciliska, D., Haynes, R. B., & Marks, S. (2008). *Evidence-based nursing: An introduction.* Hong Kong and Singapore: Blackwell.

DeNavas-Walt, C., Proctor, B., & Smith, J. (2011). *U.S. Census Bureau, Current Population Reports, P60-239, Income, Poverty, and Health Insurance Coverage in the United States: 2010.* Washington, DC: U.S. Government Printing Office.

DeWalt, D. A., Berkman, N. D., Sheridan, S., Lohr, K. N., & Pignone, M. P. (2004). Literacy and health outcomes: A systematic review of the literature. *Journal of General Internal Medicine, 19*(12), 1228–1239.

Doak, L., Doak, C., & Root, J. (1998). *Teaching patients with low literacy skills.* Philadelphia, PA: Lippincott.

Engels, R. C., Knibbe, R. A., de Vries, H., & Drop, M. J. (1998). Antecedents of smoking cessation among adolescents: Who is motivated to change? *Preventive Medicine, 27,* 348–357.

Farrelly, M., Nonnemaker, J., Davis, K., & Hussin, A. (2009). The influence of the national truth® campaign on smoking initiation. *American Journal of Preventive Medicine, 36*(5), 379–384.

Fiore, M. C., Jaén, C. R., Baker, T. B., Bailey, W. C., Benowitz, N. L., Curry, S. J.,…Wewers, M. E. (2008). *Treating tobacco use and dependence: 2008 update*. Rockville, MD: U.S. Dept. of Health and Human Services.

Gebbie, K., Rosenstock, L., & Hernandez, L. M. (Eds.), Committee on Educating Health Professionals for the 21st Century, Board on Health Promotion and Disease Prevention, Institute of Medicine of the National Academies. (2003). *Who will keep the public healthy? Educating public health professionals for the 21st century*. Washington, DC: National Academies Press.

Griener, A. C., & Knebel, E. (Eds.). Committee on the Health Professions Summit, Institute of Medicine of the National Academies. (2003). *Health professions education: A bridge to quality*. Washington, DC: National Academies Press.

Hanchate, A. D., Ash, A. S., Gasmararian, J. A., Wolf, M. A., & Paasche-Orlow, M. K. (2008). The Demographic Assessment for Health Literacy (DAHL): A new tool for estimating associations between health literacy and outcomes in national surveys. *Journal of General Internal Medicine, 23*(10), 1561–1566.

Heron, M., & Smith, B. (2007). *Deaths leading causes for 2003. National Vital Statistics Reports.* Washington, DC: Centers for Disease Control and Prevention.

Holtgrave, D., Wunderink, K., Vallone, D., & Healton, C. (2009). Cost-utility analysis of the national truth® campaign to prevent youth smoking. *American Journal of Preventive Medicine, 36*(5), 385–388.

Hughes, J. R. (2003). Motivating and helping smokers to stop smoking. *Journal of General Internal Medicine, 18*, 1053–1057.

Institute for Healthcare Advancement. (2011). Retrieved from http://www.iha4health.org/

Institute of Medicine. (2004). *Health literacy: A prescription to end confusion*. Washington, DC: National Academies Press.

Institute of Medicine. (2007). *Ending the tobacco problem: A blueprint for the nation*. Washington, DC: The National Academies Press.

Institute of Medicine. (2011). *The future of nursing: Leading change, advancing health*. Washington, DC: National Academies Press.

Kutner, M., Greenberg, E., Jin, Y., Boyle, B., Hsu, Y., & Dunleavy, E. (2007). *Literacy in everyday life: Results from the 2003 National Assessment of Adult Literacy* (NCES 2007-490). Washington, DC: National Center for Education Statistics, Institute for Education Sciences, U.S. Department of Education.

Lovato, C., Linn, G., Stead, L. F., & Best, A. (2003). Impact of tobacco advertising and promotion on increasing adolescent smoking behaviors. *Cochrane Database of Systematic Reviews*, (4), CD003439.

Maniaci, M., Heckman, M., & Dawson, N. (2008). Functional health literacy and understanding of medicines at discharge. *Mayo Clinic Proceedings, 83*(5), 554–558.

McCuller, W. J., Sussman, S., Wapner, M., Dent, C., & Weiss, D. J. (2006). Motivation to quit as a mediator of tobacco cessation among at-risk youth. *Addictive Behaviors, 31*, 880–888.

McLaughlin, G. H. (2008). *Simplified measure of gobbledygook*. Retrieved from http://www.harrymclaughlin.com/SMOG.htm

McLeod-Sordjan, R. (2011). Assessing functional health literacy: Strategy to reduce health disparities among elderly Hispanic patients with chronic disease. *Journal of Nurse Practitioners, 7*(10), 839–846.

Melnyk, B. M., & Fineout-Overholt, E. (2011). *Evidence-based practice in nursing and healthcare: A guide to best practice* (2nd ed). Philadelphia, PA: Lippincott.

Millett, C., & Glantz, S. (2010). Assigning an '18' rating to movies with tobacco imagery is essential to reduce youth smoking. *Thorax, 65*, 77–78.

Murphy-Knoll, L. (2007). Low health literacy puts patients at risk. *Journal of Nursing Care Quality, 22*(3), 205–209.

National Cancer Institute. (2008). *Tobacco control monograph 19: The role of the media in promoting and reducing tobacco use*. Bethesda, MD: U.S. Department of Health and Human Services, National Institutes of Health, National Cancer Institute. Retrieved from http://www.cancercontrol.cancer.gov/tcrb/monographs/19/index.html

National Center for Education Statistics. (2006). *The health literacy of America's adults: Results from the 2003 National Assessment of Adult Literacy*. Retrieved from http://nces.ed.gov/pubs2006/2006483.pdf

National Patient Safety Foundation. (2008). *Ask me three*. Retrieved from http://www.npsf.org/askme3/PCHC/

National Youth Tobacco Survey. (2009). Retrieved from http://www.cdc.gov/mmwr/preview/mmwrhtml/mm5412a1.htm

Nielsen-Bohlman, L., Panzer, A., Kindig, D. (Eds.). (2004). *Health literacy: A prescription to end confusion*. Washington, DC: National Academies Press.

Nightingale, F. (1893/2004). Sick-nursing and health-nursing. In L. McDonald (Ed.), *Florence Nightingale on public health care, Vol. 6. of the collected works of Florence*

Nightingale. Waterloo, Ontario: Wilfrid Laurier University Press.

Oxman, A., Sackett, D., & Guyatt, G. (1992). Evidence-based medicine workgroup. *Journal of the American Medical Association, 268*(9), 1135–1136.

Peterson, A., Kealey, P., Mann, S., Marek, P., Ludman, E., Liu, J., & Bricker, J. (2009). Group-randomized trial of a proactive, personalized telephone counseling intervention for adolescent smoking cessation. *Journal of the National Cancer Institute, 101*(20), 1378–1392.

Pfizer Clear Health Communication Initiative. (2008). Help your patients succeed: Tips for improving communication with your patients. Retrieved from http://clearhealthcommunication.com/public-health-professionals/tips-for-providers.html

Plain Writing Act of 2010 (H.R. 946), available at http://frwebgate.access.gpo.gov/cgi-bin/getdoc.cgi?dbname=111_cong_bills&docid=f:h946enr.txt.pdf

Quality and Safety Education for Nurses. (2007). *Overview.* [Online]. Retrieved from http://qsen.org/about/overview/

QuitNet. Retrieved from http://www.quitnet.com

Schillinger, D., Grumbach, K., Piette, J., Wang, F., Osmond, D., Daher, C., . . . Bindman, A. B. (2002). Association of health literacy with diabetes outcomes. *Journal of the American Medical Association, 288*(4), 475–482.

Serra, C., Bonfill, X., Pladevall-Vila, M., & Cabezas Pena, C. (2008). Interventions for preventing tobacco smoking in public places. *Cochrane Database of Systematic Reviews, (3)*, CD001294.

Shahab, L., & McEwen, A. (2009). Online support for smoking cessation: A systematic review of the literature. *Addiction, 104*(11), 1792–1804. doi: 10.1111/j.1360-0443.2009.02710.x.ADD2710

Shohet, L., & Renaud, L. (2006). Critical analysis on best practices in health literacy. *Canadian Journal of Public Health, 97*, S10.

Singleton, J., Levin, R. F., Feldman, H. R., & Truglio-Londrigan, M. (2005). Evidence for smoking cessation: Implications for gender-specific strategies. *Worldviews on Evidence-Based Nursing, 2*(2), 1–12.

Singleton, J. K., Levin, R. F., & Keefer, J. (2007). Evidence-based practice. Disciplinary perspectives on evidence-based practice: The more the merrier. *Research and Theory in Nursing Practice, 21*(4), 213–216.

Sowden, A. J. (1998). Mass media interventions for preventing smoking in young people. *Cochrane Database of Systematic Reviews, (4)*, CD001006.

Stead, L. F., & Lancaster, T. (2005). Interventions for preventing tobacco sales to minors. *Cochrane Database of Systematic Reviews, (1)*, CD001497.

Stetler, C. B., Morsi, D., Rucki, S., Broughton, S., Corrigan, B., Fitzgerald, J., . . . Sheridan, E. A. (1998). Utilization-focused integrative reviews in a nursing service. *Applied Nursing Research, 11*(4), 195–205.

Straus, S. E., Richardson, W. S., Glasziou, P., & Haynes, R. B. (2005). *Evidence-based medicine: How to practice and teach EBM* (3rd ed.). Edinburgh, UK: Elsevier.

Substance Abuse and Mental Health Services Administration. (2005). *Results from the 2005 National Survey on Drug Use and Health.* Rockville, MD: Office of Applied Studies.

Substance Abuse and Mental Health Services Administration. (2007). *Results from the 2006 National Survey on Drug Use and Health: National findings.* Rockville, MD: Office of Applied Studies.

Substance Abuse and Mental Health Services Administration. (2008). *Results from the 2008 National Survey on Drug Use and Health.* Office of Applied Studies. NSDUH Series H-36 (DHHS Publication No. SMA 09-4434).

Thomas, R. E., Baker, P. R. A., & Lorenzetti, D. (2007). Family-based programmes for preventing smoking by children and adolescents. *Cochrane Database of Systematic Reviews, (1)*, CD004493.

Thomas, R., & Perera, R. (2006). School-based programmes for preventing smoking. *Cochrane Database of Systematic Reviews, 19*, 3.

U.S. Department of Health and Human Services (U.S. DHHS). (2010a). *About healthy people.* Retrieved from http://www.healthypeople.gov/2020/about/default.aspx

U.S. Department of Health and Human Services (U.S. DHHS). (2010b). *Healthy People 2020 topics and objectives.* Retrieved from http://www.healthypeople.gov/2020/topicsobjectives2020/default.aspx

U.S. Department of Health and Human Services (U.S. DHHS). (2010c). Healthy People 2010 framework. Retrieved from http://www.healthypeople.gov/2020/Consortium/HP2020Framework.pdf

U.S. Department of Health and Human Services (U.S. DHHS). (2010d). *Ending the tobacco epidemic: A tobacco control strategic action plan for the U.S. Department of Health and Human Services.* Washington, DC: Office of the Assistant Secretary for Health.

U.S. Department of Health and Human Services (U.S. DHHS), Office of Disease Prevention and Health Promotion. (2010). National Action Plan to Improve Health Literacy. Washington, DC: Author. Retrieved from http://www.health.gov/communication/HLActionPlan/

Utah Department of Health. (2010). *Behavioral Risk Factor Surveillance System (BRFSS).* Salt Lake

City, UT: Utah Department of Health. Center for Health Data.

Vernon, J. A., Trujillo, A., Rosenbaum, S., & DeBuono, B. (2007). *Low health literacy: Implications for national health policy*. Partnership for Clear Health Communication. Retrieved from http://npsf.org/askme3/pdfs/Case_Report_10_07.pdf

Volandes, A., Paasche-Orlow, M., Gillick, M. R., Cook, E. F., Shaykevich, S., Abbo, E. D.,... Lehmann, L. (2008). Health literacy not race predicts end-of-life care preferences. *Palliative Medicine, 11*(5), 754–762.

Weiss, B. D., Mays, M. Z., Martz, W., Castro, K. M., DeWalt, D. A., Pignone, M. P.,... Hale, F. A. (2005). Quick assessment of literacy in primary care: The newest vital sign. *Annals of Family Medicine, 3*, 514–522.

Zhu, S. H., Sun, J., Billings, S. C., Choi, W. S., & Malarcher, A. (1999). Predictors of smoking cessation in U.S. adolescents. *American Journal of Preventive Medicine, 16*, 202–207.

For a full suite of assignments and additional learning activities, use the access code located in the front of your book to visit this exclusive website: http://go.jblearning.com/londrigan. If you do not have an access code, you can obtain one at the site.

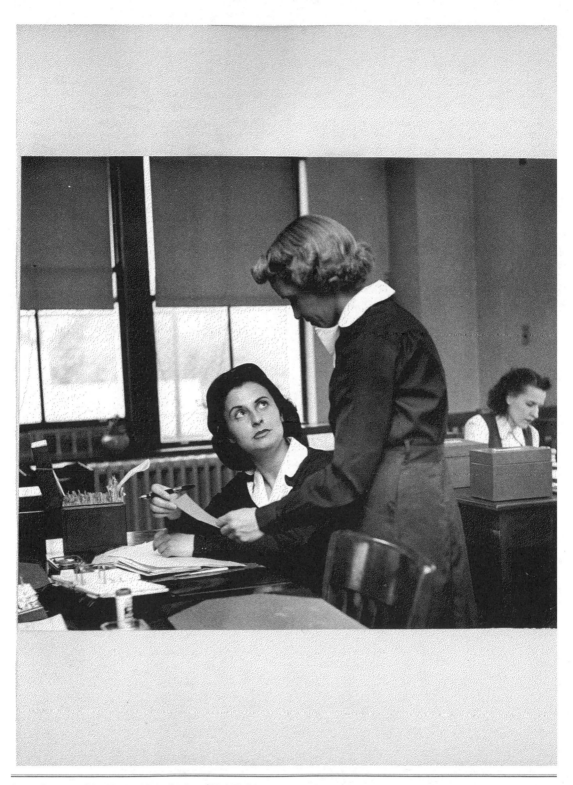

Chapter 6

Informatics in Public Health Nursing

Marisa L. Wilson
Martha Kelly
Sandra B. Lewenson
Marie Truglio-Londrigan

How impossible to portray with any justice to the subject the superb panorama of the progress of human betterment under the leadership of science through successive generations of ardent devotees blazing ever new trails, evolving ever new methods, achieving ever more outstanding results, facing ever new problems . . . (Goodrich, 1931, p. 1385).

LEARNING OBJECTIVES

At the completion of this chapter, the reader will be able to

- Define the terms used in Public Health Informatics.
- Describe the application of information technology in public health nursing practice.
- Discuss the use of nursing informatics in public health nursing.

KEY TERMS

- Data
- Database
- Data mining
- Electronic Health Records
- Informatics
- Information
- Information technology
- Knowledge
- Nursing informatics
- Personal Health Records
- Public health informatics
- Regional Health Information Exchange
- Surveillance

Public Health Informatics is the application of information science and technology to public health practice and research in order to:

1. Assess and monitor the health communities and populations at risk,
2. Identify health problems and priorities,
3. Formulate policy,
4. Assure all populations have access to appropriate care, and
5. Evaluate the effectiveness of that care. (Medterms Medical Dictionary, 2007).

The capacity to quickly gather data, to generate information from that data, and to build knowledge from the information is fundamental to all nursing, community health, and public health activities. Information management and communication are key parts of the infrastructure on which the public health system is built. Historically, public health information systems have been built using a "silo" approach—different information systems for different programs that cannot communicate with each other. The challenge for public health activities is to build integrated information systems that get the right information to the right people when they need it.

Utilizing information technology is essential to public health and, specifically, to public health nursing. Information systems, which help us to gather, manipulate, store, and process data, are an essential tool in the public health arena where accurate and up-to-date information is needed as real-time as possible. Historically, data collection has always been one of the hallmarks of public health. Florence Nightingale spoke to the need for accurate statistics about morbidity and mortality, using pie graphs and the like to demonstrate the necessity of quality nursing care (Agnew, 1958). Ozbolt and Saba (2008) recognized Nightingale's quest for this kind of data, saying, "Nightingale called for

standardized clinical records that could be analyzed to assess and improve care processes and patient outcomes. Nursing informatics thus springs from the roots of modern nursing" (p. 199). Lillian Wald, the noted public health nursing pioneer and founder of Henry Street, compared and contrasted the data collected by the visiting nurses from the Henry Street Nurses Settlement with data from four New York City hospitals. Using these data, Wald (1915) showed that care provided in the home improved patient outcomes. Nightingale and Wald valued statistical data. They collected and analyzed the data from their clinical experiences, all without the use of and speed that information technology and other forms of technology can now provide public health nurses.

This chapter highlights the use of technology as a competency that must be achieved by all practitioners (U.S. Department of Health and Human Services [DHHS], 2004). Like all nursing professionals, public health nurses need to have a basic understanding of technology and how to put that technology to use. Skiba (2008) wrote that "informatics tools can help mitigate error, provide interdisciplinary communication, promote quality, support clinical decision making, and provide the necessary infrastructure for evidenced-based practice" (p. 301). Although not specifically focused on public health nursing curricular activities, Skiba supports the case that students need to understand and use **informatics** in all healthcare settings. Skiba echoes the American Nurses Association (ANA, 2008) statement that "the evolving mandate for electronic information systems and increasing complexity of health care services and practice have raised the bar for the nursing professional. Select informatics competencies will soon be required in all undergraduate and graduate nursing curricula" (p. 17). Public health nurses must know how to use computers and information technology, as well as incorporate newer online learning technology (U.S. DHHS, 2004) into their practice. Public health nurses need to understand the importance of the Electronic Health Record (EHR), the Personal Health Record (PHR), Health Information Exchanges (HIE), and how these technologies contribute to the ability of public health nurses to assess, monitor, plan and evaluate programs for populations at need.

This chapter examines the various aspects of technology and its use in public health nursing. Throughout the chapter, vignettes from nurses who work with the public's health in mind reveal how information technology is being used, or not, in the practice setting. Their stories show the advances that have been made as well as the issues related to the diffusion of new ideas into practice (Rogers, 1983). These vignettes serve as a conduit where the true experts, those individuals working with populations in a variety of settings, tell us how they integrate information technology in the care they render. The future directions of nursing information technology for public health nursing provide the reader with additional reflections on the current status and strategies to move into the future.

Role of Technology in Public Health Nursing Practice

The need for near-real-time data and the information and knowledge that can come from this requires systems and technology. These information systems will transform public health nursing practice. Public health nurses work in health departments, clinics, visiting nurse services, ambulatory care settings, and anywhere that nursing takes place in the community. All public health workers require efficient access to near-real-time information, and their work emphasizes "population-focused services"

(ANA, 2007, p. 11). Technology affords these nurses and society a better way of systematically collecting data, analyzing those data, and then applying the data analysis in a way that informs practice and improves the health of the individual, family, population, and community.

Public health nurses have always collected data on their patients, like Lillian Wald at the Henry Street Nurses Settlement in New York City. These nurses collected data to assess the health of the patients and families they served in the community (Buhler-Wilkerson, 2001). In 1914, two years after the formation of the National Organization for Public Health Nursing, the Executive Secretary, Ella Phillips Crandall (1914), wrote a letter to the philanthropist John D. Rockefeller, explaining the success that the organization had accomplished by developing a "standardization of record cards" (n.p.). With the adoption of these record cards nationally, Crandall believed public health nurses could collect data in a way that would make previously "incoherent statistics" more "homogenous or at least comparable" (n.p.).

Public health nurses knew that records needed to be kept and somehow the statistical data needed to be collected in a way that made them useful and comparable. In 1950, Freeman wrote that "nursing will be carried on within the framework of a comprehensive program for public health" and this included maintaining "vital statistics, or the recording, tabulation, interpretation, and publication of the essential facts of births, deaths, and reportable diseases" (p. 20). In today's world, information technology assists the public health nurse to systematically collect, organize, and analyze data, as well as share it with stakeholders as they have done in the past. Now technology allows the collection and analysis to occur at a faster and more comprehensive level than ever before. Furthermore, technology affords us a way to save data and analyze large data sets that provide the needed evidence to support changes in practice. The transformative nature of technology continues now and into the future.

In today's healthcare arena, public health nurses must ask how technology can be used to:

- Provide care
- Access information to monitor the health of the public
- Identify best evidence for practice
- Enhance education for the individual, family, population, and community
- Improve public health nursing
- Communicate to others in health care
- Support research

The answers to these questions will serve to enhance the public health nurses' practice in education, research, and the delivery of care.

Information Technology

It is important for the reader to understand the concepts and terms used in **information technology** as they are applied to public health practice and public health nursing. This understanding is critical as public health nurses work toward better communication, integration, and application of information technology. Vignettes throughout this section and the chapter illustrate the technology that nurses use in their practice and how it informs practice, provides solutions, and creates challenges.

Data

Data are considered the "essential element of information" containing the "measurements and facts" (Institute of Medicine [IOM], 2003a, p. 126) that public health nurses need to make decisions in practice. According to Thede (2003), data are defined as "discrete elements that have not been interpreted" (p. 11). The ANA (2008)

uses similar language explaining that "data are discrete entities that are described objectively without interpretation" (p. 3). For example, a newly diagnosed case of tuberculosis in a small town is considered data and is reported to the local county department of health, which then reports this case to the state department of health. This case of tuberculosis singularly is considered data and is entered into a database. Certain other diseases may also be reported to the Centers for Disease Control and Prevention (CDC) and to the World Health Organization. Once reported, these data are also entered into a database.

There are many sources of data, some of which include mortality reports, vital statistics, morbidity data, and hospital data such as falls, length of stay, wounds, injuries, and occupational illnesses. Once data are reported and located in a database, analysis may be carried out. Often, the amount of data may be so overwhelming that the message the data would ordinarily convey is overlooked. It is only when the data are reported and placed into a database that patterns emerge to inform the practitioner as to what the best practice interventions may be.

Databases

Databases are systems or structures that allow for data to be stored in an organized way and that support access and retrieval (Hebda, Czar, & Mascara, 2005). Databases are collections of related records stored in a computer that permit a person or program to query in order to extract needed information (McGonigle and Mastrian, 2012). For example, in a database that maintains **surveillance** data for use by public health nurses, available data may represent patient chief complaints from an emergency visit, ambulance logs, prescriptions filled, or reportable laboratory results. The ANA (2008) explains that data become information after they are "interpreted, organized, or structured" (p. 3). The various database systems help to organize and depict the data so they can become information and eventually knowledge. The data may be accessed and shared, but the end result may be different for each user depending on who retrieves the information and how he or she interprets it. Public health nurses who note an increase in mumps, a nationally reportable disease, may see the need to develop a health education program for young families if an outbreak were to occur in their community. Immunization programs may be another intervention to consider, and yet who interprets the data, such as a private practitioner or an outpatient clinic, may direct the kind of immunization program developed. It is therefore important that public health nurses know the different types of databases available to them, how to find databases, and how to use the statistics and other vital information for their practice at the local, state, and national level. **Box 6-1**

Box 6-1 Examples of Databases

Federal Government and Health Statistics Agencies

These are federal agencies that gather, analyze, and report statistical data:

    Agency for Healthcare Research and Quality (AHRQ): http://www.ahrq.gov

        AHRQ is the lead scientific research federal agency charged with supporting research to improve quality of health care, reduce cost, improve patient safety, decrease medical errors, and broaden access to services.

Centers for Disease Control and Prevention (CDC)

    Behavioral Risk Factor Surveillance System (BRFSS): http://www.cdc.gov/brfss/

        BRFSS tracks health risks of adults in the United States.

    National Notifiable Disease Surveillance System (NNDSS): http://www.cdc.gov/epo/dphsi/nndsshis.htm

        State health departments report notifiable infectious diseases to the CDC.

    National Vital Statistics System: http://www.cdc.gov/nchs/nvss.htm

        Information from states on vital events such as births, deaths, marriages, divorces, and fetal deaths

State and Local Data Sources

Many states have their own systems for reporting data; the following are some examples:

    Arizona Public Health Services: http://www.hs.state.az.us/plan/index.htm

    California Department of Health Services: http://www.dhs.ca.gov/

International Data

    United Nations Statistics Division: http://unstats.un.org/unsd/

    World Health Organization-Statistical Information Systems (WHOSIS): http://www3.who.int/whois/menu.cfm

Hospital and Healthcare Records

    National Hospital Discharge and Ambulatory Surgery Data: http://cdc.gov/nchs/about/major/hdasd/listpubs.htm

Mortality and Morbidity Data

    Mortality Data from the National Vital Statistics System: http://www.cdc.gov/nchs/about/major/dvs/mortdata.htm

Public Health Preparedness

    Bioterrorism and Emerging Infections Site: http://www.bioterrorism-uab.ahrq.gov/

Source: Adapted from National Network of Libraries of Medicine and National Library of Medicine, 2005.

provides some examples of the types of databases that are available for the public health nurse.

Creating a Database

Public health nurses need to be comfortable enough with information technology to develop appropriate databases, such as what can be developed with products like Microsoft Access, for their nursing practice when needed. In the vignette #1, the nurse recognizes a need to collect and organize data to better assess and serve the population of interest, and she sees an opportunity to use technology from a nursing informatics perspective. Marisa Cortese-Peske, a nurse researcher, noted that the Hispanic population in the community was being overlooked in a clinical trial. Based on a concern for culturally competent and congruent care, Cortese-Peske collected data on the population of interest and initiated a database to understand patterns and trends within this population.

---

www

CASE STUDY (1)

Vignette From a Nurse Researcher

Marisa A. Cortese-Peske, RN, MS, PNP

I serve as the director of the cancer clinical trials office at a metropolitan teaching hospital in New York City. Our office offers a variety of clinical trials in both solid tumor and hematological malignancies. In the past, most clinical trials were chosen by an investigator's disease interest. Many times the investigator would not look into the population of clients that were seen or the eligibility criteria needed to enroll a patient into a study. Most clients enrolled into a clinical trial were from white, middle class backgrounds. In the past year, however, there has been a dramatic movement to enroll more clients from different cultures. This may be due in part to the fact that this hospital is applying for a National Cancer Institute designation that requires more clinical trials on populations with health disparities.

During my practice at this hospital, I have noticed many barriers in conducting clinical research properly to represent all client populations. The first barrier is actually finding clients who are eligible to participate in a clinical trial. Many of the lower socioeconomic clients are seen in a separate Medicaid clinic, so most investigators do not see the clients in this clinic because the clients are followed by the fellows. Even though the fellows do have intentions of enrolling these clients in the clinical trial, there seems to be a disconnect. I have met with clients in the clinic, and it is difficult to convince them to enroll in a clinical trial when I am not the primary provider for their care. Another problem is the language barrier. Not only am I not fluent in Spanish, but many of the investigators are not fluent in Spanish either. This creates a problem to properly explain the risks and benefits of a clinical trial. In addition, the informed consent forms are available only in English. Based on this failure to properly communicate, I believe that clients have a sense of distrust and decline to participate in a clinical trial.

At this hospital I have begun my own health initiative in expanding the number of Hispanic clients currently enrolled in clinical trials. My first step was to use the technology and create a client database to capture all cancer clients that are seen at this hospital, including a diagnosis, age, ethnicity, and prior treatments. This database went into use in January 2008, and it has already helped to identify groups of clients by disease or ethnicity.

With this database it was identified that many clients at this hospital are diagnosed with HIV-related lymphoma. In the past, however, it was never recognized exactly how many of these clients are seen at this hospital with this diagnosis.

I also realized there are numerous clients diagnosed with hepatocellular carcinoma due to hepatitis C. However, we do not have a clinical investigator at this hospital who specializes in this disease. I have expressed my concern with the director of the cancer institute, and we are currently conducting a search for a hepatocellular carcinoma specialist.

After a complete analysis of my client database, I realized that only 13% of the clients enrolled in an oncology clinical trial in 2007 were Hispanic. Hispanics account, however, for 49% of the population in the catchment area of this hospital. Whereas this disparity seems shocking, I previously recognized that many Hispanic clients who I have tried to enroll did not feel comfortable signing up for a study when they did not understand the risks and benefits of participation. I discussed this issue with the director of the cancer institute. I explained that one reason why Hispanic clients were refusing participation in a clinical trial was because they could not understand the informed consent form because it is available only in English. After months of debate I finally received the funding to translate all informed consents into Spanish. So far I have currently translated three consent forms. As a direct result, accrual numbers in the Hispanic population have increased.

With an increase in the number of Hispanic clients enrolling in clinical trials, I believe it will help to understand the physiological and/or genetic factors that cause the higher incidence of certain cancers in the Hispanic population. This information hopefully will lead to finding better treatments and preventive medicine for this population. The development of a database enabled our hospital to be more successful in this attempt.

USING DATABASES FOR TRACKING

The process of monitoring or tracking data is critical for public health nurses who want to be able to see trends and note the implication of these trends. Public health nurses may have to track data from disparate systems in order to determine trends, such as a public health nurse having to join data found in birth certificate registries with census data in a county or smaller community. The tracking of data provides important evidence for the public health nurse to support decision making and effective planning. For example, public health nurses track Lyme disease and may note an increase in a particular county. The data initially alert the public health nurse to ask critical questions. Once the proper assessment is conducted to answer these questions and the cause of the increase in the diagnoses of Lyme disease made, appropriate interventions are planned and implemented, followed by evaluation.

The public health nurse continues to track and monitor the Lyme disease in the county to determine if their planned intervention was effective.

Vignette #2 describes one nurse's experience in a home care setting that uses technology to track clients' healthcare information. In addition, the vignette shows how data tracking can be used in billing, communication, and education.

Data Mining

Another important application of technology and nursing informatics for practice is **data mining**. In 1849, the gold rush in California brought people from all over the world to small towns in northern California, like Grass Valley. The gold mine established in Grass Valley is open to visitors today. Tourists can see how the various veins of gold were identified and then extracted from the earth to create wealth and improve lives. Likewise, the rich veins of data stored in databases can be extracted to show relationships and patterns to help us develop new information and knowledge. The data collected through surveillance processes can be "mined," just as the veins of gold were mined, for any number of purposes to enhance and enrich lives in the public sphere. Data mining looks for patterns and relationships from large aggregate data sources. Data, however, have to be considered "clean" enough to be mined. Gold, when it was extracted, went through a chemical process to obtain the pure gold. The process used to clean data in preparation for effective data mining consists of "scrubbing" the data for errors that have the potential to skew any relationships or patterns. Cleansing the data, as it is called, means looking at the data for inconsistencies such as typographical errors, misspelled words, and multiple names for similar terms (e.g., "SOB" could mean "short of breath" or some other term). Abbreviations vary from institution to institution, and this can skew the data, making them difficult to use. Software packages exist to help scrub the data and remove the inconsistencies (Hebda et al., 2005).

WWW

CASE STUDY (2)

VIGNETTE OF A HOME CARE NURSE

Irene S. Rempel, BS, RN, LMSW

Home care is using computers and informatics more and more. Our intake department is able to obtain patient referral via direct telephone referrals, faxes, and two computerized systems, "Eason" and "E-discharge." Both systems are expensive but frequently used as a referral source in home care.

Patient referrals are initiated at local hospitals. Patients in need of home care are identified on either system, including their admitting diagnosis, chief complaint, demographics, insurance, medications, diagnosis, any type of procedure the patient might have had while in the hospital, physician's name, license number, National Provider Information number, and a physician's order for home care. Those orders differ from patient to patient. Some may require specific wound care. Others need diabetic teaching and intervention.

Home care companies interested in servicing a particular client make a check mark next to the patient's name and wait for confirmation from the social worker staff. Meanwhile, social workers review all companies interested in taking care of a particular patient and then make their decision as to which company they believe would take the best care of the patient. Once the decision is made, the social worker confirms electronically and provides a patient discharge date for the particular healthcare agency that has been authorized to provide care.

Once the company is approved to provide specific patient care, a registered nurse is sent out to assess the patient, his or her environment, and provide care authorized by the primary medical doctor. When making the initial assessment, the nurse always has his or her laptop provided by the agency. The company I work for uses a specific system. It is a detailed software application that covers all aspects of certified home health agency services. It generates patient information, plan of care, doctors' orders, and specific instructions for each discipline professionally involved in patient care. Our computer system provides medical and billing codes for different diagnoses and serves as a communication tool among providers. When our patients are prescribed more than one medication at the same time, the system identifies whether these medications are compatible or not. Frequently, our software identifies adverse effects and provides educational information for our patients regarding food and drug interactions as well.

Once the nurse assesses the patient in his or her own home, information is logged into our software that is specific to initial assessment, revisit forms, and discharge. If the nurse finds the information originally transmitted from the hospital differs in any way from his or her assessment, the doctor is contacted and a change of order is completed on a separate form and transmitted to the doctor and the agency for approval. Every revisit made by the nurse is recorded and transmitted to the doctor and the agency. Our system is able to generate a patient's plan of care, addendum to plan of care, and change of care. Those forms are required by the department of health and patients' insurance providers for review of medical necessity for home care, services provided, and payment to the home care agency.

Computers assist communications among all team members involved in patient care. If my patient is receiving the services of a registered nurse, physical therapist, occupational therapist, social worker, dietitian, and home health aide, the patient's progress can be analyzed and interdisciplinary conferences made without members of the team physically being in the office. Computer access has made patient information, treatment, and follow-up considerably easier than in the past. Members are communicating with each other and the doctor without leaving their offices.

McGonigle and Mastrian (2009) state that data mining "helps to identify patterns in aggregate data, gain insights, and ultimately discover and generate knowledge applicable to nursing science" (p. 148). Thede (2003) explains data mining as "the automated processes that permit the conversion of data to information and knowledge by finding hidden relationships within data" (p. 277). The use of data mining is a key concept in nursing informatics that has relevance to public health nursing. The challenge for nursing is to continue to refine and develop a standardized language that will enable data to be coded in like formats. The data then may be later mined for patterns and relationships.

Information, Knowledge, and Wisdom

The practice of public health nursing can be viewed from the nursing informatics perspective of data, information, knowledge, and wisdom (ANA, 2008). Three areas of information science that the IOM (2003a) identifies include "data, information, and knowledge" (p. 126). Data become information as they are organized and "placed in context" in information systems (IOM, 2003a, p. 126). The IOM (2003a) explains that information and information systems are essential tools that public health agencies need to monitor a population's health status and identify health hazards and risks. The information gained from these systems helps the public health nurse provide evidenced-based care to the individual, family, population, or community they serve.

Information is defined as "data that are interpreted, organized, or structured" (ANA, 2008, p. 3). **Knowledge** is information that has been "synthesized so that relationships are identified and formalized" (ANA, 2008, p. 3). Information enhances knowledge and guides decision making. The ANA (2008) further explains that wisdom is the "appropriate use of knowledge to manage and solve human problems" (p. 5). Understanding how and when to apply knowledge to make appropriate decisions is relevant to the work of public health nurses. Information technology affords public health nurses a way of making informed decisions and evaluating them to support the work they do in the community. The vignette by Cortes-Peske, above, provides an example of how information technology creates opportunities to use data that are more inclusive of populations in the community. By using the data and knowledge to gain

wisdom, public health nurses are able to understand the important influence technology plays in providing culturally competent, evidenced-based health care.

Figure 6-1 provides a visual depiction of the transformation of data, information, knowledge, wisdom, and evaluations leading to the potential for new knowledge formation. Data, information, and knowledge lead to wisdom. This data collection takes place within a context, such as a system, and can then be reviewed, organized, and synthesized to support the work of public health nurses.

For public health nurses to practice effectively and efficiently, the public health infrastructure must be designed so that the system seamlessly facilitates information input, storage, access, and management. The public healthcare system in the United States is a complex one, and the amount and types of information necessary for practice are staggering. The types of information systems necessary to facilitate the health of the public, therefore, are numerous, and each of these systems must "speak to each other": each of these systems must pass data between them and then to external points for exchange. Current strategies are supporting the development of interoperable (like plug and play) systems that are supported and realized through standards (terminological and technical). This will permit that needed sharing. According to Thede (2003), "in a well designed system, there is an interface or an exchange of information, between systems to support the sharing of data so that the data do not have to be reentered" (p. 224).

An example of such a system is the National Environmental Public Health Tracking Program. According to the CDC (2008), a lack of information needed to document links between environmental hazards and chronic disease exists. Air and water pollution are considered by the CDC (2008) as the two "most common environmental

Figure 6-1 Process of information and knowledge attainment for decision making in practice.

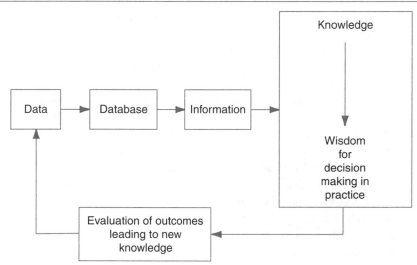

hazards" (p. 4) and "asthma, cancer, and lead poisoning . . . the most frequent adverse health effects" (p. 4). A tracking system that links these environmental hazards and chronic diseases provides a valuable tool for all public health workers and specifically for public health nurses. This facilitates an easier identification of the environmental causes of chronic illness. The National Environmental Public Health Tracking Program, developed by the CDC, is an attempt to address this issue. The national system tracks environmental hazards and the diseases they cause, updating traditional medical detective work with "computers, satellites, and geographic information systems" (CDC, 2008, p. 10). This system connects data sources, provides the tools to make sense of them, and makes that crucial information available to those who need it. In addition, the CDC has been working to develop the National Environmental Public Health Tracking Network. The CDC hopes this network

{w}ill promote information system standards to integrate local, state, and national databases of environmental hazards, environmental exposures, and health effects, will be a crucial component of the National Environmental Public Health Tracking Program. With the help of the National Environmental Public Health Tracking Network, scientists, communities, policymakers, and the public soon will have access to the information they need to make good decisions about preventing disease, keeping the American public healthy, and saving lives. (2008, p. 5)

Information Technology in Public Health Nursing

In 2001, as a result of a national crisis, it became known to the public and those responsible for policy that the public health infrastructure was lacking in a number of areas. One of those areas was the country's public health infrastructure with regard to technology and information systems (IOM, 2003a, 2003b). This realization has become even more urgent as we face threats of new emerging infections, chemical and biological terrorism, and other related and urgent health threats. Since that time, public health technology and information systems have been a priority area supported by the infusion of financial resources and technology in other areas of the healthcare arena. Under the 2009 United States Federal Health Information Technology for Economic and Clinical Health Act (HITECH), the widespread implementation of standardized and certified **Electronic Health Records** (EHRs) is being supported, and this has resulted in public health entering a much more profound era of technology-enabled information gathering. Three core functions of public health, assessment, policy development, and assurance depend on information and access to that information (IOM, 1988). Public health informatics supports this goal (IOM, 2003b). HITECH is allowing the technology infrastructure to be implemented in acute, ambulatory, and long-term care facilities. Implementation of these technologies and the development of the workflow processes to support the data collection will permit near-real-time reporting and sharing of that data, either directly into databases managed by local or state level public health departments or into **Regional Health Information Exchanges** (HIEs), which are organizations established to electronically collect and organize a core set of data from multiple organizations within a community or region, who in turn will report to local or state health departments (McGonigle & Mastrian, 2012). **Personal Health Records** (PHRs) which can be stand-alone or tethered to an EHR, allow patients to enter their own unique data (such as fingerstick readings, exercise, diet, and other self-directed health behavior results). This will

be another potential source of data for the public health nurse because this will provide data and information on patient-directed self care. Personal health records may also serve as a source of community risk assessments in the future.

Public health informatics, defined as the "systematic application of information, computer science, and technology to public health practice and learning" (IOM, 2003b, p. 63), is a key tool to support the role of the public health nurse. The IOM (2003b) document builds on the work of Yasnoff, O'Carroll, Koo, Linkins, and Kilbourne (2000), where the scope of public health informatics "includes the conceptualization, design, development, deployment, refinement, maintenance, and evaluation of communication, surveillance, and information systems relevant to public health" (p. 68). Friede, Blum, and McDonald (1995) define public health informatics as follows:

> {A}pplication of information science and technology to public health practice and research. Specifically, this means developing innovative ways to use inexpensive and powerful computers, online databases, the capacity for universal connection of people and computers, and multimedia communications to support the mission of disease prevention and health promotion. (p. 240)

The Association of Community Health Nursing Educators also defines public health informatics as the "systematic application of information, computer science, and technology to public practice" (Levin et al., 2007, p. 13).

In 2008, the ANA revised its standards and practice for **nursing informatics**, building on its earlier definition of nursing informatics to include the term "wisdom"; it defines nursing informatics as the "integration of nursing science, computer science, and information science to manage and communicate data, information, knowledge, and wisdom in nursing practice" (p. 1). The goal of nursing informatics is to "improve the health of populations, communities, families, and individuals by optimizing information management and communication" (ANA, 2008, p. 1). Informatics in public health nursing includes "the conceptualization, design, development, refinement, maintenance, and evaluation of communication, surveillance, and information systems relevant to public health" (Levin et al., 2007, p. 13).

Public health nursing practice uses technology to do more than just outreach and screening. It now encompasses areas such as consumer health, telehealth, cyberhealth, and e-Health. The use of Internet blogs and podcasts also impacts the practice of public health nursing. Technology enhances the design, conduct, and dissemination of research studies (Bakken, Stone, & Larson, 2008). It also plays a critical role in developing sustainable public health infrastructures (IOM, 2003b). For example, in the area of surveillance systems, one of the intervention strategies of the Minnesota Department of Health Population-Based Public Health Nursing Practice Intervention Wheel, the need for technology, is noted in the following citation:

> *Improved surveillance systems are likely to tax the public health system's capacity to process the growing quantity of health data required for public health improvement. Progressively, state and local governments are collecting and disseminating health status data at greater levels of detail, the number of reportable diseases is enlarging, and new developments in electronic laboratory reporting systems and electronic medical records systems will also increase the volume of data available to the public health system. Informatics methods and applications, such as decision supports and expert systems, modeling and simulation techniques, can help*

> *public health face this challenge by providing increased capacity to handle, analyze, and act on data that is likely to increase during the coming years. (IOM, 2003b, pp. 63–64)*

Other areas such as health promotion, disease prevention, and consumer health informatics are noted as having potential beneficial effects on patient and population health with the infusion of public health informatics (IOM, 2003b). Public health nurses need to note the importance of becoming involved in consumer health informatics, Web 2.0 health sources, and other e-Health systems. Our community members are using these tools in greater numbers. Eysenbach (2009) describes two phenomena of particular interest for public health nurses: Infodemiology, defined as the science of distribution and determinants of information in an electronic medium, and Apomediation, which describes how healthcare workers can stand by and guide patients and populations to correct health information on the Web. Infodemiology metrics highlight population-health-relevant events or predict them. An example of this is Google Flu Trends (http://www.google.org/flutrends/), which captures and monitors inquiries made on the Internet related to flu symptoms, which can serve as a proxy for potential outbreaks. People seek information when feeling exposed or threatened. Thus, these metrics and methods are potentially useful for public health practice and research, and should be further developed and standardized.

In addition, evidence-based practice and the development of online educational programs for the public and public health nurses serve to promote an effective and efficient public health system.

Access and Adaptability

Not only is the use of technology critical for public health nurses, but the population's ability to access information via technology is equally important. The possibility of a "digital disparity" is an issue that must be addressed. Digital disparity refers to whether or not an individual has access to information technology. This means that people who do not have access to technology for any number of social, political, or economic reasons may experience greater healthcare risks than those who do have access (Cronin, 2002). Access to technology by the public health nurse as well as the public becomes an essential part of the quality health care that can be provided. Later vignettes in this chapter demonstrate the importance of access to technology.

People, however, are not always ready to accept new technology, even if the technology is available to them. Rogers (1983) describes how innovations are accepted at varying speeds based on how people perceive the innovation. Some people embrace change and technology in nursing practice resonates with them, whereas others take a longer time to accept change (Thede, 2003). Five perceived attributes influence the speed in which an idea, like the use of computers in home care or a new information system that requires training, is accepted. Rogers (1983) identifies these five attributes as relative advantage of service, compatibility, complexity, trialability, and observability. The first attribute, relative advantage, refers to the idea that the adopter (in this instance, the public health nurse) perceives that the proposed innovation, such as using a computerized scheduling system, is better than the way previous scheduling was done. The greater the understanding of the relative advantage of the innovation, the more likely the public health nurse will quickly adopt the innovative method proposed. Second, how the public health nurse connects with or values the new system, defined as compatibility, also influences the rate of acceptance of an innovative measure. Third, if public health nurses do not

understand the use of technology in the work they do (i.e., complexity), they are less likely to accept the new innovation. Fourth, the ability to test a new product (i.e., trialability), like the use of laptops in the home or a personal digital assistant (PDA) in the field, will aid in the acceptability. And, fifth, observability occurs when, for example, the public health nurse can easily recognize how the technology adds value to his or her work and thus the innovation is more likely to be adopted and adopted earlier rather than later.

The public health workforce, of which nursing is a critical member, must be educated to ensure the healthcare needs of the population are met. Knowledge of informatics, along with epidemiology, biostatistics, environmental health, health services administration, social and behavioral sciences, informatics, genomics, communication, cultural competence, community-based participatory research, global health, policy and law, and public health ethics, are essential for all public healthcare workers (IOM, 2003b). Although all these areas are important, informatics and its use in public health nursing stands out. Informatics initiatives that will redesign the public health system are critical, and public health nurses must be ready and competent not only in their understanding of these systems but in their early adaptation and application to ensure the health of the public.

The next two vignettes presented below provide two examples of how innovative information technology has the potential to improve practice. Both show, however, how some people more readily accept innovations in practice than others.

In vignette #3, Martha Kelly reflects on acceptance of technology in a medical center, while in vignette #4, Carole Baraldi explains some of the challenges nurses face in home care settings. Technological equipment can be cumbersome, as is the collection of data. For

WWW

CASE STUDY (3)

VIGNETTE OF ADAPTING A COMPUTERIZED SCHEDULING SYSTEM
Martha Kelly, EdD, RN

My introduction into the world of nursing informatics started with the implementation of a computerized scheduling system in a large medical center in 1980. Very few hospitals had a computerized scheduling system at that time. From an informatics standpoint, the software package that was purchased allowed us to use our current staffing patterns; however, the concept of taking the control away from the role of the head nurse was a major paradigm shift. Until that time nurses did not typically have control of their unit's budget and subsequently used the time sheets as part of their reward system. The real issue was how to show nurses they still retained the decision-making portion of the schedule. The computerized system generated the first draft of the schedule, but the final decision was made by the head nurse who knew the staff and what the staffing mix should be for the unit to run well.

During this period I attended what was the first national nursing conference engaged in computer technology, entitled "Computer Technology and Nursing," that was hosted by the Clinical Center at the National Institutes of Health and held in Bethesda, Maryland. Many of the speakers at that conference addressed what we see today. Computerized patient records and computerized care plans were discussed at the conference. To my chagrin some of those in attendance seemed quite resistant to these new computer applications for nursing. For example, some were not supportive and others were critical of the concept of computerized care plans. Although the speakers were innovative, there was reluctance for early adaption on the part of some in the audience. Their reluctance was most likely reflective of this new field and the role of nursing informatics that was still being carved out. It was a time when there were mainframes but few desktop computers in a clinical setting. Even as a novice informatics nurse, it was clear that a merger of computer technology and nursing would soon come together.

technology to be supported by the very people who use it and benefit from it, adaptation to various settings may be required. Rural settings versus urban environments create different challenges for nurses using technology.

Connections

Information technology is used in a variety of settings, including hospitals, private practices, voluntary visiting nurse services, and municipal health departments. Currently, many institutions have their own data systems; however, many of the systems do not talk to each other within or between institutions. The lack of interfaces and compatibility is related to the inability to share information. The integration of systems is costly but critical for a comprehensive model of care. This is an area where focused attention will be directed in the coming years. How to develop systems that

WWW

CASE STUDY (4)

VIGNETTE OF MAKING TECHNOLOGY WORK IN HOME CARE

Carole A. Baraldi, MS, RN

I left home care more than 10 years ago, in part because of the implementation of the OASIS Tool, which created additional time on the already laborious paperwork required in home care because computers were not widely used. Furthermore, I was working fee-for-service for two agencies in New York City, and this additional work greatly impacted my financial profitability.

I decided to make a "career change" and began working in clinical trials for an international pharmaceutical company, which enhanced my computer skills. This year I reentered the home care arena and was introduced to the "tablet." My first impression was the weight of the laptop, which was necessary to ensure an extended life of the battery.

After the orientation I began making home visits with the computer and supplies stored in a luggage bag with wheels. Negotiating the New York City subways with this bag was quite challenging, because the turnstiles and stairs are antiquated and not conducive to travel.

Once in the member's home, the computer was placed on a barrier and secure table, which at times was difficult to locate. The computer frequently would crash, necessitating rebooting, which was frustrating to both me and the member. The focus of the visit was the computer and not the member and his or her environment.

Overall, I was dissatisfied with this experience and subsequently resigned after 3 months of employment. In addition, one of the nurses I met in orientation was asked to leave the agency after 6 months because her computer skills were not up to par. Several months earlier this same nurse had been mentored in the field and praised for her excellent clinical skills.

I am presently working as a consultant for a home care agency, which allows the nurses to decide how information is obtained. They can use the computer in the field or pen and paper, which is later entered into the database by administrative assistants. Information technology is vital to the healthcare industry, but I believe that in home care a certain amount of flexibility in the procurement of same should be offered, particularly with the paucity of experience.

do interface with each other will be a question to consider.

Through the Internet both the public and public health nurses gain access to a wide range of information, research, and websites. This form of communication is "reshaping how information is accessed and shared" (IOM, 2003a, p. 329). The Internet connects individuals to information that was not easily available to them before, if at all. Networking opportunities for both healthcare providers and consumers of health care abound, and the ability to disseminate information at a lower cost than more traditional means adds to the many advantages the Internet presents (IOM, 2003a).

One of the concerns when using the Internet is how one can judge the quality, accuracy, and reliability of the information that can be found on the World Wide Web (Thede, 2003). Public health nurses who work with populations must teach individuals to ask critical questions to determine the validity of the information. Thede (2003) suggests three possible ways to help the public determine the quality of a site: look for the Health on the Net Foundation logo, an organization that accredits health-related websites; check for the organizational domain (.org); and check for a copyright symbol. The use of the Internet, however, opens up many avenues that will serve public health nurses well. For example, today many home care nurses use the Internet in their practice as they apply home healthcare monitoring or seek out information and knowledge to support their clinical decisions.

In vignette #5, Teresa Haines writes about her work in student health services where Internet access is crucial to her successful decision making. The importance of using accurate and reliable sites for information is demonstrated.

---

www

CASE STUDY (5)

VIGNETTE OF INFORMATION TECHNOLOGY IN STUDENT HEALTH SERVICES
Teresa M. Haines, DNP, RN, FNP-BC

I am a family nurse practitioner and have worked at the Student Health Service at a college in New York City for 11 years. During that time I have seen dramatic change in the use of information technology at my clinical setting.

Ten years ago I purchased my first computer and started down the road toward becoming computer literate. At that time there were no computers in use at the Student Health Service. Gradually, computers were installed for use by the clerical staff to check student status and electronically convey student compliance with New York State vaccination requirements to the Registrar's office. Nurse practitioners were still using textbooks when they needed reference materials for patient care decision making. Next, computers were installed at many clerical workstations around the clinic and could be used by providers to look for online resources in lieu of potentially outdated textbook resources. Most recently, there is a computer installed in the conference room explicitly for provider resource and reference searches.

After a recent typical workday, I thought about how technology was now an integral part of my clinical practice. I saw a patient with hypothyroidism. She had blood tests on a prior visit and was returning for test results and ongoing care. Her thyroid function studies were atypical. After a brief consultation with colleagues, I went immediately to the computer to find references to aid in decision making about a treatment plan for this patient. Access to information gave a speedy resolution to an uncommon problem.

(continues)

CASE STUDY (5) (*continued*)

Later in the day I saw a patient who had an upper respiratory tract infection. She was taking an over-the-counter medication with which I was unfamiliar, and I needed to know the active ingredients. Again, consultation with colleagues did not provide the answer I needed to make an appropriate treatment plan for this patient. I looked in an over-the-counter drug reference on the shelf and could not find this particular product information because the product was only recently put on the market. Back at the computer terminal I searched and found, very quickly, the active ingredients of this product. Again, access equaled expedience and an accurate treatment plan.

In addition to my personal utilization of information technology during the workday, the Health Service has plans to grow the information technology at the clinic. A Health Service website is available for students to make electronic appointments and access health information. Educational podcasts are being developed and will soon be linked to the website to enhance patient education. Computers are planned for each examination room, and electronic medical records are also in the planning stage. Information technology in the community healthcare setting provides an invaluable resource for providers and enhances both quality and efficiency of patient care.

Using Technology to Communicate

Communication for public health is imperative. Information technology, online systems, and Internet opportunities, as well as other electronic information systems, continue to expand the volume and accessibility of information (U.S. DHHS, 2010). The use of the PDA enables one to organize information; other wireless devices, like laptop computers, tablets, iPads, and smartphones, also allow the nurse more flexibility and greater access to computers or the network. In addition, the legislative requirements for the Health Insurance Portability and Accountability Act of 1996 (HIPAA) include a privacy rule to protect patient information. Many HIPAA requirements are designed to allow for the transmissions of electronic health information, including transactions of providers, health insurance plans, and for the safeguarding and security of health data (Thede, 2003).

In any process of communication, evaluative feedback is required so that adjustments may be made. McBride and Detmar (2008) consider the need for nurses to take on a leadership role in transforming care in the community using information systems and communication. They question, however, why informatics is viewed as important for a few rather than for the entire profession. They also question why the building of feedback loops in practice is so slow when it is these feedback loops that are essential for promotion of safety and the advancement of the profession. McBride and Detmar (2008) ask, "Are we afraid that we will be regarded as less professional if we pay more attention to the context of care than to individual care plans?" (p. 195). In other words, if we are looking at individual care and the nursing process, we feel more legitimate, but when we look at nursing informatics, we are looking beyond the individual care and focusing on the environment where that care takes place; therefore, this may be perceived as not legitimate.

McBride and Detmar (2008) speak about the need for feedback loops, and technology supports the communication of the data within these loops. Online systems, for example in a health department, organize and collect data about births, deaths, and communicable diseases and then transmit these data to a regional repository and the CDC, where other public health nurses or professionals can access these data and use them to support their practice.

A method of communication is demonstrated in vignette #6. Madeline R. Cafiero describes her experiences in home care when pagers were first being introduced as a way of communication. She evaluates the use of pagers, providing the rationale for moving toward this, at the time, innovative use of technology and some of the problems it created.

The use of technology to communicate in public health also facilitates social support and social networking among populations. For example, take the time to do a Web search on your own to locate online support groups for diabetes, breast cancer, and Alzheimer's disease, just to name a few. Technology provides a forum whereby individuals may collectively "hang out," ask questions, support one another, and learn from each other. These websites and blogs may be formal and guided by professional organizations or they may be informal groups guided by laypersons. Information from these sites needs to be verified.

WWW

CASE STUDY (6)

VIGNETTE FROM CORONARY CARE TO PAGERS IN HOME CARE
Madeline R. Cafiero, MS, RN, FNP, CWOCN

Transferring to the home care department from the coronary care unit in 1986 was a culture shock. There were no cardiac monitors or automated blood pressure cuffs or arterial lines in home care; just me and my stethoscope. I soon became accustomed to this reliance on my senses and clinical judgment. It took a while to adjust to staying connected to the office while being out all day on the road.

Before each nurse left the home care office each day, the supervisors secured a list of each nurse's scheduled patients, numbered in the order they were to be visited. Patients' names were listed in the large block calendars on each nurse's desk and copied onto the supervisor's master schedule for the day. The calendar was the only way the supervisor could contact the nurse if necessary during the day. If something came up, the supervisor or office secretary would call the patient's home and ask for the nurse or leave a message for the nurse to call the office when he or she arrived. With this method, there was much reliance on the patient's memory of the call, the patient's willingness to let the nurse use the phone, and the skill of the office staff to predict what patient to call and when to actually catch the nurse in the minimum number of phone calls.

(continues)

CASE STUDY (6) (*continued*)

This system was abandoned when all the nurses received pagers in 1988. No longer dependent on the patients to find the nurse, the office would page the nurse and expect the nurse to call the office back within 15 minutes of the page. This was a lofty goal in our pre-cellular phone days. Once a page was received on the beeper, the nurse might be 20 or 30 miles between patients. In rural areas, this meant no return call until the nurse arrived at the patient's home. In urban areas if a pay phone was accessible, the nurse needed to have enough change and be in a safe enough area to park and call the office back. In the early 1990s nurses often avoided pay phones in certain neighborhoods because they were the "property" of the area drug dealers. Sometimes pages were not even received in the hill towns of our area. This caused a return to the old call-and-catch method of locating the nurse.

Pagers were known to go off multiple times during the day and usually after the nurse had gloved for a procedure. The pager would beep incessantly until a button could be pushed to silence it. Although the pager had a very wide clip to secure it, it often fell off onto the patient's driveway or stairwell, necessitating a search and rescue effort of calling the pager to locate it. Some days the pager would beep so often the nurse would place it on silent just to be able to concentrate on the patient. Of course, this meant remembering to check on the beeper afterward and return the pages received.

This system was used until I left the home care agency in 1998. Cell phones were being carried by individual nurses who chose to obtain them on their own, but most nurses continued to carry the pager. It became an essential part of their equipment, much as the cell phone and computer are today.

Applying Technology in Public Health

The next three vignettes are told by nurses who work in home care and research initiatives where a variety of tools, databases, tracking systems, cameras, and computers are used in their work. Each vignette provides a glimpse into how technology can add value to their work and offer a means to communicate, along with an increasing comfort level with the use of technology in practice.

A common tool used to collect data over the past 10 years is the Outcome and Assessment Information Set (OASIS). OASIS "is a group of data elements that: Represent core items of a comprehensive assessment for an adult home care patient; and Form the basis for measuring patient outcomes for purposes of outcome-based quality improvement (OBQI)" (U.S. DHHS, n.d.).

The collection of outcome data on all home care patients using OASIS is required by the Centers for Medicare & Medicaid Services (Schneider, Barkauskas, & Keenan, 2008). Visiting nurses collect outcome data using computers loaded with OASIS and other systems. They also use various technological tools, like digital photography and the telephone, to support their work. They gather data, place them into databases, and gain information, knowledge, and wisdom to make decisions in their practice and then evaluate the outcomes. This continuous process occurs while public health nurses care for the individual, family, community, and population. Although a systematic way of connecting all data that nurses collect may not yet exist, in vignette #7 Doreen Gallagher Wall shows how visiting nurses have been using systems like OASIS to record data sets in conjunction with other technology, such as digital photography, to support the work they do.

Vignette #8 shows how the use of information technology and informatics supports a clinical research initiative where the nurse works. Whether a common language exists,

all nurses work in collaborative roles requiring understanding of how technology supports the research process. Lois O. Carnochan provides a look at the use of large data sets, protocols generated by computer, and the need to communicate with other healthcare providers. Public health nurses work with others and need to be able to communicate and collaborate effectively.

In the final vignette #9, Lisa Seiff speaks about the need to introduce technology into practice and shows how she has made a change in the home care agency where she works.

CASE STUDY (7)

VIGNETTE OF USING TECHNOLOGY AS A VISITING NURSE
Doreen Gallagher Wall, MS, RN, BC

The use of technology in the public health, home care setting has clearly been established in the Visiting Nurse Service setting where I work. Visiting nurses use technology in the provision of care and as a support for decision making. Visiting nurses carry laptop computers where they may document and have access to important data for information and hence be connected in a wireless way. For example, Mr. J. Gomez was admitted to the Visiting Nurse Service in the summer of 2008. Part of the intake process is the gathering of information, commonly referred to as OASIS. This intake process can take up to 2 hours. Today, OASIS is fully loaded onto all laptop computers, thereby freeing nurses from being tied to paperwork. In addition, these nurses can now extract data and look for patterns and trends. Other data that are collected include care plans, finger sticks, vital signs, blood pressures, and weights.

Digital photography has also improved management of care. Visiting nurses may take a digital photo of a wound that is then sent to the primary care provider, who can view the wound and make decisions about options for treatment. This is also helpful for risk management. For example, if a nurse is conducting an intake assessment and notes an area of impaired skin integrity, he or she may take a digital photograph as evidence that this break in integrity was present before admission.

The TeleHealth program is another form of technology that supports clients to remain in their home. With the use of this technology, the visiting nurse can facilitate the management of a client's care, supporting promotion of health, and identifying problems early, thus preventing

(continues)

CASE STUDY (7) *(continued)*

acute care admissions or readmissions. For example, Mr. Gomez has a diagnosis of chronic obstructive pulmonary disease and his past history is marked by multiple emergency department visits and admissions. Since Mr. Gomez has been enrolled in the TeleHealth program, these emergency department admissions have declined. The reason for this outcome is that the nurse coordinator is able to monitor critical information on an ongoing basis without making daily home visits. The client is taught how to operate the needed technology and to transmit the objective information, such as vital signs, to the home office where the nurse coordinator monitors the data. In this way the nurse coordinator notes changes quickly in physiological functioning, thus identifying those at risk. When a client is at risk, the nurse and other primary care providers can take charge quickly, alter treatment options, and avert emergencies.

CASE STUDY (8)

VIGNETTE OF USING INFORMATION TECHNOLOGY IN RESEARCH
Lois O. Carnochan, MS, RN

I worked on a complex clinical trial/investigation in which the strategies and interventions for participants were hypothesis-driven and protocol-based. The interventions were for the prevention and control of some of the most common causes of morbidity and mortality among older women. The study was a multicentered, nationwide, clinical trial. It was designed to allow for double-blind, placebo-controlled evaluation of distinct interventions. The central focus in each of the interventions was the overall risk-to-benefit assessment of the participants.

Computerized data-based resources were essential to the conduction of the study and to the ongoing analysis of data, which continues. Strict adherence to the protocol was essential to the validity and reliability of the research. Custom data extracts and user-defined fields were used. Participants were carefully screened according to the protocol standards to be enrolled. The user-defined fields were designed to reject any participant who did not meet the criteria. Similarly, participants were randomized into the study by the computer, allowing for and ensuring that the correct interventions were assigned and that the assignments remained consistent and double-blind. Also, all visit-specific tasks were determined when the participant started in the study and the visit tasks were computer generated.

Very careful participant monitoring via custom data extracts were essential to participant safety and protocol adherence. The participant-specific data were easily determined via computer-generated reports. This information further guided nursing assessments and interventions within protocol adherence.

For example, nurses were able to assess and use the following clinical information for individuals and participant groups:

- All radiographic and laboratory results requiring follow-up.
- Dispensation of all medication by computerized number was participant-specific and ensured that the medication given remained double-blind.
- Clinical tasks specific to a particular visit type were computer determined, as were the tasks during nonroutine visits generated by untoward effects and needing immediate clinical attention.
- User-defined fields were flagged if medications were inconsistent.
- Medication-taking compliance was determined by participant adherence percentage, again computer determined.

This helped to assess if the individual could be enrolled in a medication intervention arm and also if the participant could remain in that arm.

The large database of healthcare information generated had to be protected for privacy and confidentiality. Some examples defined by HIPAA as health information that must be protected are name, Social Security number, medical record number, health plan beneficiary number, vehicle identifiers, and biometric identifiers, including finger and voice prints. Under HIPAA's "safe harbor" standard, a participant is de-identified if all identifiers have been removed and there is no reasonable basis to believe that remaining information could identify a given person. Information released by a clinical trial is done by cohort groups and never given on individuals except to the participant directly and under protocol standards.

All individuals were unblended at the end of the study and informed of the intervention in which they participated. The unblinding process could be done only by computer query. Again, user-defined fields and custom extracts yielded this information, and it was given to each participant individually to ensure confidentiality and privacy.

Challenges

Several challenges are before us as we consider the role of technology and public health nursing practice. A few of the most urgent challenges that warrant consideration are as follows:

- The creation of a standardized language, which is inclusive of nursing, that is understandable between and among all professionals.

- Funding on federal, state, and local levels to provide financial support.
- Communication between various information systems and between clinicians and the experts in informatics to help build systems that incorporate and interface systems.
- Focus on Public Health Work Force Competencies, which were developed to help educate the workforce. Categories are computer science and electronic communication,

online access, data system protection, and so on. The second group of competencies is the development and maintenance of information systems to improve the effectiveness.

- Readiness of public health nurses to accept innovation and be comfortable with applying and adapting changing technology in practice.

Although all the challenges listed above are important for consideration, the development and use of a standardized language are two of the most pressing needs for the best utilization of technology resources and practice. Standardized language and the power of its potential allow for the ability to aggregate and analyze data, which results in more timely feedback. Aggregate data

CASE STUDY (9)

Vignette of Introducing Technology as a Home Care Nurse

Lisa Seiff, RN, BSN

When I was just beginning my baccalaureate nursing education, I began working for a relatively small home care agency in New York City 6 years ago as an assistant to the Director of Nursing. I realized immediately that the agency remained in the technological Stone Age, which I knew would be a challenge for a 21-year-old who grew up with computers and technology. Five people staffed the office that ran all operations for the agency, which provided RNs, LPNs, home health aides, personal care aides, and live-ins to people requiring various levels of health care in their homes. Of the five people working in the office, only the receptionist had a computer. The minimal technology used in the office reflected the lack of technology used in the field. The nurses and aides working in patients' homes used only one type of technology—cell phones. All documentation was completed with pen and paper.

Most of my coworkers were older, which I believed at least partially explained the minimal technology being used. I soon began to question the lack of technology, specifically the lack of computers in the office. I was surprised by the receptiveness and openness that my superiors expressed in response to my suggestions. Two additional computers with Internet were quickly added to the office, but I then realized that availability of technology would not solve the problem alone. The office staff in general was averse to dedicating the time necessary to make often time-consuming changes. The agency had been in business for about 20 years, and the Director of Nursing had been there for almost 15 of those years; therefore, the attitude was "why change a model that works even if it is outdated?" I worked hard to computerize many of the forms and spreadsheets that were previously in paper format, but I often found it difficult to convince the other workers to use the technology because they had so little time to dedicate to learning the new way. They were all so proficient at doing things the old way on paper that convincing them to take the time to complete a task on the computer that could be completed without it in half or a quarter of the time was challenging.

Once I became a registered nurse and began working for the agency in that capacity, I realized quickly that I needed a way to carry with me patient information and medical reference material. I made the mistake of initially packing my nursing bag not only with the nursing items that I needed but with reference books as well. I soon realized the impracticality of my endeavor after carrying such a heavy bag for only a short period of time. I then understood the need for technology in the field. The Agency agreed to purchase for me a PDA that I could use to store all necessary patient information in addition to medical reference software. I use this PDA every day and during every nursing visit. I use it to access all necessary patient information, including diagnoses, physician information, and medication. The medical software provides me with reference information regarding medications, symptoms, diagnoses, and lab work.

Readiness and motivation to change remains a barrier, but cost is an especially difficult challenge. I sit on the agency's Performance Improvement Committee and thus am privy to conversation and debate about spending for technology. Improved patient quality of care is always a strong argument for improved technology, but where quality of care is not obviously improved by technology, the argument against investing the money remains strong. Home care nurses practice in unfamiliar and unpredictable settings every day, and technology can certainly help nurses working in the community to document faster and to share ideas and information in seconds rather than hours or days, but this comes at a large cost, especially for smaller agencies. Hopefully, with the right motivation and increasing availability of affordable technology, my agency and others can continue to expand on and improve the technology used.

can also be used for research, quality improvement, and decision-making support. Vendors need to incorporate the use of standardized language, because it is important (Ozbolt & Saba, 2008). Although not specifically directed to public health nursing practice, their implications for standardized language and practice are clear:

Clinical experts must work with terminology experts to develop computable, semantically interoperable standard language for those practice domains not adequately covered by existing standard languages. Researchers and developers must discover ways to use computable language and data to support nursing clinical and management decision at the point of need. Nursing records must be integrated with other records to support communication and retrieval of critical information. (Ozbolt & Saba, 2008, p. 204)

The need to refine the languages for nursing classification systems, such as the North American Nursing Diagnosis Association, Nursing Intervention Classifications, Nursing Outcome Classifications, or the Omaha Classification System, runs a parallel course with the need for standardized language and data mining as noted earlier in this chapter. Although beyond the scope of this chapter, the discussion about the need to standardize nursing data through minimum data sets, standardized language, and nursing classification systems is essential for the reader to explore further. In the late 1950s, nursing leaders began to classify nursing problems. In 1973, the North American Nursing Diagnosis Association began to explore the idea of establishing nursing diagnoses. This led to a movement to examine more closely nursing's need to standardize the terminology that described the work that nurses do. As public health nursing informatics gains momentum, the issues of these standardizing features will be crucial to the success of public health nursing interventions.

Conclusion

As the reader considers the public health interventions suggested in the intervention wheel, the potential for the use of technology to enhance the process becomes important. *Healthy People 2020* considers technology essential to the success of achieving the vision of a healthy society, with specific reference to the role of technology in health information and communication (U.S. DHHS, 2010). Technology, information systems, and the applications for nursing informatics play a significant role in public health nursing in enhancing practice, addressing safety, quality of care issues, as well as evidence-based practice. Throughout nursing's history data are needed, not just as a repository of information but also as a driver for knowledge generation and decision making and as a basis for evidence-based practice.

The vignettes from nurses in the field show how nurses working in home care, visiting nurse associations, research initiatives, and schools already use nursing informatics and technology in their practice. Knowledge of how nursing informatics and technology can inform and transform practice is essential for success. The rate of acceptance of the various tools and instruments may vary. The evolutionary nature of using nursing informatics and technology in practice is woven throughout the vignettes. They show how the use of the electronic medical records, pagers, cell phones, laptops, digital cameras, PDAs, systems that support clinical decision making, bar coding for medications, Internet connections, and the use of TeleHealth activities provides better access and services to their clients. Information technology has the potential to transform education and practice so that nursing care, in whatever public health setting, is delivered effectively, safely, and with the best outcomes (Ozbolt & Saba, 2008). If one considers technology as an essential part of today's social fabric, then the words of the former Dean of the Vanderbilt University's School of Nursing, Shirley C. Titus (1933/1991), resonate with us still: "Nursing, like every form of life activity, is a part of the warp and woof of the whole social fabric. Nursing cannot be an isolated, separated thing-in-itself; the flow, the interplay of social forces inevitable as day follows the night exerts an effect on nursing and nursing education" (p. 345).

References

Agnew, L. R. C. (1958). Florence Nightingale: Statistician. *American Journal of Nursing, 5*(58), 664–665.

American Nurses Association (ANA). (2007). *Public health nursing: Scope and standards of practice.* Silver Springs, MD: American Nurses Association.

American Nurses Association (ANA). (2008). *Nursing informatics: Scope and standards of practice.* Washington, DC: American Nurses Publishing.

Bakken, S., Stone, P. W., & Larson, E. (2008). A nursing informatics research agenda for 2008–18: Contextual influences and key components. *Nursing Outlook, 56*(5), 206–214.

Buhler-Wilkerson, K. (2001). *No place like home: A history of nursing and home care in the United States.* Baltimore, MD: Johns Hopkins University Press.

Centers for Disease Control and Prevention (CDC). (2008). *National Environmental Tracking Program.*

Retrieved from http://www.cdc.gov/nceh/tracking/keepingtrack.htm

Crandall, E. (1914). *Letter dated October 13, 1914, from Ella Crandall, Executive Secretary, National Organization for Public Health Nursing, to John D. Rockefeller requesting funding for the organization.* Collect RC, Record Group 1.1, Series 200, Box 121, Folder 1498, Rockefeller Archives, Pocantico, NY.

Cronin, B. (2002). The digital divide. *Library Journal, 127*(3), 48.

Eysenbach, G. (2009). Infodemiology and infoveillance: framework for an emerging set of public health informatics methods to analyze search, communication and publication behavior on the internet. *Journal of Medical Internet Research, 11*(1): e11.

Freeman, R. B. (1950). *Public health nursing practice.* Philadelphia, PA: Saunders.

Friede, A., Blum, H., & McDonald, M. (1995). Public health informatics: How information age technology can strengthen public health. *Annual Review of Public Health, 16,* 239–252.

Goodrich, A. W. (1931). The past, present, and future of nursing. *American Journal of Nursing, 31*(12), 1385–1394.

Hebda, T., Czar, P., & Mascara, C. (2005). *Handbook of informatics for nurses and health care professionals* (3rd ed.). Upper Saddle River, NJ: Pearson-Prentice Hall.

Institute of Medicine (IOM). (1988). *The future of public health.* Washington, DC: National Academy Press.

Institute of Medicine (IOM). (2003a). *The future of the public's health in the 21st century.* Washington, DC: National Academy Press.

Institute of Medicine (IOM). (2003b). *Who will keep the public healthy? Educating public health professionals for the 21st century.* Washington, DC: National Academy Press.

Levin, P., Cary, A., Kulbok, P., Leffers, J., Molle, M., & Polivka, B. (2007). *Graduate education for advanced practice public health nursing: At the crossroads.* Association of Community Health Nursing Educators (ACHNE), 1–24. Retrieved from http://www.achne.org/files/public/GraduateEducationDocument.pdf

McBride, A. B., & Detmar, D. E. (2008). Guest editorial: Using informatics to go beyond technology thinking. *Nursing Outlook, 57*(5), 195–196.

McGonigle, D., & Mastrian, K. (2009). *Nursing informatics and the foundation of knowledge.* Sudbury, MA: Jones and Bartlett.

McGonigle, D., & Mastrian, K. (2012). *Nursing informatics and the foundation of knowledge* (2nd ed.). Sudbury, MA: Jones & Bartlett Learning.

Medterms Medical Dictionary (2007). http://www.medterms.com

National Network of Libraries of Medicine and National Library of Medicine. (2005). *Public health information and data: A training manual.* Retrieved from http://phpartners.org/pdf/phmanual.pdf

Ozbolt, J., & Saba, V. (2008). A brief history of nursing informatics in the United States of America. *Nursing Outlook, 56*(5), 199–205.

Rogers, E. (1983). *Diffusion of innovation* (3rd ed., rev. ed.). London, UK: The Free Press.

Schneider, J. S., Barkauskas, V., & Keenan, G. (2008). Evaluating home health care nursing outcomes with OASIS and NOC. *Journal of Nursing Scholarship, 40*(1), 76–82.

Skiba, D. J. (2008). Moving forward: The informatics agenda. *Nursing Education Perspectives, 29*(5), 300–301.

Thede, L. Q. (2003). *Informatics and nursing: Opportunities and challenges* (2nd ed.). Philadelphia, PA: Williams & Wilkins.

Titus, S. C. (1933/1991). The new Scutari. In N. Birnbach & S. B. Lewenson (Eds.), *First words: Selected addresses from the National League for Nursing, 1894–1933* (pp. 344–353). New York, NY: National League for Nursing Press.

U.S. Department of Health and Human Services (DHHS), Centers for Medicare & Medicaid Services. (n.d.). *OASIS.* Retrieved from http://www.cms.hhs.gov/OASIS/046_DataSet.asp#TopOfPage

U.S. Department of Health and Human Services (DHHS). (2010). *Healthy People 2020 framework.* Retrieved from http://www.healthypeople.gov/2020/Consortium/HP2020Framework.pdf

U.S. Department of Health and Human Services (DHHS), Public Health Service. (2004). *The public health workforce: An agenda for the 21st century.* Retrieved from www.health.gov/phfunctions/pubhlth.pdf

Wald, L. (1915). *The house on Henry Street.* New York, NY: Henry Holt & Company.

Yasnoff, W. A., O'Carroll, P. W., Koo, D., Linkins, R. W., & Kilbourne, E. M. (2000). Public health informatics: Improving and transforming public health in the information age. *Journal of Public Health Management Practice, 6*(6), 67–75.

For a full suite of assignments and additional learning activities, use the access code located in the front of your book to visit this exclusive website: http://go.jblearning.com/londrigan. If you do not have an access code, you can obtain one at the site.

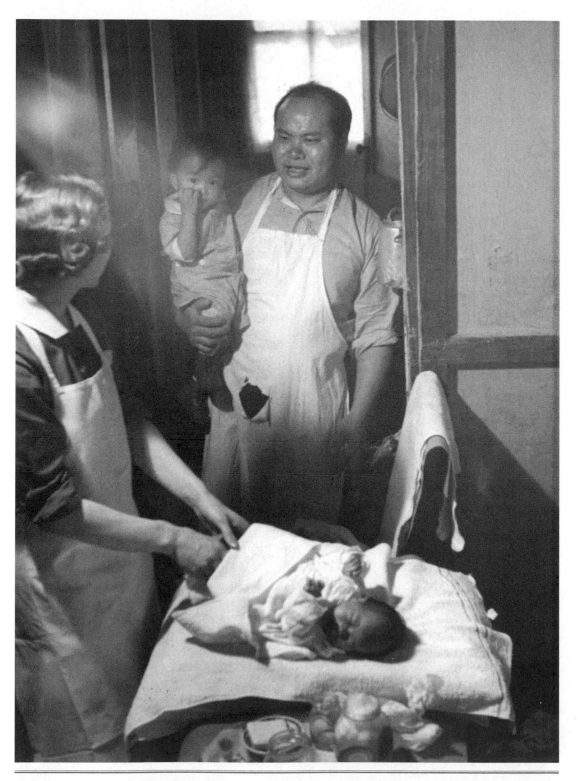

Chapter 7

Considerations of Culture in the Health of the Public

Astrid Hellier Wilson
Mary de Chesnay

These opportunities that I have so slightly touched upon bear the closest relationship to the immigrants because they are the most helpless of our population and the most exploited; the least information and instructed in the very matters that are essential to their happiness. The country needs them and uses them and it is obviously an obligation due them as well as a safe guarding of the country itself to give them intelligent conception and education of what is important to their and to our interest (Wald, 1908, p. 467).

LEARNING OBJECTIVES

At the completion of this chapter, the reader will be able to

- Define subconcepts associated with culture as a concept.
- Compare and contrast two public health issues in terms of cultural influences.
- Analyze public health nursing interventions for selected cases in terms of cultural competence.

KEY TERMS

- ❏ Culturally competent care
- ❏ Culture
- ❏ Ethnocentrism
- ❏ Participant observation
- ❏ Ritual
- ❏ Xenophobia

The purpose of this chapter is to provide a culturally based framework for public health nursing interventions. Although community health nurses certainly provide care to individuals and families, public health nursing is generally an aggregate service, and there is heavy reliance on prevention strategies directed toward populations. The chapter provides a cultural context for health care that maximizes respect for cultural diversity while accomplishing the objectives of best practices. In the first part of this chapter, basic concepts of **culture** are defined and related to important aspects of public health. In the second part of the chapter, model programs are presented that are examples of providing culturally competent care to populations.

Culture

Anthropologists specialize in the study of culture: the lifeways, folkways, **rituals**, taboos, and practices of a group of people who share symbols, values, and patterns of behavior. These shared aspects of living are socially determined and taken for granted by members of the culture. Cultural practices are learned and become ingrained in the subconscious to the extent that they become automatic. A common example is how members of the culture greet each other. In Russia, men might kiss each other on both cheeks. In corporate America executives shake hands with a firm grip. In Mediterranean countries women hug each other.

There are, however, many variations within cultural groups, particularly racial subcultural groups, and it is inappropriate to assume that all members of a group react the same in all situations. To generalize to all members of a group is considered stereotyping. For example, low-income, inner-city African Americans probably have more in common with low-income,

inner-city whites and Hispanics than they do with upper-class African Americans regardless of where they live. In this case, the culture of poverty dominates over the concept of race.

Cultural beliefs are learned and shared without conscious thought or analysis of the logic behind them. Studies that demonstrate the power of cultural beliefs are easily found in the literature (Kwong & Lam, 2008), and although some highlight the differences (Koffman, Morgan, Edmonds, Speck, & Higginson, 2008), there are examples of similarities among cultural groups that might seem to be at odds with each other. For example, Cassar (2006) studied cultural expectations about pregnancy with groups of orthodox Jews and Muslims living in the United States and found similarities in need for modesty, special diet, limited spousal role in delivery, and beliefs specific to the newborn. The two groups differed on same-sex provider, period of postpartum confinement, consulting with religious leaders, and observing the Sabbath.

Interpretation of the world according to the norms of one's own culture is called **ethnocentrism** and involves the belief that the way things are done within one's own culture is the right way. Ethnocentrism is neither good nor bad, but rather a shared perception by members of a group who have in common a set of values and mores. Ethnocentrism, however, can interfere with the ability of a person to respect different ways of doing things. For example, dogmatic assertions that prescribed rituals must be followed to maintain social control can interfere with a person's empathy for individuals who do not share one's cultural beliefs.

Ethnocentrism carried to the extreme of racism has resulted in oppression throughout modern history and the violence associated with racism justified on the basis of false conclusions about the actions and intentions of others. For example, stereotypes of African Americans as a high-crime population might lead one to fear and avoid all African Americans on the basis that some might be dangerous. A few years ago one of the authors had a young research assistant who was African American. This young man was careful to dress up for interviews (coat and tie) and to carry a briefcase to convey an image of respectability, yet he was repeatedly stopped by the police while traveling to interviews in predominantly white neighborhoods. Because he gave no signals that he might be dangerous, and because he took pains to blend in with the white, middle-class neighbors, the police actions can most reasonably be interpreted as racism.

Carried to an extreme, ethnocentrism can result in violence against those who simply do not share the cultural beliefs of the ones in power. An example in some modern-day communities is mixed marriage. Imagine, even in contemporary society, there may be difficulty with an African American and a Caucasian marrying, or two people of the same sex marrying in some areas of the United States. At the other end of the continuum of ethnocentrism is behavior that might be construed simply as rude. For example, simple greeting rituals, if not followed precisely, can be interpreted as insulting to the host. Imagine an acquaintance arriving at your home for dinner and you say "hello" but in return the person starts complaining about a problem.

Strict rules about gender-appropriate behavior apply in many countries. Women who break these rules or who are perceived by the abuser to break the rules are subjected to sanctions that often include beatings and torture. In a study of spousal abuse of pregnant women in Bangladesh, it was found that most women abused during pregnancy had a long history of prior abuse (Naved & Persson, 2008). In families in which women are regularly beaten by their male partners and relatives, the women are perceived to break rules that involve the honor of the family or the man and therefore "deserve" the beatings. This process is an internalization of blame that destroys the women's self-esteem and transcends culture or country.

Closely related to the concept of ethnocentrism is **xenophobia**, a term that describes conscious fear of foreigners. Foreigners can be interpreted as anyone of a different ethnic or racial group than one's own and can reside in close proximity to the group that is xenophobic. Xenophobia is distinguished from racism in that the phenomenon does not necessarily apply to people of minority groups. Indeed, it can be the minority group that is xenophobic about others in the community. For example, Tsai (2006) reported an ethnographic study of Taiwanese immigrant youth who settled in a Mandarin-speaking neighborhood of Seattle and who experienced xenophobia in relation to their American neighbors, excluding them from their play groups.

Critical to the study of culture is to understand the rituals associated with the culture. A ritual is a type of action that might be as simple as shaking hands when greeting a newcomer or as complex as those found in religious ceremonies. Rituals and traditions associated with key life events can enhance joy in the case of celebratory traditions such as weddings and holidays, provide a sense of comfort in the case of death and dying, and promote a gracious lifestyle as noted in table manners and the offering of food to guests.

Rituals also protect health and are especially important in public health nursing. Consider what would happen if aseptic techniques are not practiced when providing care in homes with varying degrees of cleanliness. What would happen if the sterile techniques used to package medications were not followed? Contamination of foods and drugs has been responsible for many deaths that might have been prevented if the rituals and rules about mass production were followed.

An example of a set of complex rituals is how to care for patients after death (Pattison, 2008). There are prescribed procedures, such as how to wash the body, and prescribed actions that are contraindicated. Often, prescribed actions are related to religious rituals. An example is performing a routine autopsy on a member of certain religious groups. Although sometimes autopsies must be legally mandated as in the case of murder, the process can be extremely disturbing to members of the family if their religious tradition opposes what they view as desecration of the body.

There is evidence that rituals can reduce anxiety. Often associated with religious practices, rituals provide a measure of comfort to the person who practices the rituals. In a study of 30 Catholic college students, Anastasi and Newberg (2008) found that reciting the Rosary significantly lowered anxiety as measured by the State-Trait Anxiety Inventory. In an Alcoholics Anonymous meeting, the ritual of pronouncing, "My name is _____ and I am an alcoholic," serves to let people know they are not alone.

Often, culture is viewed as the set of lifeways, rituals, and values associated with a group of people who share ethnicity and geographic territory—for example, Navajo residents of a reservation, Bantu of Africa, and Bedouin tribes of the Middle East. We also conceptualize culture, however, as transcending geographic boundaries when people share the aspects that define culture. For example, the profession of nursing might be viewed as a culture. Certainly, the culture of the country of origin of the nurse has great influence over practice. In a Taiwanese study (Chang, 2008) of 214 head nurses and 2,127 staff nurses, differences were noted

between groups in expectations of leaders. The author suggested that incorporating the most significant cultural values of personal integrity and human connectedness into the organization could help nurses function better.

Nurses around the world often seem more alike than different in terms of their shared commitment to their patients; common goals to heal and prevent illness and injury; similar rituals such as uniforms, caps, and pinning ceremonies; and specialized education. Although some countries have higher standards of education, governance, and practice, it seems reasonable to state that nursing practice in widely diverse settings has the common origin of meeting the health needs of the community. Professional organizations such as Sigma Theta Tau and International Honor Society have a mission to bring nurses from diverse countries and cultures together.

Other groups that might be viewed as subcultures within a dominant culture include patients with similar illnesses, such as HIV/AIDS, the chronically mentally ill, disabled children, pregnant adolescents, and heart attack victims. Groups of people living in close proximity can also be considered subcultures when they are a tightly knit group with shared values and rules, such as street gangs, retirees living in a gated golf community, expatriate Americans living in Oaxaca, and migrant workers on California ranches.

Participant Observation: A Skillful Technique in the Process of Becoming Culturally Competent

A key skill of public health nurses is the ability to observe and make sense of their surroundings. In a clinical sense, **participant observation** is a technique in which the nurse makes careful observations of specific processes, actions, or communications while providing care as a participant in the activity. Usually, participant observation techniques are used as research methods in ethnographies conducted over time—often a year or more. The technique, however, can be useful to public health nurses who need to pay close attention to subtle changes in their client, family, and the population and group interactions.

Participant observation is also a key method in conducting participatory action research, which is one of the best ways to design new population-based health programs. Action research involves community stakeholders in all phases of planning programs targeting that community (Brown et al., 2008; Cashman et al., 2008). For example, a public health team wants to start a program to improve psychosocial outcomes for women in a cardiac rehabilitation program. They might interview consumers in a selected program such as the "Heart Awareness for Women Program" (Davidson et al., 2008) and conduct participant observation periods to see how women move through the program.

The literature has many examples of participant observation in research, but reviewing the technique can be helpful to students who are learning observation skills to understand culture in any setting. The techniques are particularly easy to do in public settings. The following are some examples from the research literature that demonstrate how culture can be learned by an outsider. In an ethnographic study involving both participant observation and interviews, Stevens (2006) studied 15 adolescent female parents about what "being healthy" meant to them. A key finding was that although the girls were aware of public health messages about health, their fundamental needs of safe living conditions, finding food, and paying bills took precedence over practicing health promotion. For example, the girls' attention was focused on their own needs, and the key concepts that emerged from the data related to how the young

mothers were going to meet their own basic needs and the basic needs of their infants.

An example of how participant observation is a powerful supplement to interviewing in Stevens' study was food shopping. Although it seemed clear from interviews that adolescent mothers understood that good nutrition involved eating fruits and vegetables, the pressures of long hours at work and exhaustion at taking care of an infant made fast food a much easier choice. Participant observation demonstrates exactly how and under what conditions the mothers shopped for food rather than what they stated they should buy.

Similarly, Kaplan, Calman, Golub, Ruddock, and Billings (2006) conducted participatory action research in the Bronx to identify best practices of promoting public health by faith-based institutions. Addressing racial and ethnic disparities, a coalition of 40 community-based programs, including 14 churches, was mobilized to change community members' attitudes about health practices and to influence health policy on behalf of racial and ethnic minorities. Although limitations to the study were identified, the team concluded that the faith-based leaders could have an enormous positive influence on the health of their communities.

In an ethnographic study of 30 rural African American women who used cocaine, Brown and Smith (2006) found that the women tended to be either child-focused or self-focused with a wide range of responses to explain their drug use. For example, through interviews and participant observation conducted over 4 years, the researchers found that living in a rural area or small town created a sense of boredom among some of the women, who did drugs for something to do. It is one thing for someone living in a small town to say they have nothing to do, but quite another for the researcher to live there and experience firsthand what it feels like to be socially isolated.

In this study, other women used their children as an excuse, saying they felt overwhelmed with the demands of mothering. Again, participant observation makes clear to the researcher what it is like to live under the conditions required of the population being studied. Imagine a working single mother who arises at 5:00 a.m., goes to work at 6:00 a.m. as a waitress in a café until 3:00 p.m., picks up her children from school, helps them do homework, and then has to fix dinner and get them to bed by 8:00 p.m. while doing laundry and getting clothes ready for the next day. At what point in this busy day does she have time to shop for healthy food, take care of her own needs, and indulge in relaxing activities such as exercise or reading?

Similarly, in public health nursing, having a client say she is bored or overwhelmed by the demands of a growing family is much more meaningful if the nurse has visited the community and sees there are no social outlets for young mothers. An example of how the public health nurse might use this information is to start a series of group meetings about health topics (with child care provided) that could also serve as a support group for women. In the case of the population of adolescent mothers, the nurse might begin a support group that involves other professionals who could teach job training skills such as computer classes, crafts classes, or gardening. The point is that any successful intervention program can be made culturally specific by focusing on the needs and interests of the population served. Complete the field exercises in **Box 7-1** as part of your study.

Culturally Competent Care

The body of literature on cultural competence has grown since this term was determined to be the desired outcome of simple awareness of cultural differences. At its most basic level, cultural competence is a set of attitudes and behaviors

---

> ### Box 7-1 Field Exercise 1
>
> Choose one or more of the following and keep field notes about your observations and interpretations. Field notes are simply a kind of journal (use a small notebook) in which you would document the date and setting of the observation period and then describe your observations.
>
> 1. Have lunch at an ethnic restaurant in your community and observe the interactions of staff with each other and with patrons.
> 2. Identify a subcultural group within your community and visit their territory. Some examples might be an Amish farm, a Native American reservation, a juvenile court detention center, or a homeless shelter. Document your observations.
> 3. Visit a health clinic and observe the rituals of signing in, waiting room behavior, and payment processes. Document your observations.

---

by the public health nurse to take into account that the client or population has cultural beliefs, values, health practices, and ways of behaving in social interactions that may differ widely from expectations of the health providers. The public health nurse uses knowledge of the culture, which may be limited, and key informants, the client being the most important, to accomplish the goals of care without violating the rights of the client or population so as to maintain their cultural traditions.

One interpretation of cultural competence is to practice the traditions of the client population, but the danger here is that these attempts to blend into the culture are unnatural and providers might appear to be making fun of the population. Mimicry can be insulting, and so the provider inadvertently creates problems instead of preventing them. Showing respect for the other's culture does not mean trying to be someone you are not.

The American Academy of Nursing (2008) emphasizes the importance of including cultural material in nursing education. Several theorists (Campinha-Bacote, 2002; Kim-Godwin, Clarke, & Barton, 2001; Purnell, 2000, 2002; Purnell & Paulanka, 2003) have published extensively on the topic. Wells (2000) wrote that cultural competence is not sufficient and argued for cultural proficiency to replace it as the desired goal. In an attempt to clarify the definitional confusion in the literature, a descriptive study on literature in cross-cultural psychotherapy and counseling was conducted by Whaley (2008). He analyzed the two terms—cultural sensitivity and cultural competence—in a statistical literature review and proposed that cultural sensitivity is precursor to cultural competence.

Regardless of how the concept is viewed, best practice in providing culturally competent care should involve the most fundamental characteristic of respect (de Chesnay, Peil, & Pamp, 2008). Respect for differences on the part of both provider and client population leads to open communication about customs and values, and openness in the relationship leads to problem solving about how best to meet the health needs of the population. A good rule of thumb is to be as respectful, polite, and considerate as one can under the rules of one's own culture. In this way, most clients of diverse populations understand the nurse's intentions as honorable and respond accordingly.

CULTURAL COMPETENCE AND CONFLICTS

It is all well and good to say we should practice cultural competence, but what if the rights of the client population conflict seriously with the values or morals of the provider? The practice of female circumcision is an example. Abhorrent to Western practitioners, female circumcision affects millions of girls and is widely practiced in some cultures. Members of these cultures often immigrate to the United States. The United Nations has called for an end to the practice of female circumcision, also called female genital mutilation. The World Health Organization has studied the public health consequences of the procedure, and Little (2003) discussed the effects of hemorrhage, abscesses, sepsis, long-term problems with voiding, painful intercourse, and childbirth difficulties.

From a public health standpoint, it is a legitimate argument that eliminating the practice of genital mutilation is good policy. Support for the procedure, however, is ingrained in the culture and attitudes of millions of poor families who do not have access to educational programs on the public health issues and who perpetuate the practice by using a variety of practitioners who use unsterile instruments without anesthesia (Momoh, 2004; Morison, Dirir, Elmi, Warsame, & Dirir, 2004).

Even for male circumcision, which does not have the stigma associated with female circumcision, the unsterile use of implements exacerbates the spread of one of the world's most virulent pandemics, HIV/AIDS, in areas where traditional healers and religious leaders practice cutting rituals. These rituals are not only for circumcision, but also for symbolism (family bonding) and marking (curing illness), and often many boys are cut by the same tools in a short time period (Ndiwane, 2008). The cutting leads to sepsis and scarring if left untreated.

The world is becoming less a set of individual countries that are autonomous and more a global village in which there is extensive immigration and sharing of resources. Consequently, it is increasingly likely that healthcare providers and their patients find their cultural values in conflict. Respect for differences needs to be negotiated on a personal basis when providers come into conflict with clients over health issues, and education about each other's culture can certainly help prevent misunderstandings. Open discussion of these issues while maintaining the rights of the other to hold differing views is both respectful and culturally appropriate.

One way to look at whose cultural values take precedence is to view the relationship between provider and client as a contract in which the client comes to the provider as an expert to provide a specific service. The two then agree to disagree on anything not relevant to the contract. For example, a public health nurse in an inner-city immigrant neighborhood of Somali refugees wants to design a program to address diabetes management. Everyone agrees that diabetes is a major health issue for the population, but this is also a population in which female circumcision is practiced. For the nurse to try to get the women to stop this practice is inappropriate because female circumcision is a health issue that is not part of the contract. However, being open to discussing with leaders of the population the health risks without judging or trying to eliminate the cultural practice might be well received.

Complicating the issue of whose culture takes precedence is the dissonance between the rights of localities and the rights of the federal government. In a situation in which the cultural practices of a patient are in conflict with American law, the law takes precedence. For example, polygamy is illegal in the United States.

Similarly, undocumented immigrants have no legal rights that can be protected as if they were American citizens, especially in states that have enacted legislation designed to criminalize actions to help them. In the case of undocumented workers who need health care, the laws designed to eliminate services to undocumented people create a paradoxical effect by making the drain on American resources greater. If free clinics are banned from serving them, their only recourse is the emergency room, which is

10 times more expensive than visiting a clinic (de Chesnay & Chambers, 2011).

LEARNING PROCESS ON BECOMING CULTURALLY COMPETENT

Learning to provide culturally competent care is a complex process and starts with the respect for cultural differences that is fundamental to interaction with people of a different culture than one's own. One of the best ways to learn about different cultures is immersion, in which a professor takes a group of students to a foreign country or medically underserved area of the United States to practice. There are many examples of programs in which this is an integral part of nursing education (Bennett & Holtz, 2008; de Chesnay, 2005; Larson, Ott, & Miles, 2010; Nauright, 2005; Nauright & Wilson, 2012).

Although it is certainly desirable to be proficient in the language of the group with whom one is working, lack of language skill should not be used as an excuse not to interact with people, even in immersion programs in foreign countries. Adequate translators are often available in communities with large ethnic populations, and sometimes younger members of a family can translate for older members, although this practice is not often the best choice. Taking the time to learn a few words or phrases helps greatly in establishing trust and rapport.

Other approaches to consider in the process of learning and designing culturally competent programs for English-speaking ethnic minority groups within a city might include the following:

1. Project directors read as much as possible about the target population and have informal conversations with key informants. Key informants are members of the group or population of interest who are trusted members of the representative culture and who are willing to educate the staff in how

best to approach community leaders and stakeholders in a respectful way.

2. Key project staff members meet with community leaders to identify the stakeholders. Stakeholders include all those who have a vested interest in the project, such as the consumers who will be the recipient of the interventions and the gatekeepers—individuals who must give permissions for access to consumers, such as ministers for their congregations.

3. Staff members meet with stakeholders to identify issues related to the topic. An excellent way to talk about issues is in focus groups. Focus groups are conducted with small homogeneous groups of people within the target population. The focus group leader asks specific questions to elicit the group's perceptions to design appropriate aspects of the program.

4. Staff members meet with key informants or stakeholders on an ongoing basis to share developments and to plan, implement, and evaluate the unfolding process of the program together.

5. Staff members put in place evaluation measures that capture the perceptions of the stakeholders.

Complete the exercises in **Box 7-2** as part of your learning.

Culture and Public Health Nursing

Cultural considerations for public health nurses far exceed the implementation of cultural competence strategies needed to care for individuals and families. In addition to individual and family care, public health nurses focus on population health and the community as the client (Racher & Annis, 2007). The skill set necessary to integrate culture in providing health care is extended to identifying diverse cultures found in

---

BOX 7-2 FIELD EXERCISE 2

1. Assume you are a client in a community far from your home. Write a short essay on what it means to you to have a provider who is culturally competent.

2. Interview one member of an ethnic or racial minority group different from your own and ask about the person's attitude toward the practice of female circumcision. Note that it is not necessary to identify someone from a culture that practices female circumcision. Compare and contrast how your own attitude differs or is similar.

3. Imagine you are developing a diabetes education program for a group of poor African American, Asian, or Latina women in your community. How would you go about designing the program? Next, speak to a member of the cultural group you chose and ask him or her how he or she would develop the same program. What are the similarities and differences?

---

different communities. Examples of community cultures include the culture of farm workers, domestic violence, substance abuse, poverty, prisons, and rural communities.

Public health nurses are concerned with the culture and healthcare needs of underserved populations, for example, migrant farm workers and their families. Migrant farm workers make a valuable contribution to the everyday lives of the American people, and they and their "uprooted" children have numerous health problems not seen in the general population (Wilson, Pittman, & Wold, 2000). Research conducted among migrant workers and children of migrant farm workers provides insight into their perceptions of culture and health. The adults noted in the aforementioned research identify priority issues centered on the need for health information, English lessons, available community resources, and legal information, whereas the children viewed health as well-being and had a good knowledge of what to do to be healthy. The children did voice concerns about the difference in access to health care in the United States and the threat of deportation (Perilla, Wilson, Wold, & Spencer, 1998; Wilson, Wold, Spencer, & Pittman, 2000). Knowledge of the culture of migrant farm workers enables public health nurses to develop and implement community projects based on the culture of this population.

Domestic violence is no stranger to public health nurses and is present in most societies and age groups. Unfortunately, the signs of violence often go unrecognized while multiple acts of physical and psychological abuse are continually perpetrated.

Reactions to domestic violence between Latina and non-Latina women were studied, and the results showed cultural implications for the Latina women. Treatment responses that include a bicultural or bilingual counselor who focused on the family and children were demonstrated to be desirable for Latina women (Edelson, Hokoda, & Ramos-Lira, 2007). Public health nurses must consider the individual differences in women of any culture when planning programs for domestic violence.

Other types of public health programs targeting substance abuse (Hopson & Steiker, 2008; Kulis et al., 2005; Lange, 2007; Walle, 2004), poverty (Pearson, 2003; Wood, 2003), prison programs (Cervantes, Ruan, & Duenas, 2004; Devieux et al., 2005), and rural communities (Hartley, 2004; Jensen & Royeen, 2002; Savage et al., 2006) are found in the literature. The common theme in all these programs is emphasis on cultural considerations.

Substance abuse programs have been targeted at Native Americans (Walle, 2004) and women

learning to care for themselves (Lange, 2007). Two evidence-based substance abuse prevention programs targeted students in alternative schools (Hopson & Steiker, 2008) and middle school students with a Mexican heritage (Kulis et al., 2005). Both programs emphasized the importance of culturally grounded curricula. It is unlikely that curricula will be implemented or sustained if interventions are not culturally congruent with those receiving the intervention. For example, Hopson and Steiker (2008) allowed students in alternative schools to read workbook exercises and reword them to capture their lifestyles and culture to facilitate student participation.

The culture of poverty has also been reported in the literature (Pearson, 2003; Wood, 2003). Poverty is complex and encompasses many factors, such as not having basic needs like adequate food, clothing, and housing. These situations may lead children to developmental delays, dropping out of school, and giving birth during the teen years. Some examples of cultural rules of poverty are living in the present and not planning for the future, sharing money with others rather than trying to get ahead to guarantee that others will share in their need, and not expecting change because of a strong belief in fate and destiny (Pearson, 2003). Wood (2003) encourages community-based advocacy to enhance the health of children who are most vulnerable in poor families.

One intervention program for adolescent juvenile offenders provides insight into the ability to decrease recidivism and increase substance abuse resistance (Cervantes et al., 2004). Much of the success of Program Shortstop was attributed to cultural sensitivity aimed at Hispanic youth who came from low-income, immigrant families. There were four prevention/intervention sessions using videos, homework, legal education, a simulation incarceration, activities to improve family communication and conflict resolution, drug information, self-esteem building drills, parent workshops on family communication, legal rights and responsibilities, and youth mentoring. Eighty-nine percent of the youth who completed the program were not rearrested within 1 year. Also, the participants gained legal knowledge and effective ways to deal with substance abuse and delinquency at school. In a follow-up study, most parents reported that their child's high-risk behavior had decreased.

Other researchers studied the differences among African American and Cuban American adolescent juvenile offenders, predominately male, related to preventing drug and sexually risky behaviors while focusing on culture. These researchers examined levels of drug and sexually risky behaviors to determine if there were any differences among the two groups. Language in the focus groups and in-depth interviews was culturally sensitive, using the local terminology of the participants. The results in part indicated that both groups of youth engaged in risky behaviors that could lead to HIV infection and had about the same level of sexual activity and number of partners. The Cubans in this sample had higher levels of unprotected sex and higher levels of sex while using drugs than the African American youth. Some of the differences in this sample may be related to acculturation, communication with parents, and media-targeted efforts. Adolescents who are more acculturated tend to engage earlier in risky sexual behaviors, and Hispanic youth may not talk about risky behaviors at home. Specific media protective health messages may have been targeted more toward the African American youths than Cuban American youths (Devieux et al., 2005).

It is well established that rural communities may have limited resources and inadequate numbers of healthcare providers. A challenge for healthcare providers is to provide health services for vulnerable populations in rural areas (Jensen & Royeen, 2002). The Health, United States 2001 Urban and Rural Health Chartbook (Eberhardt, Ingram, & Makuc, 2001) identified risky behaviors among rural populations that may be attributed to a rural culture health determinant. There is evidence of increased risk behaviors among rural residents such as obesity, smoking, poverty, and decreased exercise and nutritional diets. In addition, environmental and cultural factors and economic issues can contribute to health behaviors and health (Hartley, 2004). Other researchers have described interdisciplinary rural health projects as "best practice" in rural health projects (Jensen & Royeen, 2002). Public health nurses can be leaders in implementing population-based models for improving the quality of health care in rural communities with particular emphasis on the unique cultural aspects of each community. Furthermore, public health nurses are uniquely positioned to partake in community-based participatory research in that they subscribe to the four principles of building trust, collaboration, excellence in science, and ethics associated with community-based participatory research (Savage et al., 2006).

Case Studies

Three case studies are presented below as examples of programs in which culturally competent interventions are predominant. Each of the case studies has populations who are targeted in *Healthy People 2020* as a result of their health disparities. Lack of availability and access to health services, lack of insurance, limited language access, and physical environments contribute to these disparities. Culturally competent interventions in each case study are aimed at achieving better health outcomes consistent with *Healthy People 2020*.

1. Migrant family project
2. Rural Georgia domestic violence project
3. Project IDEAL—diabetes

A description of the project and discussion about cultural material precedes suggested field activities that students might find useful to give a sense of the public health implications when using culturally competent interventions.

Migrant Farm Workers and Their Families Case Study

The Farm Worker Family Health Program (FWFHP) has been in existence for over 15 years in a rural area of southern Georgia. The program is a health-focused academic community partnership where faculty and students provide health screening and referrals and community organizations provide access to migrant farm workers at their work sites, trailer parks where they live, and to their children attending a county summer school program. In addition, the local Farmworker Health Clinic provides client health records, assessment forms for documentation, and some medications and serves as the referral source for clients requiring follow-up treatment from the FWFHP.

The 2-week cultural immersion program provides a unique opportunity for interdisciplinary students (undergraduate nursing, nurse practitioner, dental hygienists, physical therapy, and psychology) to gain needed cultural sensitivity while providing health-related screenings to this uninsured at-risk population. Since the inception of the program, about 10,000 episodes of care have been provided to migrant farm workers and their families. Adult screening includes vital signs, hemoglobin and glucose tests, dental screening, and physical therapy if desired. The most frequent diagnoses among adults are low back pain, dental caries, and diabetes, which is on the rise in this vulnerable population.

The child health screenings include a physical examination, height and weight measurements (body mass index), hearing and vision screening, glucose screening if indicated by increased body mass index, and hemoglobin screening. In addition, nursing students present health classes to migrant children in prekindergarten to ninth grade related to basic hygiene, dental care, nutrition, and smoking risks. The teaching strategies include discussion, lecture, videos, handout materials, games, and poster presentations. The most frequent diagnoses among the children were dental caries, anemia, vision problems, and upper respiratory tract infections.

Other students also participate. Dental hygiene students perform dental checks and fluoride treatments on all children and tooth sealants to retard decay. If needed, children are referred to a local dentist. The psychology students perform developmental assessments and provide counseling and referral if indicated. Physical therapy students assess gross motor development.

CULTURAL CONSIDERATIONS

The FWFHP noted specific cultural considerations for this particular population:

- Before attending the FWFHP, all faculty and students are required to participate in a series of modules related to the history and culture of migrant farm workers and their families.
- Communication barriers were addressed by having an interpreter available at all screenings to assist with clients who did not speak English.
- Services to be rendered in the evenings and at work sites were incorporated into the program.

- The need for educational materials in Spanish was identified and materials were made available.
- Counseling services for migrant farm workers was made available.

IMPACT ON THE HEALTH OF THE PUBLIC

The impact of this culturally congruent public health initiative included the following:

- The major impact of the FWFHP is the health care that is provided to this uninsured, vulnerable population. Even though the program runs only 2 weeks in the summer, other health programs are provided throughout the year by the local Farmworker Health Clinic. The health services are positively received by the migrant farm workers and their children.
- Community participation and resources are available for this uninsured population and for the faculty and students. Different churches in the area provide chairs and tables for the screenings and lunch for the students, faculty, and other volunteers.
- The immersion experience facilitates student understanding of the Hispanic and rural cultures. Specifically, this experience with migrant farm workers and their families can be used in students' future practice when encountering patients with a Hispanic or migrant farm worker background.
- A major positive outcome for the children is the establishment of a medical health record that is available year after year for those children who return and attend the summer program. Parents are provided with health records related to screenings and immunization schedules and are encouraged to immunize their children at appropriate times.

- Another positive outcome for the population is the referral system that is in place that enables the healthcare providers to arrange future health care in the community. One example was a man who presented with a deep laceration that had become infected and led to septicemia. The man was taken to the emergency department at a local hospital at once and treatment began immediately, thus preventing a potential amputation or death. Ultimately, the wound began healing.

Complete the exercises in **Box 7-3** as part of your learning.

BOX 7-3 FIELD EXERCISE 3

1. Interview a person whose first language is not English (or any other language you speak) about experiences with healthcare professionals who do not speak his or her language. What feelings do these experiences evoke?
2. Develop a brief training module for migrant workers or their children on a topic similar to one of the following: dental hygiene, foot care for the elderly, HIV/AIDS prevention, prenatal nutrition, infant bathing, child immunizations, anxiety prevention, substance abuse, or domestic violence. In what way(s) would you ensure that the individual or population's particular cultural values and beliefs are addressed?
3. Conduct a participant observation session at a clinic that serves the migrant population. Observe rituals, values, and folk practices. For example, who speaks for the family to the healthcare professional? How are children disciplined? Are they told to sit still or allowed to run around? Are any foods brought in, and if so, what are they? What language do they use?

Rural Domestic Violence Project Case Study

A unique program in north Georgia serves both urban and rural populations by providing assistance to victims of domestic violence for over two decades. It has grown into a center with diverse services ranging from crisis intervention, legal advocacy, transportation, child care, household establishment assistance, life skills workshops, children's programs, referral, transitional housing (hopefully leading to permanent housing), to community education.

The mission of the center is focused on the safety of women and children who are victims of domestic violence by providing the above free services. Emergency shelter and crisis intervention are paramount when domestic violence occurs, but the program provides so much more to the victims. In addition to the 24-hour hotline in English, there is now a 24-hour hotline in Spanish.

The groups receiving services include whites, African Americans, Hispanics, refugees, immigrants, and human trafficking victims. In the last 2 years, the Multi-Cultural Program has provided support services to 50 women from Mexico, 7 from Guatemala, 4 from Venezuela, 3 from Honduras, 3 from El Salvador, 2 from Peru, 2 from Brazil, 2 from Russia, 2 from Nicaragua, 1 from Honduras, 1 from Greece, 1 from Panama, 1 from the Netherlands, and 1 from Colombia. In addition, transitional housing was provided to 17 women from Mexico, 3 from Jamaica, 3 from Puerto Rico, 2 from Panama, 1 from Libya, 1 from Ghana (refugee), 2 from Haiti (human trafficking victims), 1 from Cameroon (refugee), 1 from Ethiopia (human trafficking victim), and 1 from Liberia (refugee).

The staff at the center remain sensitive to individual cultural backgrounds and try to meet needs within that framework. One example was a woman from Liberia who had walked all her life before coming to the United States and had never driven in a car, nor had anyone from her village. Nevertheless, she wanted to learn how to drive, and the center provided driving lessons, which was a life-changing event. Other life-changing events include the ability to have employment and afford and maintain an apartment, leading to a sense of achievement and self-satisfaction.

Cultural Considerations

The Rural Domestic Violence Project notes specific cultural considerations for this particular population:

- The culture of poverty is incorporated into the services provided to help the victims break their cycle of poverty. Women in the rural Domestic Violence Project who use the transitional housing and progress to long-term housing, find employment, and pay their rent and other bills expressed their satisfaction that they could maintain a home for their families and no longer had to live homeless and in adverse poverty.
- Cultural competence workshops are provided for the staff.
- Hiring of bilingual staff enhances effective communication, eliminating the need for interpreters.
- A support group was developed and implemented for the Latina population.
- Immigration and residency status information are provided.
- Sensitivity to special dietary needs, clothes, and other cultural norms is developed.
- Brochures in Spanish are provided.
- Age-appropriate services are provided for children and adolescents.

IMPACT ON THE HEALTH OF THE PUBLIC

The impact of this culturally congruent public health initiative included the following:

- Transitional housing for 3 years is available at the program's relatively new 72-unit apartment complex. The gated community consists of two-, three-, and four-bedroom units and provides low-cost housing and on-site support services. After 3 years the low-cost housing is available permanently, thus providing much-needed support for this specific population.
- Free crisis and counseling services are available for women and children who are victims of domestic abuse. The ability for women and children to have a safe shelter from an otherwise traumatic situation allows the women a respite from their immediate distress. They are in a safe place with capable counselors who can help them make necessary choices to restart their lives in an abuse-free environment.
- Legal advocacy services assist with obtaining protective orders to ensure safety for the women and their children. The advocacy services enable restraining orders to be put in place and allow the women and children to be safe at the center. Many women do not initiate these orders but are glad when someone empowers them to take necessary legal action.
- Emergency services provide for the immediate safety of the family and help the victims to develop ways to be safe and initiate these safety measures themselves.
- Immigration services are rendered to combat human trafficking and the Internet mail-order bride business.
- The special needs of children who have been living in homes with domestic violence are addressed in the program via activities such as support groups, early literacy programs, immunizations, play therapy, special outings, organized activities, and individual or group counseling sessions. Emotional distress and other psychological issues are effectively worked out among most of the children. The support groups help the children to realize they are not the cause of domestic violence in their homes and they are not alone, but rather other children experience some of the same things they do.

Complete the exercises in **Box 7-4** as part of your learning.

Project IDEAL

Project IDEAL is a program of the WellStar School of Nursing at Kennesaw State University that began in 2003 and is focused on providing diabetes prevention and self-management education for Latinos. This is a significant program because Latinos are the largest minority in Georgia, numbering almost 576,000. Latinos have a high risk for developing diabetes, and as many as 1 in 10 Latinos may have diabetes. There are ways to prevent or postpone diabetes by maintaining a healthy lifestyle, such as eating healthy foods and exercising.

Box 7-4 Field Exercise 4

1. Volunteer at a shelter and reflect upon the experience.
2. Identify and review three films about domestic violence and observe the interactions between abusers and victims. What are your observations?
3. Interview an administrator of a shelter or a therapist who specializes in violence to address the questions you have about domestic violence.

The classes are conducted in small groups and focus on maintaining a healthy lifestyle, needed medications, meal planning, blood sugar monitoring, and exercise. Coupled with the classes are the support group meetings. The support group meetings consist of special education sessions with guest speakers for adults; separate educational sessions for children; blood pressure, weight, and height screening; and follow-up, and currently participants are encouraged to take part in English as a second language classes.

Project IDEAL also provides a forum for educators and healthcare providers to study the concepts of diabetes self-management education and the American Diabetes Association criteria for recognition. Included in the program are materials for diverse Latino groups, prediabetes education materials, consultation with a Latino healthcare educator, and program development consultation and oversight.

CULTURAL CONSIDERATIONS

Project IDEAL facilitates specific cultural considerations for this particular population:

- Understanding and respecting the cultural aspects of eye contact is essential when working with Latinos, such as being aware not to get too close initially until you have eye contact and avoiding direct eye contact unless they initiate it first. This is not as critical in the younger population as it is in the older generations. With length of time and acculturation, the necessity for avoiding eye contact diminishes with some individuals.
- Understand and respect the demonstrative use of hugs in welcoming.
- Identify participants' perceptions and value of health to best foster maintenance of diabetes.

- Know that there are differences within Latino groups, and some prefer not to be in groups with Latinos from different countries, whereas others enjoy the cultural exchange that occurs.
- Consider eating habits and the cultural names of different foods in different Latino populations. The words "naranja" and "chino" can both mean orange. The use of the metric system and traditional systems can be found among Puerto Ricans, such as measuring height in inches and weight in kilograms, and the Mayans measure height in centimeters and weight in kilograms. This cultural information is essential when teaching nutrition classes such as weighing food for diets.
- Understand how people like to get information and use the "word of mouth method" in Latino populations.
- Know that some members in the Latino groups, in this project, trust individuals who survived a condition over a physician's word or teachings. Families and friends who have diabetes are trusted more than a healthcare provider, and information is sought from them.
- Many Latinos prefer health providers who speak Spanish.

IMPACT ON THE HEALTH OF THE PUBLIC

The impact of this culturally congruent public health initiative included the following:

- The major impact of this program is the reduction of HbA_{Ic} levels among participants with diabetes. This is significant because studies have shown that for every 1% reduction in HbA_{Ic} levels, an approximate 35% reduction in the risk for the microvascular complications of diabetes occurs.

- This program provides a service to an underserved population.
- Nursing students are provided with the opportunity to develop culture competence skills when participating in the program.
- Although weight reduction has not been a statistically significant benefit of the program, there is evidence that the participants are maintaining their weight and not gaining weight while in the program.
- Diabetes prevention and education to children and teens participating in the program is provided.
- Quality of life is improved for Latinos who live with diabetes.

Complete the exercises in **Box 7-5** as part of your learning.

BOX 7-5 FIELD EXERCISE 5

1. Identify a program in your community that addresses chronic illness and self-management. Ask to observe several intake interviews. How do the individual clients respond to the healthcare provider? How does the program reach out to the specific population being served?

2. Eat several meals at a local restaurant frequented by members of the Latino population and examine the types of foods on the menu. Prepare a nutritional analysis of these foods.

3. Identify a cultural group of interest and a particular health issue experienced by this group. Attend a support group meeting that addresses this particular issue and prepare a summary of the themes of the discussion.

Discussion of Cultural Issues in the Community Projects

The three projects presented are diverse and meet different health needs of selected populations, yet there are common cultural issues evident in the projects. Cultural competence is needed among those providing care to these populations. Cultural themes in common with all three projects are respect, immersion, and communication. Respect for the recipients of care encompasses allowing them to express themselves and finding ways to incorporate their desires into the plan of care. One example of respect is being sensitive to special dietary needs, clothes, and other cultural norms. Considering the farm workers' schedules by providing services in the evening and acknowledging their need for materials in Spanish illustrate respect. Respect is also shown by being conscious of the cultural aspects of eye contact and the demonstrative use of hugs in welcoming in the Hispanic culture.

Immersion in a culture helps healthcare providers understand the cultural traditions that can assist in the planning and delivering of culturally appropriate health care. Gaining an understanding of diverse cultures enhances one's own ability to practice in an appropriate, culturally sensitive manner. Much of the success of Project IDEAL can be attributed to the in-depth understanding of the Latino culture and paying attention to participants' perceptions and values about health to best foster management of their diabetes.

Providing culturally-specific workshops and preparation for staff, faculty, and students is another way to become familiar with a culture. Speakers might be invited to a panel presentation at which culturally appropriate food is served and music played.

Communication is essential in planning health care and services for diverse populations and can be a challenge because of many barriers that impede communication. Communication barriers are addressed in the case studies by the use of interpreters, hiring bilingual staff, and acknowledging the differences within Latino groups. In addition, understanding how people like to get information, such as the word-of-mouth method, in Latino populations and using key informants they trust are helpful in facilitating desired communication. Cultural considerations found in the case studies are essential for the health of the public.

Conclusion

The purpose of this chapter was to provide a cultural framework for public health nursing to best promote culturally competent health care to diverse populations. Several case studies were presented that demonstrate aspects of cultural considerations in implementing population-based projects. Public health nurses are encouraged to make use of participant observation and participatory action research methods to design programs that are culturally relevant to the stakeholders. Taking the time to learn the cultural lifeways, values, and traditions of the populations served is critical to providing health care, not only to patients and their families but also to populations.

Acknowledgments

We gratefully acknowledge the contributions of the project staff who shared information about their programs.

References

American Academy of Nursing. (2008). *Cultural competency in baccalaureate education*. Washington, DC: American Association of Colleges of Nursing.

Anastasi, M., & Newberg, A. (2008). A preliminary study of the acute effects of religious ritual on anxiety. *Journal of Alternative and Complementary Medicine, 14*(2), 163–165.

Bennett, D., & Holtz, C. (2008). Building cultural competence: A nursing practicum in Oaxaca, Mexico. In C. Holtz (Ed.), *Global health care* (pp. 601–614). Sudbury, MA: Jones and Bartlett.

Brown, D., Hernandez, A., Saint-Jean, G., Evans, S., Tafari, I., Brewster, L., . . . Page, J. (2008). A participatory action research pilot study of urban health disparities using rapid assessment response and evaluation. *Health Policy and Ethics, 98*(1), 28–38.

Brown, E. J., & Smith, F. B. (2006). Rural African American women who use cocaine: Needs and future aspirations related to their mothering role. *Community Mental Health Journal, 42*(1), 65–76.

Campinha-Bacote, J. (2002). The process of cultural competence in the delivery of health care services: A model of care. *Journal of Transcultural Nursing, 13*(3), 180–184.

Cashman, S., Adeky, S., Allen, A., Corburn, J., Israel, B., Montano, J., . . . Eng, E. (2008). The power and the promise: Working with communities to analyze data, interpret findings and get to outcomes. *American Journal of Public Health, 98*(8), 1407–1417.

Cassar, L. (2006). Cultural expectations of Muslims and Orthodox Jews in regard to pregnancy and the post-partum period: A study in comparison and contrast. *International Journal of Childbirth Education, 21*(2), 7–30.

Cervantes, R. C., Ruan, K., & Duenas, N. (2004). Program Shortstop: A culturally focused juvenile intervention for Hispanic youth. *Journal of Drug Education, 34*(4), 385–405.

Chang, Y. (2008). The impact of Chinese cultural values on Taiwan nursing leadership styles: Comparing the self-assessments of staff nurses and head nurses. *Journal of Nursing Research, 16*(2), 109–120.

Davidson, P., Digiacomo, M., Zecchin, R., Clarke, M., Paul, G., Lamb, K., . . . Daly, J. (2008). A cardiac rehabilitation program to improve psychosocial outcomes of women with heart disease. *Journal of Women's Health, 17*(1), 123–134.

de Chesnay, M. (2005). Teaching nurses about vulnerable populations. In M. de Chesnay (Ed.), *Caring for the vulnerable* (pp. 349–356). Sudbury, MA: Jones and Bartlett.

de Chesnay, M., & Chambers, D. (2011). *Free clinics as a solution to healthcare for undocumented immigrants*. Paper presented to the Society for Applied Anthropology, Seattle, WA, March 27–April 1.

de Chesnay, M., Peil, R., & Pamp, C. (2008). Cultural competence, resilience and advocacy. In M. de Chesnay and B. Anderson (Eds.), *Caring for the vulnerable* (pp. 25–35). Sudbury, MA: Jones and Bartlett.

Devieux, J. G., Malow, R. M., Ergon-Perez, E., Samuels, D., Rojas, P., Khushal, S. R., . . . Jean-Gilles, M. (2005). A comparison of African American and Cuban American adolescent juvenile offenders: Risky sexual and drug use behaviors. *Journal of Social Work Practice in the Addictions, 5*(1/2), 69–83.

Eberhardt, M. S., Ingram, D. D., & Makuc, D. M. (2001). *Health, United States 2001 urban and rural health chartbook*. Hyattsville, MD: National Center for Health Statistics.

Edelson, M. G., Hokoda, A., & Ramos-Lira, L. (2007). Differences in effects of domestic violence between Latina and Non-Latina Women. *Journal of Family Violence, 22*, 1–10.

Hartley, D. (2004). Rural health disparities, population health, and rural culture. *American Journal of Public Health, 94*(10), 1675–1678.

Hopson, L. M., & Steiker, K. H. (2008). Methodology for evaluating an adaptation of evidence-based drug abuse prevention in alternative schools. *Children & Schools, 30*(2), 116–127.

Jensen, G. M., & Royeen, C. B. (2002). Improved rural access to care: Dimensions of best practice. *Journal of Interprofessional Care, 16*(2), 117–128.

Kaplan, S., Calman, N., Golub, M., Ruddock, C., & Billings, J. (2006). The role of faith-based institutions in addressing health disparities: A case study of an initiative in the Southwest Bronx. *Journal of Health Care for the Poor and Underserved, 17*(2), 9–20.

Kim-Godwin, Y. S., Clarke, P., & Barton, L. (2001). A model for delivery of culturally competent care. *Journal of Advanced Nursing, 35*(6), 918–926.

Koffman, J., Morgan, M., Edmonds, P., Speck, P., & Higginson, I. J. (2008). Cultural meanings of pain: A qualitative study of Black Caribbean and White British patients with advanced cancer. *Palliative Medicine, 22,* 350–359.

Kulis, S., Marsiglia, F. F., Elek, E., Dustman, P., Wagstaff, D. A., & Hecht, M. L. (2005). Mexican/Mexican American adolescents and keeping it REAL: An evidence-based substance use prevention program. *Children & Schools, 27*(3), 133–145.

Kwong, E. W., & Lam, I. O. (2008). Chinese older people in Hong Kong: Health beliefs about influenza vaccination. *Nursing Older People, 20*(7), 29–33.

Lange, B. (2007). The prescriptive power of caring for self: Women in recovery from substance use disorders. *International Journal for Human Caring, 11*(2), 74–80.

Larson, K., Ott, M., & Miles, J. (2010). International cultural immersion: En vivo reflections on cultural competence. *Journal of Cultural Diversity, 17*(2), 44–50.

Little, C. M. (2003). Female genital circumcision: Medical and cultural considerations. *Journal of Cultural Diversity, 10*(1), 59–65.

Momoh, C. (2004). Attitudes to female genital mutilation. *British Journal of Midwifery, 12*(10), 631–635.

Morison, L., Dirir, A., Elmi, S., Warsame, J., & Dirir, S. (2004). How experiences and attitudes relating to female circumcision vary according to age on arrival in Britain: A study among young Somalis in London. *Ethnicity and Health, 9*(1), 75–100.

Nauright, L. (2005). Preparing nursing professionals for advocacy: Service-learning. In M. de Chesnay (Ed.), *Caring for the vulnerable* (pp. 357–362). Sudbury, MA: Jones and Bartlett.

Nauright, L., & Wilson, A. (2012). Preparing nursing professionals to be advocates: Service learning. In M. de Chesnay & B. Anderson (Eds.), *Caring for the vulnerable* (pp. 465–474). Burlington, MA: Jones & Bartlett Learning.

Naved, R. T., & Persson, L. (2008). Factors associated with physical spousal abuse of women during pregnancy in Bangladesh. *International Family Planning Perspectives, 34*(2), 71–78.

Ndiwane, A. (2008). Laying down the knife may decrease risk of HIV transmission: Cultural practices in Cameroon with implications for public health and policy. *Journal of Cultural Diversity, 15*(2), 2004–2008.

Pattison, N. (2008). Caring for patients after death. *Nursing Standard, 22*(51), 48–56.

Pearson, L. (2003). Understanding the culture of poverty. *Nurse Practitioner, 28*(4), 6.

Perilla, J., Wilson, A. H., Wold, J. L., & Spencer, L. (1998). Listening to migrant voices: Focus groups on health issues. *Journal of Community Health Nursing, 15*(4), 251–264.

Purnell, L. (2000). A description of the Purnell model for cultural competence. *Journal of Transcultural Nursing, 11*(1), 40–46.

Purnell, L. (2002). The Purnell model for cultural competence. *Journal of Transcultural Nursing, 13*(3), 193–196.

Purnell, L., & Paulanka, B. (2003). *Transcultural health care: A culturally competent approach* (2nd ed.). Philadelphia, PA: F. A. Davis.

Racher, F. E., & Annis, R. C. (2007). Respecting culture and honoring diversity in community practice. *Research and Theory for Nursing Practice: An International Journal, 21*(4), 255–270.

Savage, C. L., Xu, Y., Lee, R., Rose, B. L., Kappesser, M., & Anthony, J. S. (2006). A case study in the use of community-based participatory research in public health nursing. *Public Health Nursing, 23*(5), 472–478.

Stevens, C. A. (2006). Being healthy: Voices of adolescent women who are parenting. *Journal for Specialists in Pediatric Nursing, 11*(1), 28–41.

Tsai, J. H. (2006). Xenophobia, ethnic community, and immigrant youths' friendship network formation. *Adolescence, 41*(162), 285–299.

Turton, C. L. (1995). Spiritualized needs of hospitalized Ojibwe people. *Michigan Nurse, 68*(5), 11–12.

Wald, L. (1908). Best helps to the immigrant through the nurse. *American Journal of Nursing, 8*(6), 464–467.

Walle, A. H. (2004). Native Americans and alcoholism therapy: The example of Handsome Lake as a tool of recovery. *Journal of Ethnicity in Substance Abuse, 3*(2), 55–79.

Wells, M. (2000). Beyond cultural competence: A model for individual and institutional cultural development. *Journal of Community Health Nursing, 17*(4), 189–200.

Whaley, A. L. (2008). Cultural sensitivity and cultural competence: Toward clarity of definitions in cross-cultural counselling and psychotherapy. *Counselling Psychology Quarterly, 21*(3), 215–222.

Wilson, A. H., Pittman, K., & Wold, J. (2000). Listening to the quiet voices of Hispanic migrant children about health. *Journal of Pediatric Nursing, 15*(3), 137–147.

Wilson, A., Wold, J., Spencer, L., & Pittman, K. (2000). Primary health care for Hispanic children of migrant farm workers. *Journal of Pediatric Health Care, 14*(5), 209–215.

Wood, D. (2003). Effect of child and family poverty on child health in the United States. *Pediatrics, 112*(3), 707–711.

For a full suite of assignments and additional learning activities, use the access code located in the front of your book to visit this exclusive website: http://go.jblearning.com/londrigan. If you do not have an access code, you can obtain one at the site.

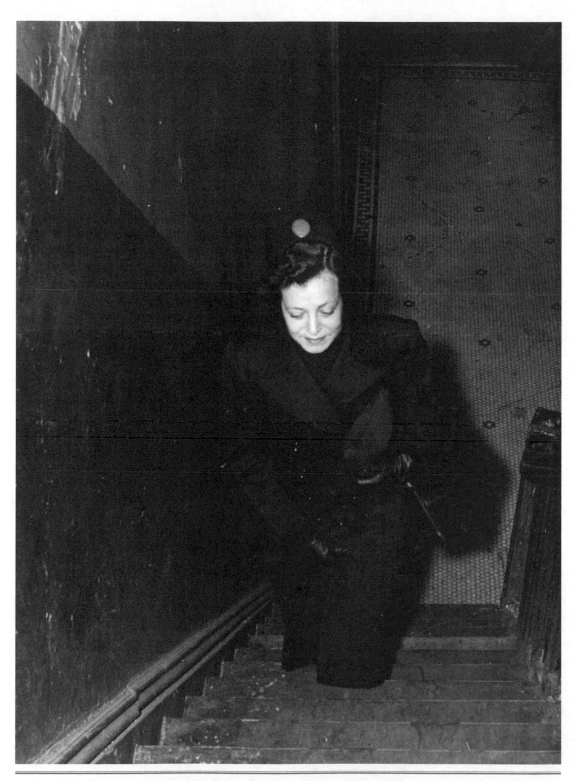

Source: Courtesy of the Visiting Nurse Service of New York.

Chapter 8

Healthcare Policy and Politics: The Risk and Rewards for Public Health Nurses

Donna M. Nickitas
Deborah Gardner

A comparison of the cost of treating tuberculosis patients in their homes and in hospitals is interesting and exceedingly important from an economic point of view. It costs no less than one dollar per day to care for one patient in a hospital. In most good hospitals the cost per day is from one dollar and fifty cents to two dollars and over. The sum so spent in caring for one patient for one year would be from four hundred to six hundred dollars. This sum is almost enough to supply a visiting nurse, who in one year, as has been shown, could and does visit from four to five hundred patients (Nutting, 1904, p. 501).

www

LEARNING OBJECTIVES

At the completion of this chapter, the reader will be able to

- Describe the relevance of healthcare policy and politics in public health nursing.
- Analyze the contextual factors that influence the development of federally funded healthcare policy.
- Identify ways in which public health nurses can participate politically in healthcare reform efforts.

www

KEY TERMS

- Advocacy
- Affordable Care Act (ACA)
- Economic Policy
- Influence

- Politics
- Public Policy
- Social policy

Why Care About Federal Policy?

While this question may seem rhetorical, perceptions of and experiences with the United States healthcare system can create the belief that to care about or try to understand federal policies on health care is fruitless. At least three issues contribute to this perspective. One prominent issue is the long-standing and interconnected problems the current system is unable to address: the rising costs of health care, the reduction in employer-based health care, the growing ranks of uninsured, and an inadequate supply of health providers. A second issue is that the U.S. healthcare system is a large and multipart healthcare complex that is rigidly hierarchical and not well coordinated or unified in purpose, scope, or values. And third, but interdependent with the previous issues, is that the politics and policies that shape the relationship between these inputs and outputs can seem extremely remote and hard to address. This chapter attempts to demonstrate that the linkages among these problems can be understood and that this knowledge is imperative for influencing and practicing public health nursing.

Public Health Nurses as a Political Force

Public health nurses have a professional obligation to articulate how intellectually demanding and complex public health nursing care is and to demonstrate the ways in which they have developed and implemented innovative models of care that promote health reform: expanding access, improving quality and safety, and reducing costs. Once public health nurses fully appreciate their political force, they are poised to influence healthcare policy. According to the U.S. Health Resources and Service Administration (2008), there are 3.1 million practicing nurses in the United States. As the largest segment of the healthcare workforce, nurses need to be full partners with other health professionals to achieve significant improvements at the local, national, and international levels in both the delivery and health policy arenas. As a professional partner, nurses have the expertise in care delivery, as well as the financial, technical, and political savvy to close clinical and financial gaps within a healthcare delivery system (Nickitas, 2011a). Yet, despite the large number of nurses in the workforce, they have not fully leveraged their strength to lead change, influence policy, and advance the health of the nation.

With more than three million members nationally, nurses can make a difference in policy and politics. For example, nurses have ranked high in public opinion polls, and the public believes that the endorsement by nurses for candidates for political office demonstrates a candidate's integrity. When divided by 435 congressional districts nationally, there are approximately 5,000 registered nurses per congressional

Lois Capps, Congresswoman from California uses her expertise as a school nurse in her political role.

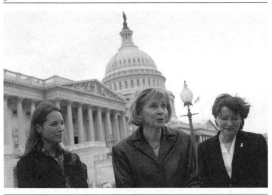

Source: © Kris Connor/Getty Images

district who can mobilize voters. The power of the "nursing numbers" has the capacity to convert votes that can make the difference in electing officials who support and endorse nursing's core values and issues.

Nursing is the most trusted profession and has been recognized as such for the past 11 years (Gallup, 2011a). Nurses continue to outrank other professions in Gallup's Annual Honesty and Ethics survey. Eighty-one percent of Americans say nurses have "very high" or "high" honesty and ethical standards, a significantly greater percentage than for the next-highest-rated professions, military officers and pharmacists.

Political Influence: A Call to Action

The recently released Institute of Medicine/ Robert Wood Johnson Foundation (IOM/RWJF) *The Future of Nursing: Leading Change, Advancing Health* strongly recommends that nurses become fully engaged in healthcare reform and policy by becoming involved with, speaking out about, and participating in the future of health care (IOM, 2011). Today's public health nurses are

pivotal in addressing population health, safety, and access to care. The opportunity to improve the health of communities and populations by understanding and influencing policy is a professional imperative.

Public health nurses have a responsibility to advocate for health care as a basic human right and ensure access to an affordable package of essential health services. They must use their collective political influence and become involved in the policymaking process. **Influence** is the ability to persuade or sway an individual or group to support or endorse a single issue (Adams, Chisari, Ditomassi, & Erickson, 2011). Adams (2009) suggests that influence is based on such factors as authority, status, knowledge-based competence, communication traits, and the use of time and timing. Learning to effectively use political influence to shape health and public policy is a key determinant in decision making, securing support and resources, as well as in motivation (Yukl & Falbe, 1990).

Policy issues affect all aspects of public health nursing, including promoting and protecting the health of population through health promotion and disease prevention. Public health nurses have had a distinguished history of **advocacy** in shaping health and public policy through the ages. For example, Lillian Wald and Lavinia Dock were early-20th century nursing leaders and activists who embraced the social issues of their day. Their professional advocacy and activism were centered in the belief that nurses were responsible for initiating and supporting action to meet the health and social needs of the public, in particular those of vulnerable populations (International Council of Nurses, 2006).

The Institute of Medicine (IOM) and the Robert Wood Johnson Foundation's (RWJF) landmark report, *The Future of Nursing: Leading Change, Advancing Health* (2011) calls for nurses to be better prepared with requisite competencies,

Early twentieth century nursing leader, Lavinia Dock advocated woman suffrage, equating the right to vote with better healthcare outcomes.

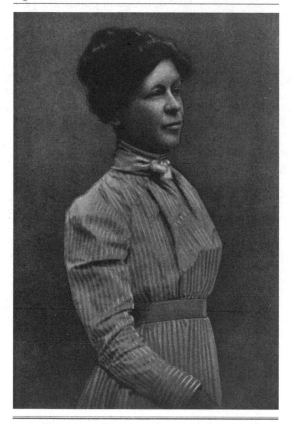

Source: Courtesy of the National Library of Medicine.

including leadership and health policy, as well as competency in specific content areas including community and public health, to deliver high-quality care. The commitment of public health nursing to societal well-being and access to health care cannot be overstated. Donna E. Shalala, Chair of the Robert Wood Johnson Foundation (RWJF) *Initiative of the Future of Nursing* at the IOM, recently stated, "...we cannot improve the quality of health care in our country without a central role for Nursing" (Nickitas, 2011b, p. 23). An example of nursing's expanded role to increase

access and provide healthcare delivery is the 2010 **Affordable Care Act.** It calls for an expanded role for nurses in the design of more efficient and cost-effective models of healthcare delivery (Daley, 2011). When public health nurses heed the call to political involvement in health and public policy, they not only advance the nursing profession but also improve the public's health (Hall-Long, 2009).

Public health nurses play a key role in shaping and influencing the delivery of health care. As a member of the healthcare workforce, public health nurses must understand the public policies and political forces creating the context for healthcare delivery in this country. While policy and politics may seem remote in day-to-day practice, they are the forces that drive the policies within a public health department, provide access to health resources for communities, and even decide who will breathe clean air. Resource constraints, policy, and politics are the levers continuously influencing consistency and change at all system levels. To serve your communities well, and to influence decision making that improves access, cost-effective quality, and safety, requires a basic understanding of this complex adaptive social system.

Defining Policy

The word *policy* is Greek in origin and is linked to citizenship (Online Dictionary of Social Sciences, n.d.). Policy represents the manifestations of ideology or belief systems about how the world should work (Rushefsky, 2008). **Public policy** is often used to describe government actions including, for example, economic and social policy. **Economic policy** promotes and regulates markets, while **social policy** seeks to improve the conditions of American society and achieve greater social equity (Aries, 2011).

Policy may be implemented through a variety of government systems, including the legislative, executive, or judicial branches of government.

Each of these systems has the authoritative capacity to direct or influence the actions, behaviors, or decisions of others (Block, 2008). As distinct systems, each branch of government plays a vital role in the formulation and regulation of health policy. It is important to know, in advance of influencing policy, which branch of government has the authority to legislate and regulate health care. For example, the legislative branch and executive branches of government had key roles in the formation and passage of the 2010 Affordable Care Act (ACA), and now the judicial branch is involved in the legality of the ACA as states challenge the federal mandate to make all Americans purchase healthcare coverage.

Policy and Values

Policy always had a moral dimension because it relates to decisions about how to act toward others. Leavitt (2009) described this moral approach as one that involves the choices a society or organization makes to reach a desired action. These actions reflect the values and beliefs of those who develop the policies. Furthermore, policy involves how and what resources should be used to achieve those policies. Thus, policies are often expressed as goals, programs, proposals, laws, and regulations that reflect the values and beliefs of those who are developing and directing the policies (Milstead, 2013).

Policies developed by nurses have frequently shown a strong belief in the importance of assisting people to care for themselves despite their illness or disability, and this belief has distinguished nursing's caring attribute from other professions. Caring is a value central to nursing. Watson (2008) suggests that to help the current healthcare system retain its most precious resource—competent, caring, professional nurses—a new generation of health professionals must ensure care and healing for the public, while learning about the value of serving others. If public health nurses want policies that reflect their nursing

A public health nurse participates in a community outreach program.

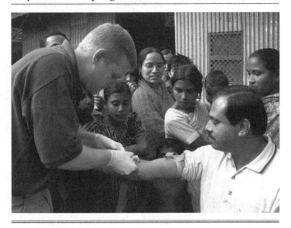

Source: Courtesy of CDC.

values, then they must get involved in the policy process to ensure their values are represented.

The long-standing interdependence of public policy, politics, and public health often makes it difficult to conceptualize or understand them separately. Public policy, like public health, is population-based. Policy encompasses the choices that a government makes regarding goals and priorities and the way it allocates resources to attain those goals. Public health is focused on society, seeking collectively to ensure the conditions in which people can be healthy. Public health, as a discipline, is interested in the equitable distribution of social and economic resources because they are such important influences on the health of populations (IOM, 1988). However, unlike public health, public policy reflects a broader array of competing values, beliefs, and attitudes espoused by those designing policy and the stiff competition for limited resources and immediate "felt" needs. Central to current debates are competing visions between public health and public policy. While the former field is increasingly cognizant of the need for a prevention focus, this approach conflicts with demands within the political field because it requires taking a shared long view and investing in the future. Paralleling this tension is a broader national policy debate that pits austerity against investment as the background of policy choices. Within the theoretical framework of The Public Health Nursing Practice Intervention Wheel, federal policy development and implementation are primary components of a public health intervention used at the system level of practice impacting the health of communities (Keller, Strohschein, & Briske, 2008).

Defining Politics

Politics is often described as the process of who gets to decide what will be done and when it will be done (Milstead, 2013). It involves power and influence for key decision making and requires significant investment in social capital. Public health nurses must understand how politics drives policy decisions and have the necessary skills and competencies to care for society and the populations they serve. Kraft and Furlong (2010) suggest that politics involves how conflicts in society are identified and resolved in favor of one set of priorities or values over another. Because resources (money, time, and personnel) are limited or finite, choices must be made. For public health nurses to have the ability to advocate resources for others and effectively shape policy, they must have the necessary political skill. This requires the ability to understand another's values and position and to use that understanding to influence others to act.

The importance of this chapter is that it will assist the reader in understanding the interface between new federal health policies that influence the public health of communities as well as public health nursing practices and the economic and political forces that are reciprocally threatening the implementation of these policies. By examining the landmark Affordable Care Act

Nursing leaders meet with President Obama.

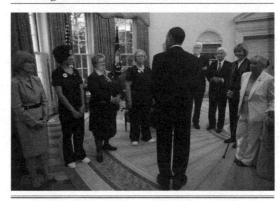

Source: Courtesy of Whitehouse.gov; official White House photo by Pete Souza.

legislation, enacted by the 111th United States Congress to remedy this nation's broken healthcare system, the challenges reformers are facing in implementing these policies will be described. The history and context that are shaping the fate of this legislation are outlined. The institutional politics at the national and state levels of government are explored. Additionally, the arguments that ushered in the new legislation, especially the critical need to control healthcare costs, connect prevention with quality care and patient safety, and to integrate technology for improving healthcare coordination will be presented. Regardless of partisan positioning, these areas provide tangible examples of issues that must be addressed in the redesign of a sustainable healthcare system that provides access to quality outcomes for all of our citizens regardless of income, race, or geographic location (Gostin, 2002).

What's Wrong With the Current U.S. Healthcare System?

In the healthcare reform debate, much has been said or written about whether or not the healthcare reform will work, what it might cost, and the impact it would have on each one of us as individuals. It has also been suggested from those who have great faith in our current system that it should be left alone. It may work well for some people, but on the whole our healthcare system ranks 37th out of 191 world health systems in the *World Health Report 2000* (World Health Organization, 2010), and our nation has the highest rate of preventable deaths among 19 industrialized nations (Cohen, 2009). In 2010, the number of nonelderly uninsured Americans reached 49.1 million, an increase reflecting a slow economy and a decline in employer-sponsored coverage. Increases in the uninsured largely reflect adults who have lost employer-based coverage and do not qualify for public coverage. This means that despite popular images of the uninsured, the majority of uninsured are working families. Low-income workers are at the greatest risk to be uninsured because job-based coverage is often not offered; even when it is, these workers are less able to afford the premiums. The lack of health insurance affects access to health care as well as increases costs. The uninsured delay or forgo needed care, making them more likely to be hospitalized for avoidable conditions. Overall, the uninsured are less likely to receive preventive care. Cost barriers to health care have been growing in the past decade, making the uninsured more likely than the insured to be unable pay for basic necessities because of their medical bills (The Henry J. Kaiser Family Foundation, 2011).

Arguably, one of the great strengths of the American healthcare system has been its strong private sector orientation, which facilitates ready access to all manner of services for those with stable coverage and strongly encourages ongoing medical innovation by product manufacturers. Our healthcare system has some of the finest medical facilities, technologies,

innovations, treatments, and human talent. Many of the world's best medical practitioners are here. Health care generates more new job opportunities than any other sector of our economy. The rapid advance of medical technology over the past 50 years has unquestionably improved the health status of millions of American citizens. Employer-sponsored insurance has played a crucial role in retaining this strong private sector presence in the U.S. health sector. However, employer-based coverage is also the Achilles' heel of American health care. One main failing is that it is not portable or owned by the worker. Moreover, because many millions of workers must change jobs and insurance frequently, there is little incentive for prevention. As employer-based health insurance costs continue to rise, those increases are being passed on to the employee through increased insurance premiums. Finally, today's open-ended federal tax exemption for some employer-paid premiums encourages expansive coverage, which further escalates cost (Capretta, 2009).

Despite its significant strengths, the U.S. healthcare system has long suffered from unequal access, disorganization, and waste (e.g., the value it provides does not match its enormous cost). Research conducted over many decades documents large disparities in the use of health care and in its cost from one location to another. These differences cannot be explained by contrasting rates or varying severity of illness among population groups. Furthermore, it is increasingly apparent that higher rates of healthcare use do not necessarily lead to better care; in fact, they sometimes lead to worse outcomes (Mechanic, 2011). Former White House advisor and bioethicist on health care, Ezekial Emanuel, notes that both political parties do agree that that our economy and our nation will not succeed if healthcare costs continue to rise. The fact that few people understand how much is spent on health care versus how much needs to be spent to provide quality care, and the difference between the two undermines the importance for needing to implement healthcare reform. He points out factually, that in 2010, the United States spent $2.6 trillion on health care, averaging over $8,000 per American, according to the Centers for Medicare & Medicaid. In comparing these costs to France, which has roughly a total gross domestic product of $2.6 trillion, the United States spent on health care what the 65 million people of France spent on everything including health care. The other important problem is growth. If healthcare costs continue to grow faster than the economy (present rate of 2% a year), it will be roughly one third of the entire economy by 2035 (Emmanuel, 2011).

How Does the Affordable Care Act Address Our Health System's Problems?

On March 23, 2010, President Barack Obama signed into law H.R. 3590, the Patient Protection and Affordable Care Act (P.L. 111-148) and seven days later signed H.R. 4872, the Health Care and Education Reconciliation Act of 2010 (P.L. 1101-152). The goals of this healthcare reform are to create a system that can provide healthcare coverage for all and no longer create personal bankruptcy. In other words, it was designed to help avoid economic disaster for employers and to hold all parties—doctors, nurses, hospitals, drug companies, and insurers—collectively responsible for making health care better, safer, and less costly (Gawande, 2009). The ACA was passed in an attempt to get policy aligned with these goals. The ACA puts in place comprehensive health

insurance reforms to increase access, guarantee more healthcare choices, invest in creating a new infrastructure that holds the potential to improve care quality, and contain costs for all Americans. Indeed, the sheer scope and complexity of the nation's healthcare system, as part of a larger political and global economic context, make the implementation of this new healthcare legislation a most formidable endeavor; this was the rationale for incremental implementation, with most changes taking place by 2014. But for the infrastructure to succeed, the tools developed by the ACA must be applied (Orszag, 2011).

Fortunately, some of the ACA provisions that increase access have been implemented and positively felt by the public. These include extending coverage for young adults to stay on their parents insurance until age 26; providing free preventive screenings to seniors on Medicare; filling in the Medicare part D "donut hole," which allows millions of seniors to receive checks for $250 (a first phase in closing the gap in drug costs thresholds), and making it illegal for insurance companies to impose lifetime limits on anyone or deny children insurance coverage for preexisting conditions. Starting in 2014, the ACA expands healthcare access for more Americans by preventing insurance companies from discriminating based on preexisting conditions, a clause particularly critical for the 13 million nonelderly adults previously denied coverage because of their medical conditions. Another step to increase access is the provision that employers with more than 50 employees will be expected to cover their employees' healthcare costs, with steep per-employee fines for violations. This legislation will require most Americans to have health insurance coverage and adds 16 million people to the Medicaid rolls. The combined legislation will extend coverage to an estimated

30 million uninsured Americans (The White House, 2011)

The law is estimated to cost the government about $938 billion over 10 years, according to the nonpartisan Congressional Budget Office (CBO, 2010). This same office has estimated that it will reduce the federal deficit by $143 billion over a decade and by $1 trillion over the next two decades by cutting government overspending and reining in waste, fraud, and abuse in Medicare, Medicaid, and Children's Health Insurance Program (CHIP). Efforts to combat fraud have returned more than $2.5 billion to the Medicare Trust Fund in fiscal year 2009 alone. The new law invests new resources and requires novel screening procedures for healthcare providers to boost these efforts (CBO, 2010).

The IOM's Quality Initiative, launched in 1996, was a tipping point in collective learning about and acknowledging how poorly the U.S. healthcare system was actually functioning. Documenting the serious nature and high costs of hospital errors on human health and safety became the foundation for clinical practice reform. For example, the IOM publication *To Err Is Human: Building a Safer Health System* found that medical error caused nearly 100,000 deaths and annually incurred an estimated $28–33 million in excess health costs. The reality that costs and quality were not aligned and that a serious chasm existed between what was known at that time to be quality care and what actually occurred in practice had a collective impact that has led to quality goals becoming institutionalized expectations (IOM, 2000).

For states to have a quality healthcare system requires a three-pronged approach: information, infrastructure and incentives (Fuchs, 2007). In line with Fuchs's three quality areas, the ACA focused on creating an infrastructure to learn what works for continuous quality improvement and to identify cost containment strategies. New institutions are in place to develop these efforts: The Patient-Centered Outcomes Research Institute (PCORI), the Center for Medicare and Medicaid Innovation (CMI), and the Independent Payment Advisory Board (IPAB, which starts in 2014). The success of this healthcare legislation in achieving quality care delivery and being affordable is critically dependent on these new centers working as intended in concert.

The PCORI, with the help of computerized records, will determine the "comparative effectiveness" of treatments. This is to strengthen evidence-based practice at a national level. As noted earlier, more health care does not necessarily equate to better health outcomes. Cost savings without compromising quality is the intention driving the strengthening of comparative effectiveness efforts. Similarly, the ACA calls for empowering an independent federal panel, the IPAB, to set Medicare rates free of pressure from providers and other interest groups. The Center for Medicare and Medicaid Innovation is providing funding to test payment models that emphasize the quality of care instead of the quantity of treatments delivered. Demonstration projects will be funded to develop models of care that are effective in the delivery of patient-centered care that is well coordinated and improves patient outcomes. One example of a new delivery system of care being developed is the Accountable Care Organization (ACO). Patient populations/communities would be provided a full spectrum of care services and proactively tracked from acute to home care experiences. But these steps may not be enough to bring about the change that many experts urge: to move away from a system in which we pay for every MRI or drug infusion on a case-by-case basis, and toward one in which salaried medical professionals are paid to do what it takes to keep the public healthy (Orszag, 2011).

What Is the Impact of the Affordable Care Act on Public Health?

One important theme of the health reform legislation is that of transforming our current medical-care system into a coordinated national healthcare system. While the ACA is about insurance coverage and costs, population health is a theme that runs through many aspects of the ACA. Among public health programs, for example, the ACA emphasizes community-based prevention. A population orientation pervades even the coverage provisions with no copay being required for evidence-based prevention service. In order to make health care available to all Americans, we would do well to remember the history of the first great expansion of coordinated public healthcare coverage when President Lyndon Johnson drove Medicare and Medicaid through Congress in 1965: "...the only sure way to bend the curve and curb the rate of increase in healthcare costs is to keep people out of the sick care system, to put as much profit in prevention as there is in acute care, and to put financial gain and pain into how individuals take (or don't take) care of themselves" (Califano, 2009).

Six months after the ACA was signed into law, the U.S. Department of Health and Human Services (U.S. DHHS) highlighted the importance of evidence-based preventive medicine by announcing nearly $100 million in grants made possible primarily by the new law's Prevention and Public Health Fund. These grants support a variety of critical public health programs in states' and local communities' efforts to fight obesity, increase HIV testing, promote tobacco cessation assistance, expand mental health and substance abuse programs, and track, monitor, and respond to disease outbreaks. The U.S. DHHS justified this effort as follows:

> *This investment in prevention and public health will pay enormous dividends both today and in the future, said HHS Secretary Kathleen Sebelius. In order to strengthen our health care system, we need to stop just focusing solely on sick care and start focusing more on proven evidence-based ways to keep people healthy in the first place. These grants made possible by the Affordable Care Act will support programs across the country that will make Americans healthier. (U.S. DHHS, 2010)*

The Prevention and Public Health Fund provides for an expanded and sustained national investment in prevention and public health programs including wellness and public health activities, prevention research, and health screenings and initiatives such as the Community Transformation Grants (CTG) program. The CTG program focuses on population health recognizing the priority health needs in communities. To reduce chronic diseases such as heart disease, cancer, stroke, and diabetes, these community programs promote prevention through healthy lifestyle practices. Almost $103 million was awarded to states and communities serving approximately 120 million Americans (CDC, 2010). The ACA also created a Council within U.S. DHHS to provide coordination and leadership at the federal level and among federal departments and agencies to develop a National Prevention Strategy. This Council sets goals and objectives for improving health through federally supported prevention, health promotion, and public health programs, in addition to making recommendations that can integrate healthcare practices.

Coverage for preventive health services is also provided by the ACA. Cost sharing is one strategy being used to control healthcare costs. The premise is that by having consumers pay a portion of their medical costs, such costs will be lowered by discouraging consumers from using care they do not really need. However, *any* copay for some would prohibit their purchasing care they did need such as not filling prescriptions and/or postponing visits to healthcare providers. As a result, basic evidence-based prevention practices will not require copayments to ensure these are available to all. For example, Medicare Part B coverage offers a personalized prevention plan with no copayment or deductible and includes a health risk assessment and other elements, such as updating family history, listing providers that regularly provide medical care to the individual, body mass index measurement, and other screenings for risk factors. The prevention plan would take into account the findings of the risk assessment and be completed prior to or as part of a visit to a health professional. Advice and referrals would be offered and might include community-based lifestyle interventions to reduce health risks and promote self-management and wellness, as well as screening schedules related to identified health risks. The new healthcare legislation also improves access to preventive services for eligible adults in Medicaid—for example, increasing access to immunizations and awarding grants to states to provide incentives to Medicaid beneficiaries with chronic illnesses who participate in healthy lifestyle programs and demonstrate changes in health risk and outcomes. The programs are currently funded for 5 years.

Other provisions in the ACA enhance funding for Community Health Centers, the National Health Service Corp (which provides care to underserved areas and populations), education and outreach campaigns regarding preventive benefits including birth control, and the operation of school-based health centers, with an emphasis on communities with barriers to accessing healthcare services. From improved nutritional labeling for standard menu items in chain restaurants to ensuring employers provide reasonable break times for nursing mothers and funding for the Childhood Obesity Demonstration Project, the new healthcare legislation is strongly focused on prevention and public health needs. The benefits for public health nursing practice are enormous (Trust for America's Health, 2010).

A note of caution: there are vulnerabilities and challenges regarding public health programs. Although the ACA has given historically high attention to prevention and public health, legislative history also shows the field's vulnerabilities, especially in funding. Historically, population-oriented public health programs have often lost out relative to other priorities. We will have to work intelligently to be sure that this history is not repeated.

What Is the Federal Government's Role in American Society: Is Health Care a Right?

The ACA has been in the eye of a political storm since its inception. Claims that health reform will fail continue to be spoken, just as threats of repeal were voiced even while President Obama was signing both Acts into law. Republicans and conservatives have continued to level criticism against the law since it was passed in March 2010, while President Obama has been vigorous in defending its objectives and future benefits. The public has heard these attacks on the reform loud and clear. According to a Gallup poll on healthcare reform taken in November 2011, 47% of Americans favored repealing the

2010 Patient Protection and Affordable Care Act, while 42% still favor keeping it. Views on this issue are highly polarized and highly partisan, with Republicans strongly in favor of repeal and the large majority of Democrats wanting the law retained. Americans' views on repealing the healthcare law mirror their reactions to its passage. In October 2010, Gallup found 40% of Americans saying passage of the healthcare law was a good plan and 48% a bad direction. Clearly, the public sentiment over the ACA reflects a deep polarization as well (Gallup Poll, 2011b).

Beyond public opinion, there are ongoing as well as new obstacles facing the implementation of the healthcare bill. For instance, opponents of the ACA have filed legal challenges and the Supreme Court has decided to review the healthcare law's constitutionality (the ruling is expected to be issued by the summer of 2012). Much of the controversy has centered on the individual mandate. Beginning January 1, 2014, most people will be required to have health insurance or pay a fine. At issue is whether the provision is constitutional; if not, can it be deleted from the rest of the law. The court will also determine whether the penalty is equivalent to a tax and therefore cannot be challenged until after it is actually levied on someone. The second issue the Supreme Court will consider is the constitutionality of expanding Medicaid. The ACA expands eligibility for the joint state–federal healthcare program to cover a greater number of poor and disabled (Barnes, November 15, 2011).

Thus, the law's ultimate fate may be in the court's hands, rather than that of the Congress. Regardless, it will be a dominant issue in the 2012 presidential campaign.

In light of the ACA's uncertainty and the reality of state budgets being cut, the states have been hesitant to set up health exchanges. Exchanges are a new kind of state-oriented health insurance market allowing individuals and small businesses access to competitive insurance rates and that offer a streamlined way to shop for insurance. In states that choose not to set exchanges, the federal government will set them up. To compromise between regulatory/public program advocates and advocates for private/market driven programs, Medicaid and state health insurance exchanges are the strategies used to increase healthcare coverage, each of which is projected to cover approximately 16 million uninsured Americans (Jacobi, Watson, & Restuccia, 2011). State-level reform is crucial to effectiveness of the ACA implementation. The House of Representatives voted to repeal the ACA and have compromised the funding necessary to administer it. In short, the obstacles appear to be expanding. Because key provisions were not slated to begin until 2014, both skeptics and supporters have time to assess the law, its prospects for success and, of course, its forecasted cost (Gallup Poll, 2011b).

Debate over the ACA before it was even passed and ever since has focused largely on its implications for the role of the federal government in American society. Americans remain divided on whether it is the federal government's responsibility to make sure all Americans have health care: 50% say yes, while 46% disagree (Gallup Poll, 2011b). Critics of the healthcare law argue that it is an example of too much government control over things that should be left to individuals and to private businesses. A majority of Americans agree that a private healthcare system is better than a government-run system, although proponents of the law can point out that it falls short of mandating a government-run healthcare system like those in Canada or European countries.

At the same time, one half of Americans say the federal government should be responsible for making sure all Americans have health insurance, underscoring the divided nature of public opinion on this issue. About one in four American adults at this point have government-provided health insurance, making it clear that the issue going forward is the degree to which government should be involved in health care in the years ahead, rather than whether the government should get out of the healthcare business altogether (Gallup Poll, 2011b).

How Does History Shape Health Care?

Healthcare reform has been long desired by Democratic presidents. President Franklin D. Roosevelt wanted national insurance included in Social Security. President Harry S Truman proposed a national healthcare program with a multi-payer insurance fund. Since then, every Democratic president and several Republican presidents have wanted to provide affordable coverage to more Americans. President Bill Clinton offered the most ambitious proposal in 1993–1994 and suffered the most spectacular failure (Stolberg & Pear, 2010). Despite these daunting precedents, the election of President Barack Obama was seen by most Democrats as a public mandate on healthcare reform. One of the most significant differences between the Clinton reform efforts and those of President Obama is that employers, corporations, and insurance companies, all alarmed at the soaring cost of health care, agreed that changes were necessary. However, as the bills were drafted, these powerful stakeholders became strong opponents of some Democratic proposals, especially one known as the "Public Option" to create a government-run insurance plan as an alternative to their offerings.

The country's economic problems, starting with those confronting President Franklin Roosevelt at the start of the Great Depression, are repeatedly evoked as a comparable historic reference. The Great Recession, prompted by overspeculation in finance and brought to light with the housing market collapse, demanded immediate and deliberate actions of risky, unprecedented proportions early in the Obama presidency. Critics argued that the U.S. economy, energy independence, major foreign policy decisions regarding the conflicts in Iraq and Afghanistan needed attention more than healthcare reform. In fact, the economy's relentless slide in late 2008 changed the Obama team's agenda. As president-elect, he was forced to contend with whether or not to bail out the financial system and how to keep General Motors and Chrysler from going under (Stolberg & Pear, 2010). The Obama administration argued that in the long-term view, the skyrocketing cost of health care was another huge domestic threat to the nation's economic balance sheet. The fact that the country's health care is the most expensive in the world and growing faster than the gross domestic product, forcing over one million people into bankruptcy, could not be ignored (Gawande, 2009). To extend medical coverage to everyone was also a way to bring costs into control, and thus healthcare reform was presented as an issue integral issue to economic stability.

President Obama's first major initiative incorporated the two inseparable issues into a stimulus package to pump money into a downward-spiraling economy. In February 2009, three weeks after President Obama's inauguration, Congress passed the massive $787 billion American Recovery and Reinvestment Act (ARRA) in an effort to create jobs, stimulate economic activity, and increase transparency in government spending. Republicans derided the bill as unaffordable and excessive. Under the aegis of economic recovery, ARRA set aside more that $149 billion, enabling extensive provisions to address both immediate and long-term deficiencies in the healthcare infrastructure. For example, $25 billion was provided to help unemployed Americans retain and extend their healthcare coverage under the Consolidated Omnibus Budget Reconciliation Act, low-income Americans were able to keep their Medicare coverage despite state budget short-falls with $87 billion marked to increase federal support for Medicaid cost million, $1 billion was allocated toward prevention and wellness programming, and $25 billion was investing for computerizing medical records to reduce costs and ensure patient privacy in records exchange. Furthermore, ARRA provided $1.1 billion for comparative effectiveness research, $500 million in training funds for the next generation of healthcare professionals, and a $2 billion investment in community health centers and healthcare technology for at-risk communities (Foundation, 2009). This impact of these efforts continues to receive strongly polarized reactions from the public and Congress.

The Economy, Polarization, Public Confusion, and Misinformation: Will the Affordable Care Act Survive?

It has been noted by leading economists that the United States is in the middle of the worst economic crisis since the 1930s (Washingtonsblog, 2010). With austerity versus investment as the background of national debate, the political budget themes of big government spending and the federal budget's mammoth deficit have

continued to take turns holding the spotlight as Congress was unable to pass a budget for Fiscal Year 2012. However, these polarizing themes of political rhetoric reflect simplistic answers to our complex economic problems. Federal fiscal policy is comprised of three main decision components: (1) the amount of money the federal government should spend on public programs; (2) the amount it should take in as tax revenues; and (3) how much of a deficit (or surplus) the federal government should run, which is the difference between (2) and (1). Similarly, three categories comprise federal spending: discretionary, mandatory, and interest paid on the nation's debt. Discretionary programs must have their funding renewed each year in order to continue operating. Examples of discretionary spending include defense, budgets for K–12 education, health research, and housing. Altogether, discretionary programs make up about one third of all federal spending. The other two thirds of government spending is for entitlement programs; such programs include Social Security, Medicare, Medicaid, and certain other programs (e.g., food stamps, federal civilian and military retirement benefits, veterans' disability benefits, and unemployment insurance). Entitlement programs are not controlled by annual appropriations (Center on Budget and Policy Priorities, 2010). The spending to continue the entitlement programs is rising dramatically, consuming an increasingly larger share of the federal budget, and for good reason. As the baby boomers age, there has been a surge in retirements, and the costs for Medicare and Social Security are increasing proportionally. Not many would call this wasteful spending. However, as the number of contributors to Social Security and Medicare is decreasing, this is creating significant cost increases with less viability for sustainment.

However, it is the discretionary programs that are consistently pointed to in budget debates, not the entitlement programs that make up two thirds of the budget costs. Only in this current recession has the idea of touching the entitlement programs received such sustained attention. When conservatives state that "deficits can be reduced and taxes cut by eliminating wasteful spending by big government," it isn't clear what discretionary spending programs are wasteful or out of control. While some government programs deserve the ax, education, transportation, and defense are already facing draconian cuts.

What is increasingly problematic is this country's ability to sustain the current benefits offered in the entitlement programs if they are not trimmed or new revenues are not sought. The current economic situation makes Medicaid, which is a joint federal–state health program for the poor and disabled (and politically powerless), most vulnerable for severe cuts. Because states cannot run deficits, many governors are straining under overstretched budgets in this recession. They argue there are more people in need and less revenue, and the plan to expand Medicaid under health reform will be too expensive; as such, they will not be able to provide matching funds. Health reformers argue that extending coverage will allow for more prevention and early interventions of care that will reduce costs in the long run (Klein, May 6, 2011). Medicare, which is the entitlement program that provides health insurance for people 65 or older and for younger people with certain disabilities, covers over 47 million people.

Then there is the issue of revenue. On the other side of the aisle, liberals are claiming that the deficit can be reduced by taxing the rich and cutting defense spending. While "taxing the rich" doesn't impact many people and raising rates can be justified, it will not do much to balance the budget. Democrats are fighting the idea of higher eligibility ages to reflect longer life expectancies. The idea that wealthier retirees

should receive less Social Security and pay more for Medicare must be considered and entitlements trimmed. The revenue side of increasing taxes is an untouchable subject with Republicans. The fact that Congress did not make tough decisions regarding how to pay for the wars in Iraq and Afghanistan is part of the deficit we now face. The truth is that both the polarized conservative and liberal rhetoric do not match reality. There is a gray area and complexity to it all. Big government is a reality and much of what it does is valued. It can also get too big. Discretionary spending can be cut, but again not to levels that will really balance the budget. Congress will need to identify justifiable spending cuts and there will be pain. Tax increases are necessary and will need to be sizeable. At the time of this writing, it is not clear if the supercommittee—12 members of Congress charged with devising a plan to deal with a mammoth deficit—will succeed (Samuelson, November 7, 2011).

As previously discussed, the ACA will cost the government about $938 billion over 10 years (CBO, 2010), but the country spends more than twice that much on health care in a single year (*U.S. Health Care,* n.d.). The debate over helping the uninsured is tangled with the other major challenge of slowing the growth of overall healthcare spending. Republicans ridicule the idea, arguing that expanding coverage and saving money is simply impossible. Reformers acknowledge the upfront expense in trying to cover the 47 million uninsured Americans but say parallel attempts to "bend the curve" on spending by implementing the other infrastructure strategies described earlier would reduce costs over the long run for everyone. The rationale is that it makes sense to do both at the same time—to provide the broader coverage with cost control.

It will be several years before the country can expect stronger economic growth to provide more revenue. Even then, the ability of economic growth to translate into more "affordable" social resources deserves skepticism, especially considering the state of health care in a previously "strong" economy. Indeed, with healthcare costs continuing to increase, health care remains a core issue in our long-term national struggle for fiscal balance.

State Responses to the Affordable Care Act

The Commonwealth Fund Commission's report, the 2009 *State Scorecard on U.S. Health System Performance*, examines trends on states' progress toward achieving systems and models of health care that meet their residents' needs. This report examines how states compare on 38 key indicators of healthcare access, quality, costs, and health outcomes. The findings of the report conclude these indicators vary significantly depending on the state that you live in. The scorecard findings reflect deteriorating coverage for adults and rising costs, with broad geographic disparities and strong evidence of poorly coordinated care (McCarthy, How, Sabrina, Schoen, Cantor, & Belloff, 2009).

States have an extensive and complicated shared-power relationship with the federal government in regulating various aspects of the health insurance market and in enacting health reforms. The passage of the ACA health insurance reform legislation was met with immediate and hostile state resistance. Members of 39 state legislatures proposed to limit, alter, or oppose selected state or federal actions, primarily targeted at single-payer provisions and mandates that require purchase of insurance (Cauchi, 2012). There is no doubt that the ACA's sprawling provisions raise a wealth of implementation challenges for states. The ACA also creates a host of opportunities for states to expand access to care, improve quality, and achieve greater efficiency in their healthcare systems. A major

challenge for state leaders is to find the resources necessary to pursue these opportunities in this current economic environment.

However, many states are moving forward with delivery system reform. For example, over 30 states have engaged in efforts to implement programs to advance medical homes in Medicaid/CHIP programs (RWJF, 2011).

Another model of care that states are developing and testing is entitled The State Action on Avoidable Rehospitalizations (STAAR). Using the state as the unit of intervention, the Institute for Healthcare Improvement initiative is providing technical assistance working in four states: Massachusetts, Michigan, Washington, and Ohio. STAAR engages clinicians and other providers across varied delivery sites with the goal of improving quality of care, the patient experience, and reducing avoidable utilization through a multi-stakeholder process to reduce rehospitalizations. Well-functioning transitions of care can reduce preventable hospital readmissions and lead to improved outcomes for patients (RWJF, 2011).

Many states are considering what potential role public health can play in a transformed health system. Leveraging the public health system with the ACA to effectively and strategically partner with the healthcare system will improve access to quality, affordable, and integrated care while also promoting chronic disease prevention. Colorado and Washington are examples of two states that are redesigning their public health efforts using a more systemic perspective. Washington has developed a state strategic road map showing how various agencies within the Department of Health will connect to local, state, federal, and private sector partners. Additional elements guiding new ways in which the department conducts business include retraining the public health workforce, modifying and modernizing business practices, and developing long-term strategies for predictable and appropriate levels of financing (Washington Department of Health, 2010). Colorado is one of four states across the country testing a chronic disease prevention integration model under a demonstration project through the Centers for Disease Control and Prevention. One significant strategy that the state is implementing in its Department of Health and Environment is to restructure its Prevention Services Division to move from disease categories (e.g., tobacco, HIV) to functions, allowing greater flexibility to respond to emerging public health issues that cross categorical program boundaries. Additionally, a new unit was also developed to identify the public health role in the new environment of health reform, taking a comprehensive approach to health outcomes (RWJF, 2011).

A considerable amount of energy and resources are focused on health information technology (HIT) and health information exchange (HIE) at both the state and federal level. The Health Information Technology for Economic and Clinical Health Act within ARRA provides states with substantial funding to support health information technology investment. Some states, like Massachusetts, Oregon, and Rhode Island, already had legislation or strategic plans in place to support the adoption of HIT and HIE before the passage of these federal provisions. While these states started early, all states are in the process of undertaking such work, and the federal government has awarded funding to all 50 states, the District of Columbia, and eligible territories through the State HIE Cooperative Agreement Program. This program is designed to support states as they develop the capacity necessary to exchange information within their state and across states (Office of the National Coordinator for Health Information Technology, 2010).

While other viable health delivery models continue to emerge at the state level, early attempts from such states as Colorado, Washington, Oregon, and Ohio demonstrate the promise of innovative state reform efforts that are attempting to improve access while actively evaluating cost-effectiveness and quality changes.

Understanding Policy Making and Public Health Nursing

Using the ACA as an example, we can see how a problem is identified and put on a policy agenda, where a plan to address said problem is developed, adopted, implemented, evaluated, and extended or modified (Hanley & Falk, 2007). This policy process is much like the nursing process: *assess, plan, implement, evaluate, assess again*. Again, using the IOM (2011) report, nurses are considered the agent who will transform the healthcare system, ensuring care is patient-centered, effective, safe, and affordable. This vision calls upon the entire nursing community to embrace this report as a blueprint for action, and requires each and every nurse to use evidence-based research and collaboration to improve health care.

Public health nurses are well positioned because their access to the community and consumer groups helps to raise public awareness about health disparities, the quality of care, or lack of access to care for the communities they serve. Public health nurses and consumers collectively can develop ideas and propose policies to solve problems of healthcare access, health disparities, safety, or quality of care.

Public Health Nurses and Political Engagement

Public health nurses' engagement in policy and politics must rise to the level of influence whereby changes in healthcare reform are fully realized. Political engagement is viewed as a continuum that extends from no engagement in politics to that of extreme activism. Individuals may choose how much they wish to engage politically throughout their lives in response to their intrinsic and external motivators, time and energy, and resources.

For the public health nurse, time is a valuable resource; therefore, investing one's time in political engagement may vary from nurse as citizen to nurse as activist. The classic description of the various levels of political activism comes from the work of Kalisch and Kalisch (1982). They have described individual political participation along the continuum ranging from spectator activities, to transitional activities, to gladiatorial activities (p. 316). For example, nurses who wonder what's happening vote occasionally or not at all; they are not involved in improving their workplace or their community. Nurses who watch things happen are spectators: they expose themselves to political stimuli, they are members of their union, they vote, sometimes they wear buttons or put bumper stickers on cars, and they participate in community activities that are important. It is essential for public health nurses to become involved in political action activities, especially to be involved in their professional or membership organizations. Numbers count and organizations that represent nurses, especially those with political action committees (PACs) and contribute to political campaigns, are valuable. Because "money talks" and buys influence, contributing to candidates that promote nursing's agenda to advance the nation's health through healthcare reform is important. It is unfortunate that campaigns are expensive, but it costs money to buy television ad time and to mail literature to people's homes.

Public health nurses must participate in the political process and not stand on the sidelines waiting for things happen. There are many ways to participate in the political process, including becoming active members of a political party; attending political meetings, forums, and rallies; helping register people to vote; or contributing and raising money for causes and campaigns through PACs; the American Nurses Association Political Action Committee (ANA-PAC) has grown over the years through nurse contributions. Song (2011) states, "ANA does not use dues dollars to support candidates. Rather, ANA-PAC raises money through the voluntary donations from member nurses across the country. ANA-PAC donates to candidates who work to implement healthy public policy for our profession" (p. 15).

Using Data to Leverage Gaps in Healthcare Quality

Public health nurses know that there are persistent quality and access gaps for minority and low-income groups. These groups have greater health disparities around specific services including cancer screening, management of diabetes, and access to care. To better assist public health nurses to address the gaps in quality and access, publicly reported sources of county and state data can inform populations, settings, and potential strategies to promote population health. These data provide information about the important problems confronting communities and compare them to other states and counties. Public health nurses then can use the data to evaluate organizational processes and outcomes to determine if there is an opportunity to improve the health of populations they serve. Using evidence to leverage interventions and actions to improve the health care of populations is how public nurses increase their influence in the public policy arena. The authors of this chapter recommend that the reader examine Chapter 13—*Getting the Word Out: Advocacy, Social Marketing, and Policy Development and Enforcement*—to explore further public health nurses' intervention strategies.

Public health nurses must ensure that their voices and interests are represented in the legislature at the state and federal levels. For example, professional nursing interest groups have seized on the public's frustration with rising healthcare costs and promoted policies that emphasize the cost-effectiveness of advanced practice nurses. It is up to the public health nurses themselves to inform and educate society about the ways in which nursing contributes to society.

Conclusion

Health and public policy continue to experience turbulent change as the Affordable Care Act moves toward full implementation. Public health nurses must use effective strategies to achieve policy goals. To accomplish these goals, public health nurses must understand policy and be familiar with sources of policy at all levels of government. Real successes for political influence and policy implementation occur when public health nurses are prepared, engaged, and respond to or lead change to advance the health of the nation.

References

Adams, J. M. (2009). *The Adams Influence Model (AIM): Understanding the factors, attributes and process of achieving influence.* Saarbrucken, Germany: VDM Verla.

Adams, J. M., Chisari, G., Ditomassi, M., & Erickson, J. I. (2011). Understanding and influencing policy: An imperative to the contemporary nurse leader. *Voice of Nursing Leadership, 9*(4), 4–7.

Aries, N. (2011). To engage or not engage: Choices confronting nurses and other health professionals. In D. Nickitas, D. Middaugh, & N. Aries (Eds.), *Policy and politics for nurses and other health professionals.* Sudbury, MA: Jones & Bartlett Publishers.

Barnes, R. (November 15, 2011). *Court to review health overhaul* (pp. A1, A16). Washington, DC: Washington Post.

Block, L. E. (2008). Health policy: What it is and how it works. In C. Harrington & C. L. Estes (Eds.), *Health policy: Crisis and reform in the U.S. health delivery system* (pp. 4–14). Sudbury, MA: Jones and Bartlett.

Califano, J. (2009). Bending the curve requires health care reform, not just sick care reform: A history lesson. *Kaiser Health News.* Retrieved from http://www.kaiserhealthnews.org/Columns/2009/August/081009Califano.aspx

Capretta, J. (2009). Healthcare in the United States: Strengths, weaknesses & the way forward. Plenary Address from CBHD's 15th Annual Conference: *Healthcare and the Common Good.* Retrieved from http://cbhd.org/content/healthcare-united-states-strengths-weaknesses-way-forward

Cauchi, R. (2012). State legislation challenging certain health reforms. National Conference of State Legislatures. Retrieved from: http://www.ncsl.org/default.aspx?tabid=18906

Center on Budget and Policy Priorities. (2010). *Policy basics: Introduction to the federal budget process.* Retrieved from http://www.cbpp.org/files/3-7-03bud.pdf

Centers for Disease Control and Prevention (CDC). (2010). *Community transformation grants: States and communities program descriptions.* Retrieved from http://www.cdc.gov/communitytransformation/funds/programs.htm

Cohen, P. (2009). How health care reform can improve public health. Retrieved from http://www.kevinmd.com/blog/2009/10/health-care-reform-improve-public-health.html

Commonwealth Fund Initiative Congressional Budget Office (CBO). (2010). *How is the Patient Protection and Affordable Care Act (ACA) funded?* Retrieved from http://www.acponline.org/advocacy/where_we_stand/access/internists_guide/i2-how-is-the-aca-funded.pdf

Daley, K. (2011). From Your ANA President: Nurses lead the way. *American Nurse Today, 6*(5), 18.

Emmanuel, E. (2011). Spending more doesn't make us healthier. *The New York Times Opinionator.* Retrieved from http://opinionator.blogs.nytimes.com/2011/10/27/spending-more-doesnt-make-us-healthier/

Foundation, T. H. (2009, March). *Kaiser Commission on Medicaid Facts.* Retrieved from Foundation, The Henry J Kaiser Family http://www.kff.org/medicaid/upload/7872.pdf

Fuchs, V. R. (2007). What are the prospects for enduring comprehensive health care reform? *Health Affairs, 26*(6), 1542–1544. Retrieved from http://content.healthaffairs.org/content/26/6/1542.full

Gallup Poll. (2011a). *Public rate nursing on most honest & ethical profession.* Retrieved from http://www.gallup.com/poll/9823/public-rates-nursing-most-honest-ethical-profession.aspx

Gallup Poll. (2011b). *Americans tilt toward favoring repeal of healthcare law.* Retrieved from http://www.gallup.com/poll/150773/Americans-Tilt-Toward-Favoring-Repeal-Healthcare-Law.aspx

Gawande, A. (2009, January 26). *Getting there from here: How should Obama reform health care? The New Yorker,* 26–33. Retrieved from The New Yorker website: http://www.newyorker.com/reporting/2009/01/26/090126fa_fact_gawande

Gostin, L. (2002). Public health law, ethics, and human rights: mapping the issues. *Public health law and ethics: A reader.* Retrieved from http://www.publichealthlaw.net/Reader/ch1/ch1.htm

Hall-Long, B. (2009). Nursing and public policy: A tool for excellence in education, practice, and research. *Nursing Outlook, 57*(2), 78–83.

Hanley, B., & Falk, N. L. (2007). Policy development and analysis: Understanding the process. In D. J. Mason, J. K. Leavitt, & M. W. Chaffee (Eds.), *Policy and politics in nursing and health care* (5th ed., pp. 75–93). St. Louis, MO: Saunders/Elsevier.

Health Resources and Services Administration. (2008). *National Sample Survey of Registered Nurses.* Retrieved from http://datawarehouse.hrsa.gov/nursingsurvey.aspx

Institute of Medicine (IOM). (1988). *The future of public health.* Retrieved from http://iom.edu/Reports/1988/The-Future-of-Public-Health.aspx

Institute of Medicine (IOM). (2000). *To err is human: Building a safer health system.* Retrieved from http://www.nap.edu/openbook.php?record_id=9728&page=1

Institute of Medicine (IOM). (2011). *The future of nursing: leading change, advancing health.* Washington, DC: National Academies Press.

International Council of Nurses. (2006). Code of ethics. Retrieved from http://www.icn.ch/ethics.htm

Jacobi, J., Watson, S., & Restuccia, R. (2011). Implementing health reform at the state level: Access and care for vulnerable populations. *Using law, policy, and research to improve the public's health.* Retrieved from http://www.aslme.org/media/downloadable/files/links/1/5/15.Jacobi.pdf

Kalisch, B., & Kalisch, P. (1982). *Politics of nursing.* Philadelphia, PA: Lippincott.

Keller, L., Strohschein, S., & Briske, L. (2008). Population-based public health nursing practice: The intervention wheel. In M. Stanhope & J. Lancaster (Eds.), *Public health nursing: Population-centered health care in the community.* Retrieved from http://www.courwareobjects.com/evolve/E2/book_pages/stanhope/pdfs/Stanhope_Ch09.pdf

Klein, E. (2011, May 6). Medicaid, no medicare, at most risk. The Washington Post, A19.

Kraft, M., & Furlong, S. (2010). *Public policy: Politics, analysis, and alternatives* (3rd ed.). Washington, DC: CQ Press.

Leavitt, J. (2009). Leaders in health policy: A critical role for nursing. *Nursing Outlook, 57*(2), 73–77.

McCarthy, D., How, S., Sabrina K., Schoen, C., Cantor, J., & Belloff, D. (2009). *Aiming higher: Results from a State Scorecard on Health System Performance, 2009.* Commonwealth Fund, October 2009. Retrieved from http://www.commonwealthfund.org/Publications/Fund-Reports/2009/Oct/2009-State-Scorecard.aspx

Mechanic, D. (2011). The brilliant, persistent pursuit of health care as a complex social system: A book review. *Health Affairs, 30*(2), 362–363.

Milstead, J. (2013). *Health policy and politics: A nurse's guide* (4th ed.). Burlington, MA: Jones & Bartlett Learning.

Nickitas, D. (2011a). Nurses. In D. Nickitas, D. Middaugh, & N. Aries (Eds.) *Policy and politics for nurses and other health professionals.* Sudbury, MA: Jones and Bartlett.

Nickitas, D. (2011b). Defining nursing's expanded role in health care: An interview with Donna Shalala. *Nursing Economic$, 29*(1), 23.

Nutting, M. A. (1904). Visiting nurses in the homes of tuberculosis patients. *American Journal of Nursing, 4*(7), 500–506.

Office of the National Coordinator for Health Information Technology. (2010). *State Health Information Exchange Cooperative Agreement Program.* Retrieved from http://healthit.hhs.gov/portal /server.pt?open=512 &objID=1488

Online Dictionary of Social Sciences. (n.d.). *Politics.* Retrieved from http://bitbucket.icaap.org/dict.pl?alpha=P

Orszag, P. (2011). How health care can save or sink America: The case for reform and fiscal sustainability. *Foreign Affairs, 90*(4), 42–56.

Robert Wood Johnson Foundation. (2011). Chapter 8: State efforts improve quality, contain costs and improve health. *State of the states initiatives.*

Retrieved from http://www.statecoverage.org/stateofthestates2011

Rushefsky, M. (2008). *Public policy in the United States: At the dawn of the 21st century* (4th ed.). Armonk, NY: M. E. Sharpe.

Samuelson, R. (2011, November 7). Busting the budget myths. *The Washington Post*, A19.

Song, A. (2011). Defining ANA-PAC's role in the political process. *American Nurse, 43*(3), 15.

Stolberg, S. G., and Pear, R. (2010). Obama signs health care overhaul bill, with a flourish. *The New York Times Online*. Retrieved from http://www.nytimes.com/2010/03/24/health/policy/24health.html

The Henry J. Kaiser Family Foundation. (2011). *The uninsured and the difference health insurance makes*. Retrieved from www.kff.org/uninsured/upload/1420-13.pdf

The White House. (2011). Get the facts straight on health reform. *Health Reform in Action.* Retrieved from http://www.whitehouse.gov/healthreform/myths-and-facts#healthcare-menu

Trust for America's Health. (2010). *Patient Protection and Affordable Care Act (HR 3590) Selected Prevention, Public Health & Workforce Provisions.* Retrieved from http://healthyamericans.org/assets/files/Summary.pdf

U.S. Department of Health and Human Services (U.S. DHHS). (2010). HHS awards nearly $100 million in grants for public health and prevention priorities. *News Release.* Retrieved from http://www.hhs.gov/news/press/2010pres/09/20100924a.html

US Health Care. (n.d.). Retrieved from Politics Central.com http://politicscentral.com/us-health-care/

Washingtonsblog. (2010, February 23). *Naked capitalism.* Retrieved from Guestpost http://www.nakedcapitalism.com/2010/02/guest-post-greenspan-says-greenspan-worst-financial-crisis-ever-including-the-great-depression.html

Washington Department of Health. (2010). *An agenda for change.* Retrieved from http://www.doh.wa.gov/PHSD/doc/AgendaForChange.pdf

Watson, J. (2008). Social justice and human caring: A model of caring science as a hopeful paradigm for moral justice and humanity. *Creative Nursing, 14*, 54–61.

World Health Organization (WHO). (2000). *World Health Organization assesses the world's health systems.* Retrieved from http://www.who.int/whr/2000/media_centre/press_release/en/

Yukl, G., & Falbe, C. M. (1990). Influence tactics in upward, downward, and lateral influence attempts. *Journal of Applied Psychology, 75*, 132–140.

For a full suite of assignments and additional learning activities, use the access code located in the front of your book to visit this exclusive website: http://go.jblearning.com/londrigan. If you do not have an access code, you can obtain one at the site.

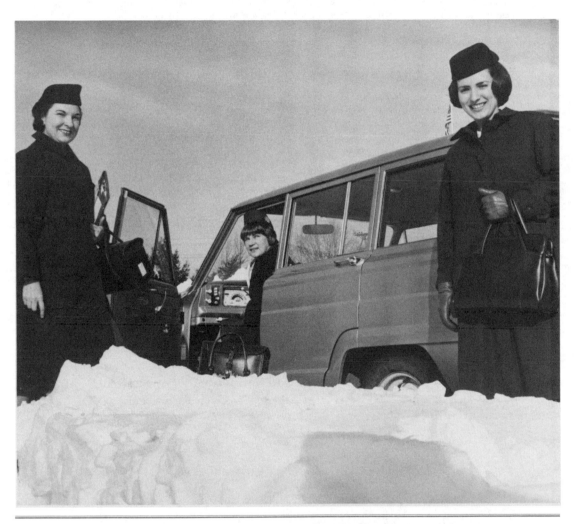

Source: Charlottesville-Albemarle Public Health Nursing, Imogene Bunn Collection: University of Virginia.

Chapter 9

Hitting the Pavement: Intervention of Case Finding: Outreach, Screening, Surveillance, and Disease and Health Event Investigation

Margaret Macali
Marie Truglio-Londrigan

While visiting in a home recently to look up a case of a one-year-old child that was blind (and will be so permanently, but could have been given its sight if the proper medical care had been given it when born) I also found a seven-year-old boy whose leg was drawn up in a V-shape with the knee quite rigid. I found the child had fallen, broken the leg at the knee, and, never having had a physician, the bones knit in the position described. I referred the case to a specialist on children who performed an operation and, after lying in a hospital six months, the boy left using both his legs. . . . The great work of the visiting nurse, socially, lies in this field, not only relieving petty ailments and dealing with the common diseases, but searching out the cases that other wise go unattended (Steel, 1910, p. 341).

LEARNING OBJECTIVES

At the completion of this chapter, the reader will be able to

- Describe the red wedge of the Minnesota Department of Health Population-Based Public Health Nursing Practice Intervention Wheel Strategies, which includes case finding, outreach, screening, surveillance, and disease and health investigation.

- Verbalize culturally appropriate and congruent ways to initiate these intervention strategies.

- Explore the various ways that public health nurses apply and perform the strategies of case finding, outreach, screening, surveillance, and disease and health investigation.

www

KEY TERMS

- ❑ Case finding
- ❑ Disease and health event investigation
- ❑ Outreach
- ❑ Screening

- ❑ Surveillance
  - ○ Directly Observed Therapy
  - ○ Index case

The strength of the Minnesota Department of Health Population-Based Public Health Nursing Practice Intervention Wheel Strategies (Keller, Strohschein, & Briske, 2008; Minnesota Department of Health, 2001) is in the identification of specific intervention strategies and the level of practice (systems, community, and individual/family) that are applied by public health nurses who are charged with protecting the public's health. "Protecting the public" are words that have historically inspired a few so that the many may live healthy lives. The purpose of this chapter is to present to the reader one section of the intervention wheel (red section), which includes case finding, outreach, screening, surveillance, and disease and health event investigation. **Case finding**, as an intervention strategy, takes place at the individual/family level of practice.

This chapter is divided into several sections. The first is the description of these key intervention strategies. The second is a demonstration of how these intervention strategies are applied within the context of several public health issues. The third is the presentation of a case study, so that readers may understand the

process of these interventions. The final section is a look at the case study and the application of the intervention strategies to the various levels of practice, including individual/family, community, and system.

Minnesota Department of Health Population-Based Public Health Nursing Practice Intervention Wheel Strategies

Case Finding

Case finding is exactly what the words imply: to find new cases for early identification of a client with a particular disease or to find cases where particular contact person(s) may be at risk for developing a certain disease. Liebman, Lamberti, and Altice (2002) noted that case finding is important from several points of view. First, by identifying individuals with a particular disease, treatment may be provided in a timely way, thus resulting in reduced morbidity. Second, the identification of individual(s) prevents further transmission of the disease. Finally, in addition to the early identification of individual(s) with a disease through case finding, the process of case finding is also significant in the identification of high-risk individual(s) and "serves as an important opportunity for health education and teaching to promote primary prevention of disease, even among those found not to be infected" (p. 345).

Case finding is essential to identify individuals at risk for disease. Case finding is also important for early diagnosis of those with infectious and noninfectious disease(s), including food-borne and waterborne illnesses. In recent years the process of case finding has also been instrumental in the identification of individuals experiencing still other noninfectious disease(s), including chronic illness; mental health issues such as anxiety and depression; and social, spiritual, emotional, or environmental issues including abuse, violence, and addictions. Skjerve et al. (2007), for example, studied the use of a cognitive case-finding instrument known as the seven-minute screen in a population of older adults for the identification of dementia. Jack, Jamuson, Wathen, and MacMillan (2008) explored public health nurse perceptions of **screening** for intimate partner violence (IPV) and noted that "screening using a standard set of questions is difficult to implement . . . the standard practice is to assess for mothers' exposure to IPV during in-depth assessment of the family; the nature of in-depth assessment having a case-finding rather than screening approach" (p. 150). Puddifoot et al. (2007) looked at anxiety as a treatable condition that frequently goes untreated because it is not diagnosed; the key question here is how to find the unidentified case. These researchers studied whether two simple written questions would aid in the identification of anxiety in a particular person, thus facilitating case finding and ultimately treatment. Similarly, Damush et al. (2008) noted how post-stroke depression is often undiagnosed and ultimately untreated, resulting in an increase in morbidity

and mortality. The purpose of this study was to determine if detecting patients with post-stroke depression in administrative databases using a case-finding algorithm among veteran stroke survivors would be possible. The essence of case finding in these particular situations is that this process identifies individuals in need and connects those individuals to resources such as treatments, support groups, agencies, counseling, and other support services. This echoes the words of Keller and colleagues (2008), who stated, "case finding locates individuals and families with identified risk and connects them with resources" (p. 199). There are various strategies that the public health nurse may use that facilitate and sustain this case-finding process. One needs only to ask how to find these cases. The answer is outreach, screening, surveillance, and disease and health event investigation.

OUTREACH

The public health nurse may use various strategies to engage in case finding. One of these strategies is **outreach**. The word "outreach" creates a vision for us in which the public health nurse or other public health practitioner actually reaches out into the community and connects with and helps those in need. Keller et al. (2008) noted that "outreach locates populations of interest or populations at risk and provides information about the nature of the concern, what can be done about it, and how services can be obtained" (p. 199). Rajabiun et al. (2007) described a qualitative study in which they investigated the process of engagement in HIV medical care. Analysis of the data demonstrated that the participants frequently cycled in and out of care based on a number of influences. The researchers identified that those individuals who had cycled out of care must be found so that care could be reestablished. Outreach, however, was identified as an intervention that played a significant role in connecting participants back to the needed care, thus enhancing care of the individual and in the process protecting the public.

The process of outreach is not a simple one. The public health nurse must take into account the specific population of interest, the demographics of that population, the particular problem that needs to be addressed, where they live, the resources available to them, that particular population's values and beliefs, how they live in the world, and whether or not they want to be found. Although the entire process is rather complicated, the actual enactment requires four important steps.

The first is how the outreach will be carried out so that the public health nurse can gain access to the population and find those in need, hence case finding. Is it via mobile van, motorcycle, walking in the community, telephone calls, knocking on doors, or any other method of connecting with the population of interest? In a school-based community health course, Truglio-Londrigan et al. (2000) worked with community health nursing students in a senior housing project. To gain access to the population of older adults to identify their individual needs, the students knocked on the 99 doors of the building. The students in this course believed that the doors in the apartment buildings were there for protection by keeping people out, but they were actually a barrier to care and services. Their answer to this was to knock on every single door and meet every single person living in the apartment complex. Nandi et al. (2008) assessed access to and use of health services in Mexican-born, undocumented individuals in New York City. To gain access to this population, recruitment took place in communities with large populations of Mexican immigrants. Areas were selected in two phases. In the first, the U.S. Census data were used to identify neighborhoods with the highest numbers of the targeted population. The

second step in the process was a walk-through of the key identified neighborhoods to conduct interviews. Finally, Liebman et al. (2002) noted that a mobile van was an innovative approach to case finding. The authors identified that the use of the van was a way for professionals to move out into communities and gain access to hard-to-reach populations who may not come into traditional health clinics.

The photo on this page provides an example of how one particular public health nurse reached out and gained access to populations of interest. As you examine this photo, look at the nurse and imagine that it is you in the photo. What are you thinking? Who are you visiting? Where do they live? What do you suppose you will find when you reach the end of your destination? What type of services do you suppose you will provide?

A second important consideration is the person who will be doing the outreach. Will the person be a lay worker who lives in the community and is a member of the population of

---

A public health nurse with an Eskimo and a dog team preparing to make a call on local residents.

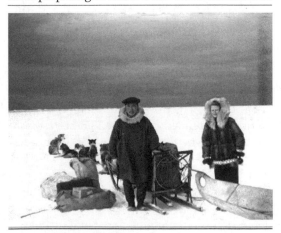

Source: Courtesy of the CDC.

interest? Mock et al. (2007) wanted to promote cervical cancer screening among Vietnamese American women. To determine the effectiveness of this approach, a study was designed to look at lay workers who did the outreach plus media-based education (combined intervention) and media-based education only. Vietnamese woman acted in the role of lay outreach coordinators and lay health workers. Ultimately, the combined intervention motivated more Vietnamese American women to obtain their Pap tests than did media education alone, thus identifying that the person doing the outreach may have a significant impact on whether or not individuals in need will be found and ultimately connected with the needed care and/or resources. Findley et al. (2008) presented a coalition-led childhood immunization program that included an outreach component in which trained peer educators were used. Other elements of this initiative included bilingual and community-appropriate materials as well as reminders to parents. Results demonstrated that students enrolled in this program were more likely to receive timely immunizations than children not enrolled in the program, again demonstrating the importance of finding cases and connecting those cases to needed care and resources. Toole et al. (2007) wanted to conduct a survey of homeless individuals to determine their needs. The difficult part of this type of research is how to find these homeless individuals, so the researchers enlisted formerly homeless, trained, research assistants to aid in the process.

A third consideration is how the message will be delivered to the population once the connection is established. Is it via the newspaper, flyers, booklets, television ads, songs, radio announcements, Internet advertisement, text messaging, or some other technological advancement not yet discovered? The importance of knowing the target population is critical. The public health

nurse may have a plan for an outreach process that is well developed and the population is identified and accessible, but if the message is developed in a way that is not congruent with the population, the message will miss its mark. For example, several years ago community health nursing students identified a need in conjunction with a county department of health and the office on aging in a local county. That need was to deliver nutritional education to the population of older adults living in a particular community. The community students went to the nutrition center and spoke with the older adults, and indeed these older adults concurred that programs on nutrition would be very beneficial for those who used the nutrition center. The community students spent a great deal of time in the development of the program. On the day in which the program was delivered, this author was conducting an observation and noted that students arrived in costumes of the "Fruit of the Loom Guys" traditionally seen on the television undergarment commercials. The costumes were great and the older adults loved them. When the students progressed up to the stage to deliver the message, it was very clear that while their presentation was intriguing to the older adults, the minute they began to deliver their message they lost the attention of their population. The community students had developed a rap song about the food groups. In the audience the older adults began to look confused, many asking, "What are they saying?" The message was lost because the connection was lost. The message that the students developed was not congruent with the population they were targeting. This is similar to concepts pertaining to health teaching and educational programming, covered later in this text.

Finally, the fourth component for consideration is where the final point of contact or service in the outreach process is being rendered. The example given above concerning the presentation of a nutritional program for older adults in a community nutrition site is an example of the final point of contact for the program delivery. Toole et al. (2007) discussed the dilemma of the homeless and raised the question of where they may go when they first become homeless. The lack of access to services creates a situation where the homeless person will increasingly be more likely to experience poor health. The investigators of this research had to think about how they could access this population to hear the voices of these vulnerable people. The researchers knew if they were going to be successful in gaining access to this population and to find individuals, they must go to where they were. These areas included "(i) unsheltered enclaves (including abandoned buildings, cars and outdoors) and congregate eating facilities without sleeping quarters; (ii) emergency shelters; and (iii) transitional housing or single room occupancy (SRO) dwellings" (p. 448). It is not unheard of for public health nurses to ride city buses day and night into neighborhoods where they know their clients travel, in an attempt

to find them and give the care they may need. **Table 9-1** provides examples of points-of-contact for targeted populations.

SCREENING

Another strategy that public health nurses may decide to use in their process of case finding is screening. Keller et al. (2008) stated that "screening identifies individuals with unrecognized health risk factors or asymptomatic disease conditions in populations" (p. 199). Leavell and Clark (1965) addressed the concept of screening as an intervention strategy that is beneficial in its ability to engage in case finding for individual(s); it can provide early identification of a disease, thus facilitating prompt treatment. This early identification is considered in the secondary level of prevention during the early pathogenesis period when the person(s) is asymptomatic. The benefits of screening and early identification of disease are numerous:

- Early detection and diagnosis, leading to early treatment

Table 9-1 EXAMPLES OF OUTREACH AND GAINING ACCESS TO TARGETED POPULATIONS

Targeted Individuals, Families, and Populations	Mechanism of Outreach and Access
Mothers and caretakers of preschool-age children	Health promotion safety educational programs in park settings as children engage in play
Heads of households responsible for purchasing food and cooking	Health promotion educational programs on nutrition outside food stores and accompanying the person as they shop up and down the food aisle
Day workers waiting to begin their day	Health promotion programs on immunizations and the provision of such at pick-up sites
Adolescents engaging in extreme sports	Health promotion programs on use of safety pads at a skate park

- Early detection breaking the chain of transmission and development of new cases
- Early detection leading to a decrease in morbidity and mortality
- Early detection leading to lower costs pertaining to treatments
- Early detection protecting the community and/or the targeted population

This improvement in health and well-being is documented in the literature. Hartge and Berg (2007) noted that "women can improve their prospects for long-term health by being screened for several cancers with tests proved to decrease morbidity and mortality from colorectal, breast, and cervical cancer" (p. 66). Liebman and coworkers (2002) identified that case finding via screening not only is significant because it breaks the chain of further transmission, but it also may identify individuals who present with high-risk behavior. This knowledge therefore provides opportunities for education that focuses on primary prevention and health promotion. This identification of individuals at risk for a disease through screening presents with the same benefits listed above and also includes the following:

- Early detection of high-risk behaviors and modifiable risk factors, leading to prevention of disease
- Early detection leading to empowerment of the person or the population being targeted
- Early detection leading to improvement in lifestyle and quality of life

The application of screening to identify individuals at risk for developing disease takes us closer to health promotion and disease prevention. Wimbush and Peters (2000) described the implementation of a cardiovascular-specific genogram that may be used to identify persons at risk for cerebrovascular disease within families. These authors further described the complex array of risk factors associated with cerebrovascular disease and noted the differences between modifiable risk factors, such as lack of exercise, high fat and high sodium diets, high blood cholesterol, obesity, smoking, high blood pressure, and stress, as compared with nonmodifiable risk factors, such as age, gender, and genetic predisposition. The application of the genogram, a tool used to illustrate family health and relationship patterns over generations, facilitates the public health nurse's understanding of risks present in a family and which of those risks are modifiable. The use of the genogram, in this way, demonstrated promise as a tool to obtain data to inform the public health nurse as to individuals at risk for cerebrovascular disease. Fedder, Desai, and Maciunskaite (2006) similarly presented a strategy that was based on an infectious disease management model that would improve early detection. The authors proposed that practitioners consider "a chronic disease event—e.g., a heart attack, breast cancer diagnosis, or diabetes mellitus diagnosis—as the index case and then screen the siblings and progeny (their brothers, sisters, and children), who are predictably at higher risk" (p. 331). Again, the overall goal is to increase awareness and target risky behavior in others, facilitating prevention and health promotion.

Screening takes place in individual and mass screening models. Screening for the individual involves working with one person and performing a screening test such as taking a blood pressure reading. Conversely, a mass screening may be a situation where a particular group is targeted for a particular screening program pertaining to one or even multiple diseases. The reason the particular group may be targeted has to do with data derived either from an assessment or surveillance data. These data are a source of information for the public health nurse and inform the nurses' decision making.

The data may indicate that the group in question is at greater risk for the development of a particular disease, such as diabetes. In this case, the public health nurse may engage in an initiative to develop and implement a mass screening to identify new cases of this disease.

The benefits of screening are well documented; however, there are limitations as well. One such limitation is what happens to the individual once he or she is informed that the screening test is positive. For example, in the mass screening above, what happens to an individual who is told that his or her blood sugar level is elevated? What type of follow-up is provided? What good is this type of mass screening if the public health nurse finds a case but there is no mechanism to ensure that the individual has access to care for diagnosis, treatment, and follow-up? The University of Medicine and Dentistry of New Jersey's Mobile Health Care Project addressed this issue. They established a collaborative, joint partnership initiative with the Children's Health Fund where a nurse–faculty-managed mobile healthcare unit provided care to the underserved population of Newark, New Jersey. One of the goals of this initiative was to provide health promotion services in the form of screenings. Individuals with positive findings were referred to the University of Medicine and Dentistry of New Jersey hospitals and affiliates for treatment and additional referrals (McNeal, 2008), thus making sure people had access to the care they needed.

Although the benefits of screening are well known, the public health nurse and other public health practitioners must engage in continual dialogue in terms of deciding if a disease is in fact screenable. Escriba-Aguir, Ruiz-Perez, and Saurel-Cubizolles (2007) discussed this issue and identified that if a screening program is to be undertaken, several assumptions must be met: "(a) existence of a test with good sensibility and specificity, (b) high incidence of the problem, (c) existence of appropriate intervention and support measures..., and (d) the diagnostic tool should be acceptable for the population to whom it is aimed and for professionals who apply it" (p. 133).

The issue of sensibility and specificity is an important one. The UK National Screening Committee (2008) offers advice and recommendations about screening based on evidence: "In any screening program, there is an irreducible minimum of false positive results (wrongly reported as having the condition) and false negative results (wrongly reported as not having the condition)" (n.p.). This concern is further defined by others when they speak to the concepts of sensitivity and specificity to address this issue. "Sensitivity quantifies how accurately the test identifies those with the condition or trait . . . . Specificity indicates how accurately the test identifies those without the condition or trait" (McKeown & Hilfinger Messias, 2008, p. 261).

It is evident that there are also ethical and economic considerations to be considered in these cases. For example, the public health nurse and other public health practitioners need to consider the following questions with regard to these possibilities. How ethical is it to conduct screening tests that may inform people they have a disease when they do not? Will these individuals engage in unnecessary testing? Who will pay for the cost of this unnecessary testing? Are there any adverse effects of this unnecessary testing? What is the emotional trauma that the individual will experience and is this important to consider? How ethical is it to conduct screening tests that may inform people that they do not have a disease when in fact they do? What will happen to these individuals? How much later will they be diagnosed and will the diagnosis be too late for any effective treatment modality? What is the emotional trauma that this individual will experience? Will the screening produce positive health outcomes, i.e., a healthier population? The Public Health Action Support Team (2010) posted an online tutorial entitled *Health Knowledge: Screening,* which addresses many of these questions and speaks about screening not as a singular test but as a process and a program. This tutorial discusses the importance of commissioning high-quality screening "programs" that are efficient, coordinated, and of good value. Taking the time to access this video will provide you with a comprehensive understanding of screening that also considers cultural nuances.

Public health nurses and other public health practitioners may also refer to the work of the U.S. Preventive Services Task Force (USPSTF) for practice decisions with regard to the above. The USPSTF, sponsored by the Agency for Healthcare Research and Quality, is a panel of experts in prevention and primary care. The USPSTF conducts rigorous systematic assessments of evidence for the effectiveness of preventive services such as screening, counseling, and preventive medications. The mission of the USPSTF is to "evaluate the benefits of individual services based on age, gender, and risk factor for disease; make recommendations about which preventive services should be incorporated routinely into primary medical care and for which populations and identify a research agenda for clinical preventive care" (USPSTF, 2010, n.p). Based on these evaluations the USPSTF assigns one of five letter grades to each of its recommendations (A, B, C, D, or I). **Box 9-1** provides an explanation of this grading system and its application for practice.

As of October 2008 there were new screening guidelines for colorectal cancer. The USPSTF recommends screening for colorectal cancer using fecal occult blood testing, sigmoidoscopy, or colonoscopy in adults beginning at age 50 years and continuing until age 75 years. This guideline was given a grade A recommendation. As seen in Box 9-1, the grade A means that the USPSTF strongly recommends that clinicians routinely provide the service to eligible patients, thus providing guidance to healthcare providers in the clinical practice setting. The guidelines for this particular situation are listed as grade A recommendations for the age group 50 to 75 years, but not for those ages 76 to 85 years. The USPSTF recommends against routine screening for colorectal cancer in adults ages 76 to 85 years; however, there may be considerations that support colorectal cancer screening in an individual patient. In this situation the grade of C recommendation means the USPSTF makes no recommendation for or against routine provision of the service. Finally, the USPSTF recommends against screening for colorectal cancer in adults older than age 85 years. This recommendation was given a grade of D meaning that the evidence is insufficient to assess the benefits and harms (USPSTF, 2008). Again, these recommendations provide guidance to the healthcare provider in the clinical practice setting. These guidelines also state that the USPSTF concludes that the evidence is insufficient to assess the benefits and harms of computed tomographic colonography and fecal DNA testing as screening modalities for colorectal cancer. In this situation the grade of I is recommended.

Screening is an important strategy for case finding; however, as identified above there are challenges that must be addressed. Wald (2007) addressed these challenges in an editorial, noting that the type of quantitative information needed on the screening performance of a test is usually not even known. "The culture needs to change, so that screening is subject to professional scientific assessment before it is promoted to the public" (Wald, 2007, p. 1).

Box 9-1 USPSTF Grade Definitions

The USPSTF grades its recommendations according to one of five classifications (A, B, C, D, I), reflecting the strength of evidence and magnitude of net benefit (benefits minus harms).

A: The USPSTF strongly recommends that clinicians provide [the service] to eligible patients. The USPSTF found good evidence that [the service] improves important health outcomes and concludes that benefits substantially outweigh harms.

B: The USPSTF recommends that clinicians provide [this service] to eligible patients. The USPSTF found at least fair evidence that [the service] improves important health outcomes and concludes that benefits outweigh harms.

C: The USPSTF makes no recommendation for or against routine provision of [the service]. The USPSTF found at least fair evidence that [the service] can improve health outcomes but concludes that the balance of benefits and harms is too close to justify a general recommendation.

D: The USPSTF recommends against routinely providing [the service] to asymptomatic patients. The USPSTF found at least fair evidence that [the service] is ineffective or that harms outweigh benefits.

I: The USPSTF concludes that the evidence is insufficient to recommend for or against routinely providing [the service]. Evidence that [the service] is effective is lacking, of poor quality, or conflicting and the balance of benefits and harms cannot be determined.

Source: Adapted from U.S. Department of Health and Human Services (DHHS), Agency for Healthcare Research and Quality, U.S. Preventive Services Task Force (2000–2003).

Surveillance

The oldest **surveillance** systems date back centuries. John Snow's work with cholera in London in 1854 is an example of public health surveillance and disease and health investigation, discussed later in this chapter. These past surveillance processes focused on communicable diseases, leading to interventions such as quarantine. Today, public health surveillance includes the monitoring of communicable diseases and chronic illness, birth defects, behaviors, and injury. Interventions have expanded to include disease control and prevention.

Klaucke et al. (1988) stated, "Epidemiologic surveillance is the ongoing and systematic collection, analysis, and interpretation of health data in the process of describing and monitoring a health event" (p. 1). The application of public health surveillance data is noted by the U.S. Department of Health and Human Services and Centers for Disease Control and Prevention (U.S. DHHS/CDC, 2006) as data that can be "useful in setting priorities, planning, and conducting disease control programs, and in assessing the effectiveness of control efforts" (p. 337). This public health surveillance provides data that inform the public health nurse about patterns of disease occurrence and the potential for disease in a population, thus facilitating initiatives in disease prevention. The term "public health surveillance" is presently used in reference to the monitoring of health events in populations, as opposed to medical surveillance, which describes the monitoring of individuals (U.S. DHHS/CDC, 1992, 2006).

A review of the definition of public health surveillance informs the public health nurse of the exact nature of the process. This process may be viewed in **Box 9-2.**

The first step in the systematic public health surveillance process is that of data collection. This

Box 9-2 Systematic Public Health Surveillance Process

Collection of data

Analysis of data

Interpretation of data

Dissemination of data

Public health action

Source: U.S. DHHS/CDC, 2006.

collection takes place as data are reported by those individuals in practice. Each state has a system of reporting that guides those in practice as to the disease and/or conditions that must be reported, who is responsible for reporting, what information is reported, and to whom and how quickly the information must be reported (U.S. DHHS/CDC, 1992, 2006). Diseases that are reported are known as notifiable diseases. These diseases are revised periodically, with diseases being added to the list while others are deleted depending on trends, patterns that are being manifested by the data, and the health of the public. **Box 9-3** gives examples of notifiable diseases.

Those responsible for reporting notifiable diseases generally include physicians, dentists, nurses, medical examiners, and administrators of hospitals, clinics, nursing homes, schools, and nurseries, to name a few. The type of disease and the threat to the public determine how quickly the person doing the reporting has to submit the case report. For example, a disease that poses great threat may have to be reported immediately, whereas others may allow a longer period of time. The case report is usually sent to the local department of health, which then forwards the case report to the state department of health. In some cases information may then be sent to the CDC and the World Health Organization (WHO). When the healthcare provider sends the case report to the department of health, this is called passive surveillance; if a member of the department of health goes out into the community to obtain information, it is known as active surveillance.

The second step in the surveillance process is the analysis of data. As data are collected, they are continually being monitored and analyzed. Sources of data that may be analyzed include those listed in **Box 9-4**.

According to the U.S. DHHS/CDC (1992, 2006), the data are first monitored and analyzed for descriptive information such as time, place, and person. In addition, the public health nurse and other public health practitioners, such as the epidemiologist, must monitor and analyze the data and determine if what they are viewing is expected or different. They must also be able to determine what that difference is. One way of doing this is to look at the recently reported data and to compare those data to previous years, looking for trends and patterns.

The interpretation of data is the next step in the surveillance process. As the public health nurse and/or the epidemiologist notes a difference in the expected pattern in a particular population, this is a signal to those involved that additional investigation is necessary and that the information must be disseminated to those in practice for action.

The dissemination of this surveillance data, the fourth step, takes place as information is sent to those in the practice setting to "inform and motivate" (U.S. DHHS/CDC, 2006, p. 367). During an outbreak, epidemic, natural disaster, or potential terror event, interpretation and dissemination of data are both ongoing and circular, thus affecting public health actions.

The final step in the systematic public health surveillance process is that of action. The entire process would be useless if no action was taken. The action signifies the response to the data, and

BOX 9-3 NATIONALLY NOTIFIABLE INFECTIOUS DISEASES: UNITED STATES 2012

Infectious Diseases Designated as Notifiable at the National Level During 2012

Anthrax

Arboviral diseases, neuroinvasive and nonneuroinvasive
- California serogroup virus disease
- Eastern equine encephalitis virus disease
- Powassan virus disease
- St. Louis encephalitis virus disease
- West Nile virus disease
- Western equine encephalitis virus disease

Babesiosis

Botulism
- Foodborne
- Infant
- Other (wound and unspecified)

Brucellosis

Chancroid

Chlamydia trachomatis infections

Cholera

Coccidioidomycosis

Cryptosporidiosis

Cyclosporiasis

Dengue
- Dengue Fever
- Dengue Hemorrhagic Fever
- Dengue Shock Syndrome

Diphtheria

Ehrlichiosis/Anaplasmosis
- *Ehrlichia chaffeensis*
- *Ehrlichia ewingii*
- *Anaplasma phagocytophilum*
- Undetermined

Giardiasis

Gonorrhea

Haemophilus influenzae, invasive disease

Hansen disease (Leprosy)

Hantavirus pulmonary syndrome

Hemolytic uremic syndrome, post-diarrheal

Hepatitis
- Hepatitis A, acute
- Hepatitis B, acute
- Hepatitis B, chronic
- Hepatitis B virus, perinatal infection
- Hepatitis C, acute
- Hepatitis C (past or present)

HIV infection (*AIDS has been reclassified as HIV stage III*)

HIV infection, adult/adolescent (age $>=13$ years)

HIV infection, child (age $>=18$ months and <13 years)

HIV infection, pediatric (age <18 months)

Influenza-associated pediatric mortality

Legionellosis

Listeriosis

Lyme disease

Malaria

Measles

Meningococcal disease

Mumps

Novel influenza A virus infections

Pertussis

Plague

Poliomyelitis, paralytic

Poliovirus infection, nonparalytic

Psittacosis

Q fever
- Acute
- Chronic

Rabies
- Animal
- Human

Rubella (German Measles)

Rubella, congenital syndrome

Salmonellosis

Severe acute respiratory syndrome-associated coronavirus (SARS-CoV) disease

Shiga toxin-producing *Escherichia coli* (STEC)

Shigellosis

Smallpox

Spotted Fever Rickettsiosis

Streptococcal disease, invasive, Group A

Streptococcal toxic-shock syndrome

Streptococcus pneumoniae, drug resistant, all ages, invasive disease

Syphilis
- Primary
- Secondary
- Latent
- Early latent
- Late latent
- Latent, unknown duration
- Neurosyphilis
- Late, non-neurological
- Stillbirth
- Congenital

Tetanus

Toxic-shock syndrome (other than streptococcal)

Trichinellosis (Trichinosis)

Tuberculosis

Tularemia

Typhoid fever

Vancomycin-intermediate *Staphylococcus aureus* (VISA) infection

Vancomycin-resistant *Staphylococcus aureus* (VRSA) infection

Varicella (morbidity)

Varicella (mortality)

Viral Hemorrhagic Fevers, due to:
- Ebola virus
- Marburg virus
- Crimean-Congo Hemorrhagic Fever virus
- Lassa virus
- Lujo virus
- New world arenaviruses (Gunarito, Machupo, Junin, and Sabia viruses)
- Yellow fever

Source: Adapted from Centers for Disease Control and Prevention. (2012).

this response is in the form of an intervention for change. These interventions may be in the form of a coalition whose members work together in a partnership to target a particular population and pool their resources for action and change. The action for change may also be in the form of targeting of monies for programming, research, and policy development.

The material presented above signifies that the public health surveillance process is really a circular process. **Figure 9-1** is a pictorial of this process.

Effectiveness/Technology

The World Health Organization (2003, p. vii) identified key factors that are essential if a

Figure 9-1 Information loop.

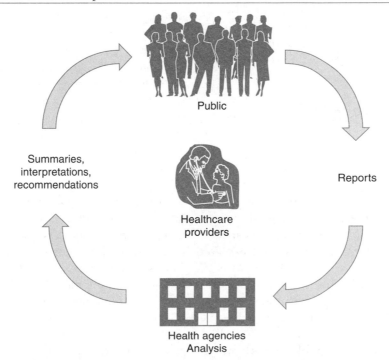

Source: Adapted from U.S. DHHS/CDC (1992, 2006).

systematic public health surveillance system is to be effective; the system must be:

1. Useful
2. Efficient
3. Flexible
4. Representative
5. Simple

The use of technology is critical to this. Technology, as a tool that facilitates, tracks, and disseminates data and other sources of health information, is addressed by the WHO (2008, p. 86) in the following statement: "A well-functioning health information system is one that generates reliable and timely strategic health information on which to base decisions at different levels of the health system." In the *Healthy People 2020* Framework Document, technology is addressed with specific reference to health information technology and health communication. The need to be vigilant in the building and sustaining of this technology is critical to meet the goals and objectives of this national health initiative.

Disease and Health Event Investigation

The final intervention is that of disease and health investigation. Keller et al. (2008) noted that disease and health investigation "systematically gathers and analyzes data regarding threats to the health of populations, ascertains the source of the threat, identifies cases and others at risk, and determines control measures" (p. 199). The entire process may be viewed in **Box 9-5**.

For public health nurses and other public health practitioners, the start of any investigation begins with an event, such as disease, that presents in an individual(s) (this is called the **index case**). The public health nurse and/or other public health practitioner begin the

---

Box 9-5　Process of Disease and Health Event Investigation

Identifying the source of the threat
Identifying cases
Identifying the contacts
Identifying others at risk
Determining control measures
Communication with individuals, families, and populations

Source: Adapted from Minnesota Department of Health, 2001.

---

investigation by asking questions. These questions serve as a reminder to the epidemiological concepts of the agent, host, and the environment discussed earlier in this text. For example, the investigator may ask these questions: Who is affected? Are there any other people affected? Have these people anything in common or are they connected in any way? Where do the people live? Did they venture into any other areas that they do not commonly go to? Where do they live, work, go to school, play, etc.? Is there a particular time that is presenting as a pattern, for example during the summer when it is very humid with much rain?

Other data are essential to gather in this systematic process. For example, the public health nurse and other public health practitioners need to go out into the field, conduct direct observation, and speak to people in the communities. This is critical to the process because subjective information from individuals in the community may bring forth information that is important to the success of the investigation. Collecting specimens is also important in determining what the offending agent is. It is very important to realize that this process is not a one-time deal. In other words, as the public health nurse engages in this investigation, he or she may have to go out into the field not once or twice but multiple times to ensure that the data gathered are reliable and valid. The nurse must share the information with others and confer findings. Critical thinking is key to the success of the investigation.

At the completion of the investigation, the public health nurse will come to know what the problem is and which intervention will correct the issue. Because the public health nurse is dealing with a population, any education and communication that take place must be done from a population perspective. Of course, as with any process, once the interventions are initiated there must be careful monitoring and surveillance to see what the outcome is and if the intervention is a success or not. One of the most famous examples of this **disease and health event investigation** took place in the middle of the 19th century, carried out by an anesthesiologist named John Snow. **Box 9-6** describes the disease and health investigation of cholera.

Public Health Issues in Practice

Public health nursing combines nursing practice and public health sciences, focuses on populations even when dealing with individuals, and is always connected with government at a local, county, state, and/or federal level. Public health nursing may start at the population level, working down to the individual index case, which Venes (2005) defined as "the individual whose condition leads to an investigation" (p. 1090); or it may start with the index case, working up to the population at risk. Either way, the population is always the main focus and the governmental and/or legal relationship is always a part of what guides the practice. Keller, Strohschein, Lia-Hoagberg, and Schaffer (2004) described public health nursing services to "individuals

Box 9-6 Disease and Health Investigation of Cholera by John Snow

In 1854, John Snow conducted an investigation of a cholera outbreak in London's Golden Square. Initially, John Snow determined who was afflicted with the signs and symptoms of cholera, then he identified where they lived. Next, Snow took this information and placed it on a map of Golden Square. By doing so, he had a clear picture of all the cases of cholera in front of him. The picture with all the spots created a visual image that permitted him to "see" more clearly the patterns and clusters of cases. The map is shown here.

Snow believed that the source of the cholera was water, and because of this he also marked on the map the locations of water pumps used by the population of Golden Square to get their daily water supply. He immediately noted that more cases were around pump A than around pumps B and C.

Snow knew he must talk with the people of Golden Square, so he went out into the community and asked questions. What he found was that the people of Golden Square knew that something was wrong with pump B and as a result they stayed away from it and would not use the water. He also found out that pump C was not accessible to the people of Golden Square; thus they did not use it. At that point he had an idea. He thought that pump A, known as the Broad Street Pump, might be the source for the cholera. But, he also noticed that directly east of pump A there were no cholera cases.

(continues)

BOX 9-6 (*continued*)

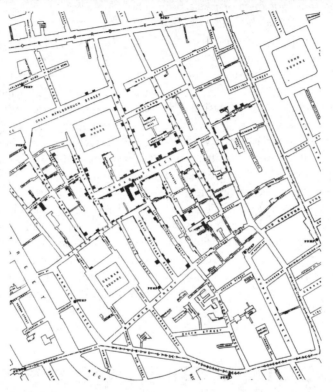

This did not make any sense to him, so once again he investigated by asking key questions and making observations. He discovered that the people directly to the east of pump A obtained their water from a very deep well situated in a local brewery. He also found that people who worked in the brewery had a daily allotment of malt liquor. Thus, these people were protected because their source of water was derived from two safe supplies. To further his investigation, Snow then returned to those who were afflicted with cholera or who had lost loved ones and determined that the one item that all these individuals had was that they obtained their water from pump A. This investigation led to changes in that people who knew that pump A was the contaminated source ceased using this pump and therefore halted the cholera outbreak.

Source: From U.S. DHHS/CDC, 1992, 2006.

or families as population based because those individuals are part of a targeted constituency" and services to them "clearly contribute to improving the overall health status of that population" (p. 457). Much of public health practice, including public health nursing practice, is based on legislation such as sanitary and communicable disease laws. It is because federal, state, and local laws require enforcement that public health nursing can be described as a combination of nursing practice and public health sciences, including the enforcement of federal, state, or local health laws. The U.S. DHHS and the CDC guide public health practice, including public health nursing at the federal level, whereas the State Commissioner of Health and each state's legislated Standards of Performance for Local Boards of Health guide the practice at a local level. As a result, many public health nurses may find they first consult with their state health department rather than the CDC for direction in case finding, surveillance, outreach, and disease investigation. Because of this, certain examples provided within this chapter relate to the specific state health departments within which the writers function.

Tuberculosis (TB) control; investigation of foodborne illnesses; and rabies prevention, exposure, and follow-up are examples of practice areas guided by the aforementioned federal regulatory agencies and each state's legislative practice standards. Tuberculosis, foodborne illness, and rabies are all listed as notifiable at the federal level (see Box 9-3), but enforcement of this mandate occurs at the local and state levels. Public health nurses participate in this mandate by ensuring that those individuals already ill receive the appropriate treatment, by checking that contacts to index cases are adequately managed, and by investigating and intervening in outbreaks (CDC, 2006). A presentation of these diseases, along with an exploration on the application of the Minnesota Department of Health intervention wheel, follows.

Public Health Issue: Tuberculosis

The New Jersey Department of Health and Senior Services (NJDHSS, 2011a) defines *Mycobacterium tuberculosis* as the causative agent for the communicable disease of TB. Tuberculosis is most often a pulmonary disease, but it can also affect other organ systems such as the spine, kidneys, or brain (NJDHSS, 2011a). In concert with the CDC and the WHO, NJDHSS (2011a) describes

the occurrence of TB as a result of contact with the infectious organism found in droplets from infectious persons when they cough or sneeze.

Mantoux tuberculin skin testing (TST) continues to be the recommended screening technique to identify exposure to infection by *M. tuberculosis* when a significant reaction occurs. If this reaction is combined with a negative chest X-ray and lack of symptoms, the person has latent TB infection, is not ill, and is not infectious (NJDHSS, 2011b). Tuberculosis disease is considered when *Mocobacterium tuberculosis*, an acid-fast bacilli, is found in a stained smear from a pulmonary source (NJDHSS, 2011b). Acute pulmonary TB is a result of reactivation of the latent TB infection or a reinfection.

The NJDHSS (2007) provides case definitions of TB as confirmed and presumptive. Confirmed pulmonary TB disease requires a positive sputum/pulmonary culture for *M. tuberculosis* and abnormal chest X-ray along with presenting clinical symptoms of TB disease (NJDHSS, 2007). If "cultures are negative or if no specimen could be obtained for culture identification/confirmation," the case is presumptive (NJDHSS, 2007, Standard #3, p. 2). "A presumptive diagnosis of TB must meet the clinical case definition for pulmonary TB to be confirmed" (NJDHSS, 2007, Standard #3, p. 2). A clinical case definition (NJDHSS, 2007) requires the following:

1. Tuberculin skin test reading was significant or positive, indicating latent TB infection
2. Effective anti-tuberculosis therapy was prescribed and taken
3. Radiographic change (improvement or worsening) occurred

Health providers are expected to report to the state department of health any confirmed or probable TB case(s) within 24 hours. This type of reporting, as mentioned earlier, is considered passive surveillance because the state receives the report without any specific action on its part. This reporting then initiates a series of activities such as case finding, outreach, active surveillance, and disease investigation, all located under the banner of TB control.

Tuberculosis control starts with an individual index case; moves to outreaches to family and other close contacts; expands to workplace, school, or other potential exposure sites; and ultimately relates to the population at large. It is the larger population that public health nursing wants to keep safe. In helping specific individuals achieve health, the public health nurse protects the population.

During the case finding and contact disease investigation stages, population groups are considered at risk based on their exposure to the index case. Each person's closeness to the index case, length of exposure time, and the specific exposure environment are all factored into determination of risk. During the ensuing disease and health event investigation, at-risk populations are interviewed and skin tested (screened) to determine their health status. Data information is circular as viewed in Figure 9-1; during this process, surveillance is considered active.

For pulmonary and laryngeal TB cases, treatment is required by law and includes medical management and the potential for **directly observed therapy** (DOT). Directly observed therapy is based on standards of care developed from practice-based research. NJDHSS (2007) defined directly observed therapy as the "direct observation by a healthcare worker of a patient's ingestion of anti-TB medications at a frequency prescribed by the treating physician" (Standard #6, p. 19). In addition, it "provides the opportunity to identify previously unknown contacts to infectious TB cases, [may help to] identify undisclosed substance abuse [and] allows [for] the health care worker to build a therapeutic

relationship with the client" (NJDHSS, 2007, Standard #6, p. 19).

Treatment is based on the diagnosis and on the state of resistance exhibited by the bacilli on culture. In addition, the answers to the following questions are important: Is this an active case or a latent TB infection? Is it infectious or noninfectious? Pulmonary or nonpulmonary? Is the person co-infected with HIV? Is the individual pregnant or a child 6 years of age or younger? Goals of treatment are to cure the case and prevent transmission to other individuals, and in doing so the public health nurse may again need to engage in the process of outreach. It is important to note that noncompliance by the individual can result in court-ordered confinement until a noninfectious state is achieved.

Public Health Issue: Foodborne Illnesses

Although TB is an example of airborne transmission of disease, foodborne illness is usually transmitted person to person via the fecal–oral route, although vector transmission can occur. Vector transmission takes place, for example, if a fly lands on food after being contaminated by the causative agent. If that food then becomes contaminated, it could become a vehicle for foodborne illnesses such as *Escherichia coli*, *Salmonella*, *Shigella*, or hepatitis A if ingested into the human system.

Foodborne illnesses may be reported as a singular event (one individual) or a family/community event (individuals who attended a family picnic, specific restaurant, or day care). Foodborne illness surveillance is passive until a report(s) comes in. Depending on the specific event, surveillance quickly becomes active. The resulting disease and health event investigation begins with the reported event (index case); extends to potential contacts; outreaches to the food supplier, restaurant, day care agency, school, and/or treating hospital; is screened and diagnosed by stool and food samples; and ends with remedial methods to prevent further illness. When commercial food handlers are involved, registered environmental health specialists or sanitarians are also involved. The sanitarian is a state-licensed individual responsible for environmental health inspections and ensuring that compliance is upheld with public health laws. These environmental health specialists work with the food supplier, restaurant, and/or food handler by providing food management education, conducting inspections, and collecting food samples. Legal interventions that may occur include fines, suspension of license, and/or food-handlers course requirements.

The public health nurse works with all public health practitioners throughout the entire process outlined above, including the strategies noted in the intervention wheel. To illustrate this involvement, the specifics of shigellosis are examined.

Transmitted by the fecal–oral route and usually person to person, shigellosis is caused by the *Shigella* bacteria (NJDHSS, 2008b). Its most common symptoms are diarrhea that can be bloody, nausea, vomiting, stomach cramps, and a fever that usually develops between 1 and 4 days after swallowing the bacteria but may not occur for up to one week. It is important to note that "asymptomatic infections can also occur" (NJDHSS, 2008b, p. 2). Its spread usually occurs among household contacts, children in preschools or day care, persons living in residential facilities, men who have sex with men, and via contact with a contaminated object or food through ingestion or direct contact with an infected person (NJDHSS, 2008b). Diagnosis occurs after finding the *Shigella* bacteria in the stool. "A person may continue to transmit the *Shigella* bacteria as long as bacteria are present and excreted in stool" (NJDHSS, 2008b, p. 3), which can last approximately 4 weeks from

illness onset. Asymptomatic carriers may be infected for much longer.

As noted in Box 9-3, shigellosis is a reportable illness. Many states, including New Jersey, use the same shigellosis surveillance case definition as the CDC, which is classified as confirmed or probable. Confirmed requires "isolation of *Shigella* from a clinical specimen from any site of the human body, regardless of symptoms" and probable requires a "clinically compatible case that is epidemiologically linked to a confirmed case" (NJDHSS, 2008b, p. 4).

When the local health department receives a *Shigella* report, the case finding, outreach, surveillance, and disease investigation processes are initiated. Although the responsibility in this case primarily lies with the health officer, it is often the public health nurse who outreaches to the index case to obtain the history and gather important information pertaining to the signs and symptom. The date when symptoms first appeared is critical because it informs the public health nurse as to the incubation period. For shigellosis, the incubation period may vary from 1 to 4 days but can also range from 12 to 50 hours and up to 1 week (NJDHSS, 2008b, p. 3. This disease investigation would then need to include specific index case information up to 4 days before symptom onset. Other important information the public health nurse needs to secure includes a food history (what foods were eaten, when they were eaten, where they were eaten), travel history, types and location of outside activity, work history, and inclusion of household contacts. The public health nurse also needs to ask additional questions: Did others eat the same food? Have they also become ill? Did they need to see a doctor? What are the foods common to all who became ill? Are the numbers of reported cases increasing and are they part of a community group, such as day care or school? Is the index case or subsequent cases a person who directly prepares or handles food? The answers to these questions then direct the continued processes of disease investigation, case finding, outreach, and surveillance. As shown in Figure 9-1, the informational loop is circular. Surveillance continues to be active until all aspects of the disease or outbreak are closed.

Primary prevention is always a first priority in public health practice when it comes to foodborne illness. For example, when an environmental health specialist conducts a restaurant inspection, he or she also provides food handling education. Both practices are meant to prevent any contamination with the management of food. Public health nurses frequently find themselves in situations where the provision of health education is essential for prevention. The following example illustrates this point.

Public health nurses conduct immunization school audits, and at the same time they may find themselves in the position of providing education in infection control and prevention of communicable diseases. In this one particular circumstance, a public health nurse was provided a table located in the dining area of the preschool to review the infants'/children's immunization records. While conducting this audit, the public health nurse observed one of the child care workers changing a baby's diaper on a changing table located in the same room near the food preparation area. In addition, before-and-after diaper change hand washing was not observed. What educational and prevention opportunities presented themselves with this observation? Besides what the public health nurse should do, what type(s) of referrals could be made to further enhance the infection control interventions for this nursery/preschool?

Public Health Issue: Rabies

Whereas TB and *Shigella* are communicable diseases for which no preventive vaccination exists, rabies can be prevented by vaccination, but not by the vaccination of humans; it is the routine vaccination of domestic animals that can help prevent rabies. "Pre-exposure vaccination [for humans] should [only] be offered to persons in high-risk groups, such as veterinarians and their staff, animal handlers, rabies researchers, and certain laboratory workers" (CDC, 2008a, p. 21).

Rabies can be described as "a rhabdovirus of the Genus *Lyssavirus*" (NJDHSS, 2008a, p. 2) that is typically present in the saliva of clinically ill mammals and is transmitted through a bite. Although all warm-blooded hosts can be susceptible to the virus, in the United States distinct variants have been found in coyotes, foxes, raccoons, skunks, and several species of bats (CDC, 2007).

The CDC (2008a) report on human rabies prevention indicated that improved dog vaccination programs, coupled with enhanced stray animal control, has resulted in a considerable decrease of rabies cases in domestic animals since World War II:

> In 1946, a total of 8,384 indigenous rabies cases were reported among dogs and 33 cases in humans. In 2006, a total of 79 cases of rabies were reported in domestic dogs, none of which was attributed to enzootic dog-to-dog transmission, and three cases were reported in humans, {none of which} was acquired from indigenous domestic animals. (p. 2)

Even with this decline, rabies still causes concern among public health professionals because confirmed human exposure to the rabies virus is generally always fatal unless appropriate postexposure prophylaxis (PEP) is provided.

The management of potential human exposure requires an accurately assessed risk for infection (CDC, 2008a). Human incubation for rabies may range from days to years but is usually weeks to months. Because of this, the CDC (2008a) considers "administration of rabies post-exposure prophylaxis [as] a medical urgency, not a medical emergency, but [stresses] that decisions must not be delayed" (p. 3). The application of the intervention wheel strategies is presented here to demonstrate the processes that the public health nurse is involved with in cases of human exposure to rabies.

Rabies postexposure follow-up starts with receiving the report of a bite, scratch, or exposure to saliva from a potentially infected animal and extends to outreach and case finding with the individual(s) exposed. Determination of risk often falls to the public health nurse, especially if the victim did not present to a medical care provider. Other times the assessment may be shared when an emergency room primary care provider reports to the local health department. Containment and quarantine of the domestic animal falls to animal control with enforcement shared by the licensed environmental specialist or sanitarian. The animal is quarantined and observed for "10 days after a bite" (CDC, 2008a, p. 18) to ensure it is not rabid. This quarantine occurs whether the animal was vaccinated or not. Any untoward signs and symptoms compatible with rabies result in the animal being euthanized and the head removed and sent to the state laboratory for testing. Should the exposure be a result of a wild animal, the capture and securing of the head for testing comes under the jurisdiction of animal control and veterinarian services.

The public health nurse's responsibility includes obtaining health/event information; providing postexposure-related information to the individual(s) involved; and securing, tracking, and documenting the required postexposure treatment for the exposed client. As with foodborne illness, surveillance is passive until the report is received, at which time it becomes active. Recommendations for PEP include the prompt and thorough cleansing of the wound, followed by passive rabies

immunization with human rabies immune globulin and vaccination with a cell culture rabies vaccine (CDC, 2008a, p. 2). Furthermore, recommendations include the use of a reduced four-dose vaccine schedule:

These new recommendations reduce the number of vaccine doses to four. The reduction in doses recommended for PEP was based in part on evidence from rabies virus pathogenesis data, experimental animal work, clinical studies, and epidemiologic surveillance. These studies indicated that 4 vaccine doses in combination with rabies immune globulin (RIG) elicited adequate immune responses and that a fifth dose of vaccine did not contribute to more favorable outcomes. For persons previously unvaccinated with rabies vaccine, the reduced regimen of 4 1-ml doses of HDCV or PCECV should be administered intramuscularly. The first dose of the 4-dose course should be administered as soon as possible after exposure (day 0). Additional doses then should be administered on days 3, 7, and 14 after the first vaccination. (CDC, 2010, p. 1)

As mentioned above, the disease and health event investigation is shared with health officers, environmental sanitarians, animal control officers, and veterinary professionals who control the animal-related sequence of events. It may also be shared with the state departments of health and the CDC. An example of this occurrence happened in July 2007, during the South Atlantic Summer Showdown softball tournament held in Spartanburg County, North Carolina. The CDC (2008b) provided a report regarding this interstate public health response to a rabid kitten. A summation of that report is as follows.

From July 13 through 15, 2007, approximately 60 teams, with 12 players each, from multiple states participated in the South Atlantic Summer Showdown softball tournament. On July 14, one of the North Carolina coaches, upon finding "an apparently healthy and alert kitten" (CDC, 2008b, p. 1337) in a garbage bin, placed the kitten in a box, brought it to six or more different games at two different facilities, and at the end of the day took the kitten to her home. On July 15, the coach's housemate took the kitten to an emergency animal hospital because it had become increasingly lethargic, was behaving abnormally, and had bitten her. When the housemate presented the kitten to the attending veterinarian, however, she did not report the bite. Instead, she signed a routine release form that indicated "the kitten had not bitten anyone during the preceding 10 days" (CDC, 2008b, p. 1337). Because the kitten was severely ill, this release allowed for the kitten to be euthanized with cremation scheduled for July 18.

On July 18, a softball player's mother contacted the emergency animal hospital upon learning the kitten had become sick. Because this mother had also been bitten by the kitten when it was at the tournament, she asked whether the kitten had been tested for rabies. Learning that it had not, she picked up the cat's body and brought it to the local health department, which sent the head to North Carolina's State Laboratory for rabies testing. A positive rabies diagnosis was made. That fact became the starting point for what was eventually a four-state rabies investigation. "Of the approximately 60 teams participating in the tournament, 38 had players and associated family and friends who reported exposure to the rabid kitten" (CDC, 2008b, p. 1338). Of that number, 27 individuals were assessed as having exposures that warranted postexposure prophylaxis because they "had reported actual exposure to the kitten's saliva, either through a bite, a lick on the oral or nasal mucosa, or a claw scratch" (CDC, 2008b, pp. 1338–1339). Cooperation of investigators within the four affected states and the CDC "enabled the expeditious identification

and prophylactic treatment of exposed persons while preventing unnecessary administration of PEP" (CDC, 2008b, p. 1339).

Case Study Application: When Time Is of Importance

Thus far, this chapter has presented for the reader three different public health issues. The case described here is a detailed account of one of the issues presented, TB, and the application of the intervention wheel strategies of case finding, surveillance, disease and health event investigation, outreach, and screening.

The Case

On June 14, a 39-year-old woman was admitted to the hospital with complaints of cough, fever, decreased appetite, night sweats, and a weight loss of 23 pounds over the last month. The admission chest X-ray revealed bilateral upper lobe infiltrates. The physician ordered immediate respiratory isolation and a bronchoscope with bronchial wash. The latter took place on June 17 and was 3+ positive for acid-fast bacillus. A probable diagnosis of pulmonary *M. tuberculosis* was made; treatment was started on June 19 with first-line anti-TB medications. A report to the local health department occurred on June 21, 7 days after the hospital admission, thus initiating an active surveillance. One month later, the final culture was identified as *M. tuberculosis* with pan-sensitivity to the TB medications that had been prescribed.

Tuberculosis Interview and Plan

On June 22, the public health nurse began the disease and health event investigation when she reached out into the community as she arrived at the hospital to interview the newly reported TB index case. During this communication, she learned the patient had been a part-time volunteer for a local day care center, working approximately 2 to 5 hours per week. Reporting that her sister was the center's director, the patient stated her work was mostly secretarial with little exposure to the children. The public health nurse also learned the index case had been coughing for approximately 2 months—1 month longer than noted on admission. Therefore, she may have been infectious longer than previously thought. As a result of this important information, further investigation was needed and in a timely manner.

The state TB nurse manager was called in. Both public health professionals realized that the first steps in the subsequent contact investigation were to identify the infectious period, develop a list of contacts, and then visit the day care center, again signaling the importance of outreach. In talking to the public health nurse and reviewing the medical record, the state TB nurse manager determined the infectious period to be February 17 to June 14. This conclusion set the beginning of the infectious period at 3 months before the cough onset and ended it when the patient was hospitalized in respiratory isolation. The following day both the public health nurse and TB nurse manager met with the day care director to discuss potential exposure to children and staff, conduct an on-site assessment of environmental factors, identify high-priority contacts during the infectious period, and provide TB education to the key individuals involved.

On-Site Assessment and Identification of Contacts

Because index case confidentiality is always a consideration in work site or congregate setting investigations, the state TB nurse manager obtained a signed written statement from the director of the day care center indicating her obligation to respect the issues of confidentiality as related to the index case and this investigation. The index case also signed a written consent for

the health department to conduct the investigation at her work site.

The on-site assessment, which is so important to this disease and health event investigation, again demonstrated the importance of outreach. This assessment revealed a small day care center with low ceilings and only one window, located in the kitchen. The play area room measured 17 by 23 feet; ceiling height was 6 feet 5 inches. There were 35 children, 4 years of age or younger, all born in the United States; there were five staff members. The director reported that the index case had spent most of her time in the play area room.

Given the size of the rooms, poor ventilation, the age of the children, and the infectiousness of the index case, all children and staff were considered high-priority contacts. During the meeting the director also indicated she had a 6-month-old infant who did not attend the day care but spent approximately 5 to 6 hours with the index case on weekends. This infant, also considered a high-priority contact, was available for the public health nurse to plant a TST that same day. When the screening test was read 48 hours later, the reaction was 15 mm, a reaction considered positive. A follow-up chest X-ray revealed infiltrates. The infant was admitted to the hospital with a tentative diagnosis of probable pulmonary TB, and anti-TB medications were started.

Contact Investigation Continues

The disease and health event investigation process continued as the public health professionals collected the names and located information of all identified contacts, in all exposure settings, including household, social, and workplace. Outreach and notification of all contacts were required because they needed TSTs and screening. Educational sessions were also provided to parents of all day care children. In addition to the 39 children and staff contacts at the day care center, the index case also named nine other high-priority contacts, seven household and two social. Active surveillance and outreach continued as the public health nurse visited the patient's household to verify the contacts, provide education, and conduct TST screening. This visit determined that all household contacts had been identified, and none was immune compromised. The nurse then conducted a home visit to the identified social contacts' residences. There it was discovered that one social contact had a 6-month-old infant not named on the initial index case interview. During this home visit and contact interview, the nurse realized this baby had approximately 70 hours of exposure per week to the index case during the determined infectious period. Furthermore, the infant had been presenting with signs and symptoms of what the mom thought were a "cold"; she was thinking of calling the baby's doctor. The TB clinic was called, and the infant was referred to the emergency room and then subsequently admitted to the hospital. Probable pulmonary TB was the diagnosis, and treatment was started.

Summary

In the day care center, 14 of 35 children were TST positive; 50%, or 7 of these children, were diagnosed with confirmed pulmonary TB disease. All TB cases were treated and later placed on DOT upon hospital discharge. The remaining seven children were placed on treatment for latent TB infection.

Of the household and social contact population, 70% were found to be TST positive; the two infants were diagnosed with confirmed pulmonary TB disease and treated in the same manner as the day care children. The remaining TST-positive adults were placed on treatment for latent TB infection.

As you reflect on this case study, do you see the intervention strategies discussed in this chapter being carried out by the two public health nurses? What exactly did they do and how did they do it?

Minnesota Department of Health Population-Based Public Health Nursing Practice Intervention Wheel: Levels of Practice

As public health nurses work with their target populations, they must always keep in mind the cultural context of those they serve. With TB, *Shigella*, and rabies, they are concerned about the individual, family, and population's relationship to the index case and how best to reach out to all in the most effective way so that outreach, case finding, screening, surveillance, and disease intervention may take place. It is important to note that for these interventions to be effective, the nurse must be a part of the community, not in an office behind a desk. The public health nurse must combine nursing practice and public health sciences, including the enforcement of federal, state, or local laws. The public health nurse must be able to apply and perform the 17 intervention strategies of the intervention wheel and also apply those skills and initiate change at the individual/family, community, and system levels of public health practice. How may the public health nurse apply these 17 strategies at the 3 various levels of practice? Public health nurses need to examine and explore what ways are best received by the individual/family, population, and community.

Consideration of the case study above illustrates how the public health nurse worked on the individual and family level. On the individual/family level, the public health nurse developed a trusting relationship with each person.

Considering the fear that is often associated with a diagnosis of TB, the public health nurse's ability to reach out and connect with the index case, especially in the questioning phase, was critical. The case study also illustrates the importance of working with each individual, given the sensitivity and the need for confidentiality. This again highlights the importance of trust development in the public health nurse's relationship with each individual contacted during the investigation. Once this relationship is established, the public health nurse may engage in health teaching and counseling, two additional strategies discussed in other chapters, which assist with the disease and health investigation.

On the community level, the public health nurse worked with multiple community organizations. For example, the emergency department, hospital, day care center, state department of health, and the local department of health were all actively involved in the disease and health investigation. This particular case study does not delve into the way the educational sessions were provided; however, this may be a potential example of how a community may step in to assist in this process. For example, if the population involved did not speak English and the public health nurses were not fluent in the population's primary language, this would have been an opportunity to reach out into the community and receive outside assistance from another agency or organization.

On the systems level, policy and law sustain the process in the case study. For example, TB is one of the many diseases presented on the Nationally Notifiable Infectious Diseases list. This system-level strategy ensures that newly diagnosed cases are sent to the departments of health, local and state, for follow-up and case finding via disease event investigation. This ensures the identification of others at risk or active cases yet to be diagnosed, thus protecting the public.

Conclusion

This chapter presents the red sections of the Minnesota Department of Health Population-Based Public Health Nursing Practice Intervention Wheel. The section discussed is that of case finding, outreach, screening, surveillance, and disease and health event investigation. The chapter was divided in a way that permitted the reader to first learn about these four particular public health nursing interventions. The second section presented various public health issues: TB, foodborne illnesses, and rabies. A third section presented a case study that demonstrated how the public health nurse applied these interventions throughout the levels of public health practice. Public health nursing is not a linear practice. It is a challenging practice that requires the public health nurse to think, apply, and do on multiple levels and spheres. It is forever changing and challenging.

References

Centers for Disease Control and Prevention (CDC). (2006). Summary of notifiable diseases—United States, 2006. *Morbidity and Mortality Weekly Report, 55*, 1–9. Retrieved from http://www.cdc.gob/mmwr/preview/mmwrhtml/mm5553al.htm

Centers for Disease Control and Prevention (CDC). (2007). *Natural history of rabies*. Retrieved from http://www.cdc.gov/rabies/history.html

Centers for Disease Control and Prevention (CDC). (2008a). Human rabies prevention—United States. *Morbidity and Mortality Weekly Report, 57*(RR03), 1–26, 28. Retrieved from http://www.cdc.gov/mmwr/preview/mmwrhtml/rr5703al.htm

Centers for Disease Control and Prevention (CDC). (2008b). Public health response to a rabid kitten—four states. *Morbidity and Mortality Weekly Report, 56*(51),

1337–1340. Retrieved from http://www.cdc.gov /mmwr/preview/mmwrhtml/mm5651a1.htm

Centers for Disease Control and Prevention (CDC). (2012). Nationally Notifiable Conditions Infectious and Non-Infectious Case. Atlanta, GA: Centers for Disease Control and Prevention. Retrieved from http://www. cdc.gov/nndss/document/2012_Case%20Definitions.pdf

Centers for Disease Control and Prevention (CDC). (2010). Use of a reduced (4-dose) vaccine schedule for postexposure prophylaxis to prevent human rabies. *Morbidity and Mortality Weekly Report, 59* (RR-20), 1–9.

Damush, T. M., Huanguang, J., Ried, L. D., Quin, H., Cameon, R., Plue, L., & Williams, L. S. (2008). Case-finding algorithm for post-stroke depression in veterans health administration. *International Journal of Geriatric Psychiatry, 23*, 517–522.

Escriba-Aguir, V., Ruiz-Perez, I., & Saurel-Cubizolles, M. J. (2007). Screening for domestic violence during pregnancy. *Journal of Psychosomatic Obstetrics & Gynecology, 28*(3), 133–134.

Fedder, D., Desai, H., & Maciunskaite, M. (2006). Putting a public health face on clinical practice: Potential for using an infectious disease management model for chronic disease prevention. *Disease Management Health Outcome, 14*(6), 329–333.

Findley, S. E., Irigoyen, M., Sanchez, M., Stockwell, M. S., Mejia, M., Guzman, L., . . . Andres-Martinez, R. (2008). Effectiveness of a community coalition for improving child vaccination rates in New York City. *American Journal of Public Health, 98*(11), 1959–1962.

Hartge, P., & Berg, C. (2007). Improving uptake of cancer screening in women. *Journal of Women's Health, 16*(1), 66–67.

Jack, S. M., Jamuson, E., Wathen, C. N., & MacMillan, H. L. (2008). The feasibility of screening for intimate partner violence during postpartum home visits. *Canadian Journal of Nursing Research, 40*(2), 150–170.

Keller, L., Strohschein, S., & Briske, L. (2008). Population-based public health nursing practice: The intervention wheel. In M. Stanhope & J. Lancaster (Eds.), *Public health nursing: Population-centered health care in the community* (pp. 186–214). St. Louis, MO: Mosby Elsevier.

Keller, L. O., Strohschein, S., Lia-Hoagberg, B., & Schaffer, M. A. (2004). Population-based public health interventions: Practice-based and evidence-supported. Part 1. *Public Health Nursing, 21*(5), 453–468

Klaucke, D. N., Buehler, J. W., Thacker, S. B., Parrish, R. G., Trowbridge, F. L., Berkelman, R. L., & the Surveillance Coordination Group. (1988). Guidelines for evaluation surveillance systems. *Morbidity and Mortality Weekly Report, Supplements, 37*(S-5), 1–18.

Leavell, H., & Clark, E. (1965). *Preventive medicine for the doctor in his community: An epidemiologic approach.* New York, NY: McGraw-Hill.

Liebman, J., Lamberti, M. P., & Altice, F. (2002). Effectiveness of a mobile medical van in providing screening in services for STDs and HIV. *Public Health Nursing, 19*(5), 345–353.

McKeown, R., & Hilfinger Messias, D. K. (2008). Epidemiology. In M. Stanhope & J. Lancaster (Eds.), *Public health nursing: Population-centered health care in the community* (7th ed., pp. 241–277). St. Louis, MO: Mosby Elsevier.

McNeal, G. (2008). UMDNJ School of Nursing mobile healthcare project: A component of The New Jersey Children's Health Project. *The ABNF Journal, Fall,* 121–128.

Minnesota Department of Health, Division of Community Health Services, Public Health Nursing Section. (2001). *Public health interventions: Application for public health nursing practice.* St. Paul, MN: Minnesota Department of Health.

Mock, J., McPhee, S., Nguyen, T., Wong, C., Doan, H., Lai, K. Q., . . . Bui-Tong, N. (2007). Effective lay health worker outreach and media-based education for promoting cervical cancer screening among Vietnamese American women. *American Journal of Public Health, 97*(9), 1693–1700.

Nandi, A., Galea, S., Lopez, G., Nandi, V., Strongarone, S., & Ompad, D. C. (2008). Access to and use of health services among undocumented Mexican immigrants in a US urban area. *American Journal of Public Health, 98*(11), 2011–2020.

New Jersey Department of Health and Senior Services (NJDHSS). (2007). *Standards of care for tuberculosis disease and latent TB infection.* Retrieved from http:// www.state.nj.us/health/cd/documents/complete _standards_of_care.pdf

New Jersey Department of Health and Senior Services (NJDHSS). (2008a). *Rabies (human and animal).* Retrieved from http://www.state.nj.us/health/cd /manual/rabies.pdf

New Jersey Department of Health and Senior Services (NJDHSS). (2008b). *Shigellosis.* Retrieved from http://www.state.nj.us/health/cd/documents/chapters /shigellosis_ch.pdf

New Jersey Department of Health and Senior Services (NJDHSS). (2011a). *Tuberculosis: Frequently asked questions.* Retrieved from http://www.state.nj.us/health /tb/tbqa.shtml

New Jersey Department of Health and Senior Services (NJDHSS). (2011b). *New Jersey Administrative Code Department of Health and Senior Services Title 8, Chapter 57, Communicable Disease*. Retrieved from http://www.state.nj.us/health/tb/documents /njac8-57_tb_regulation

Public Health Action Support Team. (2010). *Health knowledge: Screening {online tutorial}*. Retrieved from http://www.healthknowledge.org.uk/interactive-learning/screening

Puddifoot, S., Arroll, B., Goodyear-Smith, F. A., Kerse, N. M., Fishman, T. G., & Gunn, J. M. (2007). A new case-finding tool for anxiety: A pragmatic diagnostic validity study in primary care. *International Journal of Psychiatry in Medicine, 37*(4), 371–381.

Rajabiun, S., Mallinson, R. K., McCoy, K., Coleman, S., Drainoni, M., Rebholz, C., & Holbert, T. (2007). The public health approach to eliminating disparities in health. *American Journal of Public Health, 98*(3), 400–403.

Skjerve, A., Nordhus, I. H., Engedal, K., Pallesen, S., Braekhus, A., & Nygoord, H. A. (2007). The seven minute screen (7MS). *International Journal of Geriatric Psychiatry, 8,* 764–769.

Steel, A. (1910). Neighborhood nursing. *American Journal of Nursing, 10*(5), 340–342.

Toole, T., Conde-Martel, A., Gibbon, J., Hanusa, B., Freyder, P., & Fine, M. (2007). Where do people go when they first become homeless? A survey of homeless adults in the USA. *Health and Social Care in the Community, 15*(5), 446–453.

Truglio-Londrigan, M., Arnold, J., Santiao, M., De Sevo, M., Higgins Donius, M. A., & Valencia Go, G. (2000). "Knocking on 99 doors": The experience of The College of New Rochelle (New York). In P. S. Matteson (Ed.), *Community-based nursing education: The experience of eight schools of nursing* (pp. 57–75). New York, NY: Springer.

UK National Screening Committee. (2008). *What is screening?* Retrieved from http://www.nsc.nhs.uk /whatscreening/whatscreen_ind.htm

U.S. Department of Health and Human Services (DHHS) Public Health Service, Centers for Disease Control and Prevention (CDC). (1992). *Principles of epidemiology: An introduction to applied epidemiology and biostatistics* (2nd ed.). Washington, DC: American Public Health Association.

U.S. Department of Health and Human Services (DHHS), Centers for Disease Control and Prevention (CDC). (2006). *Principles of epidemiology: An introduction to applied epidemiology and biostatistics* (3rd ed.). Washington, DC: American Public Health Association.

U.S. Department of Health and Human Services (DHHS). (2010). *Healthy People 2020 framework*. Retrieved from http://www.healthypeople.gov/2020/ Consortium/HP2020Framework.pdf

U.S. Preventive Services Task Force (USPSTF). (2000–2003). *Grade definitions: Strength of recommendations*. Retrieved from http://www.uspreventiveservicestaskforce .org/3rduspstf/ratings.htm

U.S. Preventive Services Task Force (USPSTF). (2008). *Screening for colorectal cancer*. Retrieved from http://www .uspreventivetaskforce.org/uspstf/uspscolo.htm

U.S. Preventive Services Task Force (USPSTF). (2010). *USPSTF introduction*. Retrieved from http://www .uspreventivetaskforce.org/intro.htm

Venes, D. (2005). *Taber's cyclopedic medical dictionary* (20th ed.). Philadelphia, PA: F. A. Davis.

Wald, N. J. (2007). Screening: A step too far. A matter of concern. *Journal of Medical Screening, 14*(4), 163–164.

Wimbush, F., & Peters, R. (2000). Identification of cardiovascular risk: Use of a cardiovascular-specific genogram. *Public Health Nursing, 17*(3), 148–154.

World Health Organization (WHO). (2003). *WHO-recommended standards for surveillance of selected vaccine-preventable diseases*. Geneva, Switzerland: Author.

World Health Organization (WHO). (2008). *Priority interventions: HIV/AIDS prevention, treatment and care in the health sector*. Geneva, Switzerland: Author.

For a full suite of assignments and additional learning activities, use the access code located in the front of your book to visit this exclusive website: http://go.jblearning .com/londrigan. If you do not have an access code, you can obtain one at the site.

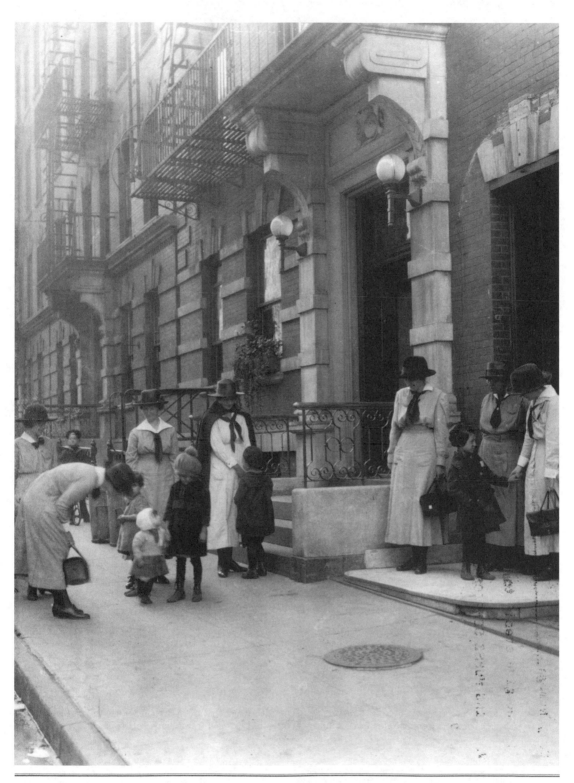

Chapter 10

Running the Show: Referral and Follow-up, Case Management, and Delegated Functions

Janna L. Dieckmann

To meet the rightful demand of the children for play, we conducted in our back yards one of the first playgrounds in the city. It was an experimental station in a way, as well as an enlightenment of the general public, and was instrumental in helping to develop public feeling in the matter. After a time the interests of the residents of the settlement were directed to the "Out-Door Recreation League," share being taken in its executive work... (Wald, 1902, p. 569).

LEARNING OBJECTIVES

At the completion of this chapter, the reader will be able to

- Describe the public health intervention strategies of referral and follow-up, case management, and delegation.
- Discuss how intervention strategies may be implemented at the individual/family, community, and system levels.

- Describe the steps of the referral and follow-up process.
- Describe the case management process.
- Apply the public health intervention strategies of referral and follow-up, case management, and delegation to the case study presented in the chapter.

KEY TERMS

❑ Case management
❑ Delegation

❑ Referral and follow-up

The public health nurse designs and implements interventions within a complex network of health, social welfare, housing, and other services. Maximizing nursing services requires nurses' comprehensive knowledge and effective interface with a complex and well-functioning system of multiple services that are available, accessible, and culturally competent. Public health nurses have understood that the determinants of health and the multiple causation of disease mean that individual change must have multiple foci. Public health nursing services work best by collaborating with other community-based caring and helping systems. Our clients—patients, families, populations of interest, systems, and communities—require more than public health nurses can directly provide. We have become experts in identifying client needs and connecting clients to community services providers and services systems.

This chapter addresses three important public health interventions in the green wedge of the Minnesota Department of Health Population-Based Public Health Nursing Practice Intervention Wheel: referral and follow-up, case management, and delegated functions. These interventions have similarities, may overlap, and may be addressed toward similar objectives. All three interventions draw the public health nurse to working beyond the nurse–client dyad, as the nurse seeks to add the contributions of other community services and health providers to improve the system for client support and change. At the community practice level, this means public health nurse participation in initiating services or expanding availability and access to meet an identified need. At the systems practice level, the public health nurse modifies organizations and policies that shape systems of care. At the individual/family practice level, this

includes interventions to change knowledge, attitudes, beliefs, practices, and behaviors (Rippke, Briske, Keller, Strohschein, & Simonetti, 2001).

The first of the three public health interventions addressed in this chapter, referral and follow-up, "assists individuals, families, groups, organizations, and/or communities to identify and access necessary resources in order to prevent or resolve problems or concerns" (Keller, Strohschein, & Briske, 2008, p. 199). Case management "optimizes self-care capabilities of individuals and families and the capacity of systems and communities to coordinate and provide services" (Keller et al., 2008, p. 199). Delegated functions, the third intervention, "are direct care tasks a registered professional nurse carries out under the authority of a health-care practitioner as allowed by law. Delegated functions also include any direct care tasks a registered professional nurse entrusts to other appropriate personnel to perform" (Keller et al., 2008, p. 199).

Minnesota Department of Health Population-Based Public Health Nursing Practice Intervention Wheel Strategies and Levels of Practice

Referral and Follow-Up

Referral and follow-up interventions are hallmarks of public health nursing. The referral process is defined as "a systematic problem-solving approach involving a series of actions that help clients use resources for the purpose of resolving needs" (Clemen-Stone, McGuire, & Eigsti, 2002, p. 316). As a practice expectation and as an ongoing intervention, the public health nurse seeks to link individuals/families, populations, communities, and systems to resources. New public health nurses quickly gain knowledge of the interfaces between target populations and assistive resources. Experienced public health nurses have extensive information, experiences, and facility in establishing linkages between and among community members, groups, and organizations. Individuals/families, populations, communities, and systems often seek the knowledge and advice of public health nurses when they want to know where to go for help or when they want to improve systems and services that provide resources (Rippke et al., 2001, p. 81).

Referral and follow-up interventions are related to other public health nurse interventions and generally occur in the context of ongoing nursing service. For example, health teaching for weight reduction provided by the public health nurse to a group of adults at a community center may encourage group members' interest in increasing their physical activity and muscle strength. Based on group members' expressed need, the public health nurse would seek and explore appropriate resources and provide group members with a tailored recommendation of relevant resources. At a later point the public health nurse would evaluate or follow up on the referral to determine the extent and character of the contacts between group members and the resources to which they were referred. In this example, referral and follow-up interventions further the goals of the health teaching intervention but remain a separate intervention characterized by unique guidelines, practices, and values. The referral process is most effective when it is linked to other public health nurse interventions.

Referral and follow-up interventions may be applied with counseling or consultation interventions to link the individual/family, population, community, or system to a resource to prevent or resolve a problem or concern. The more information the public health nurse has about the expressed concern and the targeted intervention, the better and more sustainable the referral and follow-up is likely to be. Referral and follow-up is also used after screening and case finding (related to surveillance, disease investigation, and/or outreach) to address a need identified by this particular public health nurse intervention. The ethics of both screening and case finding direct the public health nurse to make formal plans to respond to newly identified needs. For example, when the individual or family has a positive screening result or a "case" is identified, linkage to a relevant resource is required. Advocacy interventions also generally demand linkage(s) to services and resources to address aspirations and needs at any practice level.

The two other intervention approaches addressed in this chapter, case management and delegated functions, are also interrelated with the referral and follow-up intervention. Case management is a goal-oriented process that uses available resources to achieve case management objectives. Referral and follow-up interventions occur jointly with the case management plan. Delegated function interventions shift care responsibility to an eligible resource or provider of care. The interface with this resource requires the public health nurse to apply referral and follow-up strategies. Additional elements of case management and delegated functions interventions are described in later sections of this chapter.

PUBLIC HEALTH NURSES AS "SENDERS" AND "RECEIVERS" OF REFERRALS

Public health nurses make and receive referrals. They may send or initiate a referral on behalf of a client or may receive a referral for a new or already known client. The process of receiving referrals at a public health nursing organization is generally formal to accommodate the frequency of requests and to provide a means to track data and referral outcomes. Referrals—both formal referrals from organizations and professionals and informal referrals from the client or the client's network—are received as part of an intake process at the public health nurse organization. In some agencies, public health nurses are permanently assigned to receive referrals, and in some agencies the intake function rotates among nurses. For cost or effectiveness reasons, intake may be alternatively delegated to skilled non-nurse staff members under the direction of a public health nurse. Once a referral is received, it is weighed and a plan to respond is established. The referral may be accepted for services from the public health nurse organization, or it may be determined that the needed resources or services are not available from the public health nurse organization. In this situation, the referral may be declined and the referring agency or person promptly notified by intake public health nurses.

The intake public health nurse may also make recommendations for more appropriate, alternate agencies to receive the referral. Most communities have organized systems of information and referral, generally directed by social workers educated in this specialty area. Contacts with information and referral systems, sometimes called "First Call for Help," are available by telephone and increasingly online for specific geographic communities. Many states now have a "211" switchboard to connect callers to community resources. These systems request specific information about the client and the need to closely match the request with an appropriate resource. Information and referral differs from the public health nurse intervention of referral and follow-up in that information and referral provides only information on available resources.

Even though information and referral agencies may provide comprehensive information, information and referral does not make a referral or conduct follow-up. Based on information provided by the information and referral agency, the public health nurse or the group/family must select a possible resource and contact the suggested service agency to initiate a request for assistance.

It is important to note that the intake function of public health nurse agencies provides nurses and organizations with information about community needs and about gaps in resource availability, affordability, and appropriateness. Even when a public health nurse organization is unable to respond to an intake request, each request helps build a description of current community needs. When a mismatch between community need and existing resources is found, public health nurses and public health nurse organizations will seek to meet emerging or newly defined needs by developing new resources or by modifying or improving existing resources. Analysis of the needs may also suggest that resources exist but that there is a barrier to access. For example, a community organization providing HIV/AIDS prevention and care services has historically targeted a defined geographic area. Now, a neighboring area requires resources because it has experienced increased HIV incidence and AIDS prevalence. One solution would be to expand the existing HIV/AIDS service area into the neighboring community.

GAINING KNOWLEDGE ABOUT AVAILABLE FORMAL RESOURCES

Public health nurses must gain a working knowledge of available community resources to make effective referrals and must develop working relationships with resource organizations to fulfill follow-up obligations. How does a public health nurse build knowledge of community agencies and resources? Descriptive and contact information about community agencies and resources should be included in the public health agency orientation and public health staff development programs. Information can be shared in print or electronic formats, especially when there are changes in eligibility or availability of services. Many public health nurses maintain contact lists or active files of potential community resources. Public health nurse agencies may also develop relationships with specific resources, which may include formal strategies for interagency contact, referral, and follow-up (Allender & Spradley, 2005). Consultations with public health nurse supervisors or agency social workers can assist public health nurses to identify relevant resources.

In addition to formal structures for gaining information about community agencies, organizations, and resources, public health nurses learn about agencies through their informal networks. Informal networking with other public health nurses is often the most fruitful source of resource identification. Clients, families, and other health professionals can provide information about resources, which is especially helpful when it is from the resource user's viewpoint. Observing the presence and activities of other agencies and organizations in a community also suggests who is operating in an area and the types of services offered. For example, home-delivered meals are a strategic service for homebound elders and the chronically ill. Before referring a client, a public health nurse would pose questions about the service to colleagues and clients. Perhaps a home-delivered meal program provides excellent meals at the promised time at an inexpensive cost. On the other hand, perhaps the service's waiting list is 10 months, meals are too salty for many recipients, and delivery drivers get lost and miss deliveries. Knowing what to expect from a potential resource, as well as whether the client can accept the pros and cons of resource operations, enables the public health nurse to weigh the value of the actual referral.

IDENTIFYING REFERRAL NEEDS: WHEN AND WHO?

A referral must have merit. "Merit" takes into consideration whether a referral is the right referral at the right time for the right client. Determining the merit of a referral is heavily influenced by community values and expectations and (1) whether or not referrals are an effective strategy, (2) the timing of a referral, (3) whether the referral is to prevent a problem or address an existing problem, and (4) the nature of the "match" between the referral resource and the client.

Among public health nurses in some agencies, developing and making referrals is an infrequent activity. Client needs may have been overlooked, resources are scanty, or the nurses are overwhelmed. On the other hand, most public health nurses would agree that use of community resources extends the effectiveness and quality of public health nurse interventions and is well worth the time and attention required to prepare and complete a referral.

The actual timing of making referrals may vary among public health nurses and across public health nurse organizations. Some public health nurses wrap referrals into case closure activities, whereas others ensure that referrals are made early enough in the nurse–client relationship that new community resources have begun client services before public health nurse service termination; this makes it easier to conduct follow-up activities as the nurse maintains contact with the client before case closure. The public health nurse can both observe the impact of the community resource's contacts with the client and directly ask the client about the use and success of the referral agency's services.

Public health nursing approaches also vary in whether community resources are applied early to prevent client crises or in a more targeted fashion to address client crises once present. Many public health nurses prefer to engage in preventive activities to avoid crises, although some would rather reserve community resources to address emergent problems. Both perspectives are based in ethical judgments about when and how services are best involved, and both raise questions about cost-effectiveness. In prevention, lower cost can be spread over a wider population whose members may or may not be at risk. Public health nurses often base interventions on the ethic that suffering should be prevented whenever possible. When addressing crises that have already occurred, individual costs are likely higher, but these costs are directed only at individuals experiencing actual health problems.

Some client groups are seen as more deserving than others of receiving resources. Some clients can be viewed in a more favorable light than other clients, because their concerns or needs are interpreted in a more sympathetic manner. For example, a person with alcoholism, living on the street, might be viewed less sympathetically than a stable couple with a young child. Or those making every effort to improve their health would be viewed more positively than those with the same health concern but who make no effort to help themselves. Society is more willing to provide aid and assistance when clients are sympathetic, are deemed "moral," and are seen as attempting self-improvement. When the public views a client group as being more "deserving," they are willing to provide greater resources for resolving their needs and are more open to paying for more expensive resources (Dieckmann, 1999; Katz, 1996). For example, as AIDS has become more mainstream since the mid-1980s, communities are more willing to commit resources to people living with HIV/AIDS. When clients are viewed as sympathetic and deserving, it is more acceptable to fund services and more resources become available. These principles not only have implications for individual/family use of referral resources but also for the overall availability of resources at the community and systems practice levels.

STEPS TO CONDUCTING REFERRAL AND FOLLOW-UP

Implementing the steps of the referral and follow-up intervention assumes active client participation and client control. Assistance in planning is offered to the client, and the public health nurse collaborates with the client. Because the referral process is client-centered, the public health nurse avoids making decisions for the client but seeks to establish a working partnership that uses a problem-solving approach to achieve shared goals.

Individual/family clients, populations, communities, and systems vary across a continuum as to their ability to contribute to the referral process. Some clients are dependent on the public health nurse for gathering information, weighing options, and requesting the referral. In these situations, public health nurses use referral planning and implementation to build relevant skills and independence in clients. Other clients are more independent in considering and implementing referrals, placing the public health nurse in almost a consultative role. Here, the public health nurse validates and extends these clients' independent problem-solving behaviors. The public health nurse provides clients with the opportunity to learn and adopt new behaviors to achieve their next steps to full independence.

The steps to conduct referral and follow-up are sequential; these steps are based on the outline provided by Clemen-Stone and colleagues

(2002) and McGuire, Gerber, and Clemen-Stone (1996). If a need or resource cannot be identified or if the client declines referral, it may be useful to revisit earlier steps. These steps are appropriate for individuals/families, populations, communities, and systems. Additional comments about the implications of the referral and follow-up intervention for communities and systems are found at the end of this section (see Referrals and Follow-Up at Systems and Community Practice Levels, below).

Step 1: Establish a Nursing Relationship With the Client. Nursing interventions begin with establishing a respectful working relationship with the client, which serves as a basis for individualizing or targeting care. The referral and follow-up intervention is often used with existing clients for whom the public health nurse has provided other public health interventions. Here, the professional relationship has already been established. On the other hand, a public health nurse may initiate a professional relationship with a new client solely to develop and implement a referral and follow-up. Whether based in an ongoing collaborative intervention or in a brief encounter, the public health nurse must similarly establish trust and gain the client's agreement to engage in the referral process. Public health nurses may quickly assess and develop working hypotheses about the client that may later be confirmed, but the nurse should not establish fixed assumptions in the initial step.

Step 2: Identify Client Need and Set Objectives for Referral. Based on a caring, professional relationship with the client, the public health nurse gathers information about the client and the client's context. Listening to the client's perspective on his or her current situation and larger context is crucial (Wolfe, 1962). What is the client's need and what are the parameters of the need? Clients may benefit from a thorough discussion of the need. Allowing the client to review and describe a need provides essential information for the nurse, but the process of verbally articulating needs also enhances client comprehension of the need, investment in the referral process, and self-efficacy in securing a solution. Because one intention of the referral process is to increase client independence, incorporating strategies that facilitate client empowerment are beneficial to strengthening current decisions for self-care and later self-determination.

When the public health nurse has secured an apparent understanding of the client's needs, the nurse reflects a synthesis of the need back to the client to confirm that what has been heard is what the client meant to convey. Probing for further client information or perspective may be helpful. After brief consideration, the public health nurse presents his or her summary of the client's expressed need and proposes options for addressing this need. Critically important at this point is the nurse's determination whether the client's need is in practice one need or several. If several, then the public health nurse proposes at least two ways of posing the need and gains client agreement with one interpretive approach. Given a favored approach, the nurse and client work collaboratively to establish objectives for the referral.

This give-and-take process may be quite brief, or it may be lengthy. If the referral and follow-up intervention is conducted with an individual/family, organization, community, or system, more than one well-organized meeting may be required to share information, make decisions, and gain a working consensus about objectives. As the process of making a referral proceeds, the nurse and client may choose to return to this step for further clarification of need(s) and redetermination of objectives.

Step 3: Search for Resources and Explore Resource Availability. A systematic search for resources to meet the need and the identified referral objectives is conducted by the nurse, sometimes with participation of the client. Public health nurses familiar with meeting needs similar to the client's may quickly establish a group of options, either from personal experience or from consulting personal or agency resource files. Addressing more complex client needs may require consultation with professional colleagues or with information and referral specialists. Although the principles of making a good referral can guide the public health nurse, a nurse's experience and confidence in making referrals contributes to a prompt and personalized outcome. A nurse's ability to apply the art of nursing is especially relevant in the selection of potential referral resources. The client and the resource must fit together in both tangible and intangible ways for the referral to effectively accomplish the identified goals.

Step 4: Client Decides Whether to Agree to Referral. Information about potential referral resources is presented and discussed with the client. The client may select a resource(s), may wish to consider the resource(s), or may decline to agree to any referral. It can be helpful to provide clients with written information to allow later review of potential resources or later communication with the resource by the client. Application of the referral and follow-up intervention is based on ethical principles of client self-determination that places decision making in the hands of the client (McGuire et al., 1996). When a client is uncertain or declines referral, the public health nurse may explore the client's feelings and reasons, identify factors that might facilitate or deter resource use, negotiate use of identified resources, propose a wider variety of referral resources, and/or reassess the client's needs and objectives for service. If a client declines referral at any point, no referral is made. The nurse must balance encouragement with an open ear that the client does not wish a referral.

Step 5: Public Health Nurse Matches Client With Resource and Makes the Referral to the Resource. The client and the nurse select a resource or resources that best match the client's needs and preferences. Does the client believe the resource will work for him or her? The public health nurse's knowledge of the client and client's needs is important in making the referral to the identified resource and in explaining the client to the agency. If the client is a population, community, or a system, a referral might be a grant application or similar application to secure program funding. When clients are more experienced or skilled, they may make the referral themselves; this increased skill in self-managing care is a factor in client empowerment. Other clients may lack experience, be self-doubting, or be overwhelmed and emotionally fragile. As the nurse makes the referral, he or she asks questions and gains more information to assist the client to maximize interactions with the resource. The public health nurse also provides the client with tailored information about the resource and with anticipatory guidance on using the agency's resources.

Some agencies require detailed application information; the nurse gathers information and confirms with the client what information should be shared. Some communities use written interagency referral forms that have been developed to address system and resource needs for sharing information. Although patient privacy laws now prevent their use, in the past the agency that received a written referral would respond in writing to the referral source to describe initial contacts and plans for the referred individual or family (Cady, 1952; Kraus, 1944).

Step 6: Follow-Up to Facilitate Client Utilization of Resource. Nursing interventions at this step, alternatively called "following along," can ease the client's experience with the resource. Soon after the client follows through and contacts the resource, the public health nurse contacts the client to determine the client's progress and engagement with the resource. Is the client using the resource as planned? Is the resource agency engaged with the client? The public health nurse can reemphasize the purpose of the referral, interpret the resource to the client and the client to the resource, and promote linkages between client and resource. If signs of a weak linkage are found, the nurse may advocate for the client with the resource. The public health nurse can also directly address any barriers to seeking or using the resource (Will, 1977).

Step 7: Evaluation of Referral Process and Outcome, Client Outcome, and Resource Assistance. Did the client receive services and what was provided by the resource? In what ways did the client's status change as a result of working with the resource? Obtaining adequate information and data for evaluation can be challenging but is an essential element in the ongoing process of making referrals. Whether the client is an individual/family, population, community, or system, evaluation of referral and client outcomes has system-level implications. Lack of resources or poor service from resources in the community suggests gaps that public health nurses should address. Because the referral and follow-up intervention is a continuous process, public health nurses learn from each referral and provide feedback to improve the system itself and nurses' utilization of system resources.

BARRIERS TO SUCCESSFUL REFERRAL AND FOLLOW-UP

Successful follow-through on any referral frequently depends on the resources of clients and is based on several factors. Wolfe's (1962) classic analysis identified the central role of client motivation in initiating resource utilization: To what extent does the client see the referral and resource use as important? Does the referral appear to be practical and relevant to the client's situation? Individualizing the referral for the client or the family and tailoring the referral to the client's expressed preferences enhance referral utilization.

The concepts of perceived benefits and perceived barriers in the health belief model can assist in facilitating client follow-through for resource use. Clients accept a recommended referral only when they expect a benefit that is greater than the perceived barriers. Public health nurse interventions are designed to enhance perceived benefits by clarifying the expected positive impact of accepting the referral and by explaining specific actions to engage with the referral resource. At the same time, public health nurse interventions are directed toward reducing perceived "tangible and psychological costs" of accepting the referral by identifying perceived barriers and reducing their impact through clarifying misinformation and applying reassurance, incentives, and concrete assistance to use the resource (Champion & Skinner, 2008, pp. 47–49). For example, referral follow-through by patients at risk for cancer was improved when diagnostic/treatment appointments were scheduled within 2 weeks, when patients received clear instructions, and when patients received careful attention from the clinic staff (Manfredi, Lacey, & Warnecke, 1990).

Public health nurse interventions at the system and community practice levels seek to reduce institutional and systemic barriers; for example, adding evening and weekend service hours or providing more trained interpreters can increase the accessibility of programs offered at public health nurse clinics (Office of Minority Health, 2001).

A wide variety of factors may delay or obstruct clients' participation in the referral process or in using the referred resource, despite initial agreement with the significance of the problem, plans for solution, and selection of and referral to the resource. From an individual or family viewpoint, differences in religious/cultural beliefs or practices can increase uncertainty and reduce trust of a new resource. Or clients may become uncertain about why they were referred to a resource or doubt that it is a priority and so postpone or forget to engage with services. Structural barriers, such as geographic barriers, may make certain resources unusable, or resources may

simply be unavailable. Appointment times may be inconvenient or require a long wait. Financial barriers may place good resources outside clients' reach or may delay the resource's acceptance of the client so long that clients lose motivation to make change.

These barriers may also suggest ineffective or flawed systems because of lack of financial or professional resources or a lack of consensus to address individual/family or community problems or concerns. Public health nurses may need to advocate at the community or system levels; for example, this advocacy may include screening services or enhancing existing services to improve utilization, such as translation or handicap accessibility.

An example of the complexity and importance of making referrals is the practice of partner counseling and referral services, provided as part of the spectrum of care for HIV-positive individuals and their partners. Community interventions related to *Healthy People 2020* recommendations for HIV (U.S. Department of Health and Human Services [U.S. DHHS], 2011a) includes a link to "Interventions to identify HIV-positive people through partner counseling and referral services," as analyzed and developed by the Task Force on Community Preventive Services (U.S. DHHS, 2011b). The role of referral here is to notify sexual partners of HIV-positive persons of their exposure and of the need to visit health services for counseling, screening, and/or medical treatment (Hogben, McNally, McPheeters, & Hutchinson, 2007).

STRATEGIES FOR FOLLOW-UP

Several effective strategies are helpful to use in following up on client referrals. If resources are limited, public health nurses may establish priorities for whom to contact based on complexity of need or family situation, or on frequency or intensity of client contacts during the referral process. On the other hand, it may be helpful to invest in following up on all referrals. For example, until 1937, public health nurses in New York City delivered infants' birth certificates directly to the family home, because this provided an opportunity to refer newborns for prompt health supervision (Bokhaut & Mahoney, 1960).

Follow-up postcards or letters can be sent to clients, but responding to mailed forms can require significant effort. Electronic mail may provide easier communication exchanges, but this technique may not be available to all. Telephone calls provide a framework for effective intervention, with a focus on reviewing the referral and its outcomes, supportive listening, additional teaching, or identifying/making additional referrals (Cave, 1989). This additional contact can reconfirm the appropriateness of the referral and resource for the client and allows for additional assessment of the client and context. Rather than promoting dependence, follow-up telephone calls promote independent decision making and critical thinking by encouraging client reflection and providing a means to reinforce client choices and actions (Donaldson, 1977). Follow-up home visits can be extremely useful but are also expensive in staff time and travel costs; reserving this approach for higher-risk groups requiring intensive services and multiple referrals may best balance costs (Brooten, 1995; Wingert, Teberg, Bergman, & Hodgman, 1980). One teen pregnancy program found that home visiting led to significant increases in the proportion of prenatal adolescents who identified and kept prenatal appointments; enrolled in the Women, Infants, and Children program; and applied for Medicaid (Flynn, Budd, & Modelski, 2008). Additionally, the technological advancements of today's healthcare environment provide additional

evidence of how this technology may be put to use with regard to follow-up (Lillibridge & Hanna, 2008).

ETHICS OF REFERRAL AND FOLLOW-UP

Public health nurses must also navigate several ethical conflicts or challenges embedded in referral and follow-up intervention at any practice level. The first conflict lies in the potential gap between what the client wishes/wants and the public health nurse's professional determination of need. Should the client's view or the nurse's view prevail? Some conflicts may arise from a lack of communication or misunderstanding. In this situation, the public health nurse may have to revisit the process of determining need and selecting objectives to meet the need. Perhaps the client's need has become more complex or multifaceted than originally determined, or perhaps, as a result of the referral process, the client has become more sophisticated in self-identifying the need and has now become more assertive in directing criteria for a reasonable solution. Clients may also be surprised at the lack of actual resources to meet their need or feel a right to "their share" out of a belief that others with similar needs have received more assistance.

A second type of ethical conflict in referral and follow-up is determining whether society can or should provide the resources or services that clients want. Many resources have eligibility criteria that can seem arcane to clients and families or even to communities. Is a client's selected option a need or a want? Differentiating between needs and wants is often a matter of perspective of our "needs" contrasted against their "wants," but public health nurses may have ethical obligations to both the client and the wider societal system. On what basis do public health nurses make judgments about resource access and distribution? Balancing individual rights to resources against ensuring the wider public good is difficult. The public health nurse must recognize when to protect limited resources and when to strongly advocate for meeting client needs.

Mandated or legally required referrals are a third type of ethical conflict for the public health nurse. In contrast to a voluntary referral that clients themselves decide whether to accept or reject, public health nurses must make legal reports or referrals to protect individuals or society from certain diseases and health conditions or from violence, abuse, or neglect; for example, parents may neglect immunizations or physically abuse their child, an individual may receive a positive screen for a reportable disease, or a frail older adult may have money stolen by a relative. When referral is mandated, it may be better to directly discuss the mandated referral with the individual/family. If a threat to the nurse is a concern, the discussion may take the form of notification through telephone or written formats. The nurse–client relationship can survive a mandated referral, thus allowing the public health nurse to be in an excellent position to contribute to and support a solution.

The last ethical conflict occurs when clients firmly decline a referral. Based on the ethic of self-determination, the solution is extremely clear: the client always and at any time maintains a right to decline referral. Coercive referrals, or referrals based on subterfuge, have no place in an ethical nursing practice. On the practical side, if clients oppose a referral, they are very unlikely to engage with or use a resource effectively. Unwelcome referrals are more likely to waste the referral agency's staff time and financial resources. Certainly, public health nurses may provide these clients with written information about a referral or may call back to check on clients' subsequent status, but

client refusals of referral are clear and must be respected.

REFERRALS AND FOLLOW-UP AT SYSTEMS AND COMMUNITY PRACTICE LEVELS

The principles of referral and follow-up for the individual/family level of practice have been discussed previously in this text. However, referral and follow-up also have implications for public health nursing interventions at the systems and community levels. Community- and systems-focused practices contribute to the context of referral and follow-up for individuals, families, and populations. Public health nurse engagement at the community and systems practice levels is often based on direct knowledge gained from individuals/families, of the strengths and weakness of referral, and of follow-up practices in a particular geographic area. Experienced public health nurses often identify weak areas that have potential to be strengthened through community and systems changes.

Public health nurses must move outside familiar programs and agencies to build linkages with both health and nonhealth resources that seek to monitor and address neighborhood and community needs at the systems level. Thinking broadly and creatively can increase the potential for problem solution, through modification of organizations, policies, laws, and/or power relationships. Public health nurse participation in these groups can lead to involvement in community assessment and intervention to reduce or remedy barriers to client/family access of resources. Perhaps new resources and services will be established in the community, or perhaps nursing organizations will seek support and broaden their existing services. The search for effective and appropriate resources to meet local, contemporary needs is ongoing; evaluation of existing programs and systems is a useful first step.

Acknowledging a need for additional resources and/or greater coordination and linkages among existing agencies may result from careful assessment but also from events that capture community concern. Our daily news often includes tragic reports; one community responded to the murder of a 7-year-old girl by her 12-year-old sister by first gathering and reflecting on the events and on how this might have been prevented. Several agencies had known and worked with this family, but breakdowns in referral and follow-up resulted in inadequate assistance. As a short-term system response, the community nursing service coordinated monthly interagency conferences to discuss cases, problems, and linkages. As a long-term system change, community agencies agreed to work toward improving county mental health services.

The public health nurse also has a role in shaping community norms, attitudes, awareness, practices, and behaviors for referral and follow-up. Are referral systems working well enough that individuals, families, and populations who require assistance are able to locate and use appropriate resources? Public and private health insurance does not address this expense, but do communities acknowledge these needs? Voluntary charitable groups, such as United Way, provide funding for information and referral services, but many community residents are unfamiliar with this resource and its use. Economic retrenchment in healthcare facilities and agencies discourages building and maintaining referral and follow-up systems, even when there is evidence that costs of care can be reduced. Individuals, families, and populations who require referral are often those who least know how to navigate contemporary community resources. Public health nurses have a role in raising their clients' needs and in reflecting the deficits of the current referral and follow-up system

to the widest community audience. Individuals do need help—and want help—to change, although community attitudes may frame this positive, optimistic quality as overburdening services. Community attitudes and community willingness to make financial commitments are key to improving linkages between those needing resources and existing resources.

Case Management

Case management "optimizes self-care capabilities of individuals and families and the capacity of systems and communities to coordinate and provide services" (Keller et al., 2008, p. 199). The American Nurses Credentialing Center (2008–2009) described case managers in the following manner:

> *Nurse case managers actively participate with their clients to identify and facilitate options and services, providing and coordinating comprehensive care to meet patient/client health needs, with the goal of decreasing fragmentation and duplication of care, and enhancing quality, cost-effective clinical outcomes. Nursing case management is a dynamic and systematic collaborative approach to provide and coordinate health care services to a defined population. Nurse case managers continually evaluate each individual's health plan and specific challenges and then seek to overcome obstacles that affect outcomes. A nurse case manager uses a framework that includes interaction, assessment, planning, implementation, and evaluation. . . . To facilitate patient outcomes, the nurse case manager may fulfill the roles of advocate, collaborator, facilitator, risk manager, educator, mentor, liaison, negotiator, consultant, coordinator, evaluator, and/or researcher. (para. 1)*

Case management takes place in a variety of settings. Some of these settings may include acute care, school-based programs, public health such as departments of health and/or visiting nurse practices, long-term care, and independent practices. Additionally, the individuals, families, and populations served generally present with complex needs and are vulnerable in their ability to access needed services. As such, a model of case management where there is a care manager who advocates for the client and family serves the system as well as clients, families, and populations (Bower, 1992).

Case management is often conducted in conjunction with other public health nursing interventions, including both the referral and follow-up intervention and the delegated functions intervention. Depending on client/family need, a public health nurse using the case management intervention may apply the delegated functions intervention to shift care provision to achieve improved quality or reduced costs or perhaps to secure more culturally relevant care providers fluent in the family's preferred language and knowledgeable of their cultural practices.

The case management intervention shares some aspects with the referral and follow-up intervention; some have suggested that referral is a component of case management, and others see case management as a more intensive application of referral. This chapter interprets case management and referral/follow-up as separate practices that share some elements. For example, the timeline of nurse–client interactions is quite different between the two. In referral, the public health nurse may have limited contacts with the individual/family; after implementing the referral plan, the public health nurse conducts follow-up to facilitate referral resource utilization, and to conduct evaluation. Case management, in contrast, suggests frequent interactions over a long period. Ongoing nurse–family

interactions permit the case manager to shadow the individual/family as they use resources to work toward their goal; this approach can be conceptualized as "following along" with the family to facilitate individual/family change.

Case management relates to several other public health nursing interventions. Outreach or case finding interventions may precede case management to identify individuals/families in need of services; case finding may also follow case management. Case management implementation may include the public health interventions of advocacy, collaboration, consultation, counseling, and health teaching. At the provider level of intervention, case management may lead to advocacy or collaboration and is closely associated with provider education (Rippke et al., 2001).

Framing Case Management

The characteristics of case management can be seen through two contrasting "frames." One approach to framing case management relies on its objective financial outcomes, which are driven by goals of cost containment, efficient use of resources, and reduced fragmentation of care. Case management may be focused "primarily on maintaining quality while controlling costs of health care through coordination and management of care" (Kersbergen, 1996, p. 169), through programs in which services are managed rather than cases. Because it is difficult to resist societal pressures to restrain spending, cost containment can easily become the driving force in case management. But care rationing may be structurally and ethically inconsistent with nursing's professional precepts and with the goals of quality care and thus possibly compromise the professional values of its nurse case managers (Beilman, Sowell, Knox, & Phillips, 1998). Knollmueller (1989) cautions about the risk of "turning case management into a scheme for rationing services if we limit the scope of service to a management of the benefit or a funding package and disregard the human faces behind the service" (p. 42).

The second contrasting frame for case management relies on meeting the needs and enhancing quality of life for individuals, families, populations, and communities; increasing service quality across the continuum and developing new services when needs are revealed; and developing the capacity of systems and communities to coordinate and provide services (Rippke et al., 2001). This approach to case management reflects public health nursing values in that it is client centered and relationship based but may yet be a vision rather than a working model.

CASE MANAGEMENT AT THE
INDIVIDUAL/FAMILY PRACTICE LEVEL

Case management "describes a process more than it defines a structure or an outcome" (Knollmueller, 1989, p. 38) and is frequently directed toward particular populations, especially populations with multiple needs, such as the frail elderly, people living with HIV/AIDS, or children with congenital illness (Tahan, 1998). As such, the first step in case management at the individual/family practice level is to conduct outreach and case finding to all individuals/families considered at risk and to offer case management services. As this step unfolds, the public health nurse seeks to develop a trusting professional relationship as a basis for effective case management. With the involvement of clients and families who respond to outreach and meet priority criteria for the agency's case management services, the nurse assesses their functional level to identify their needs. How and what do individuals and families

identify as an adequate quality of life, and what is the gap between these goals and their current status? Note that this step should include assessment of financial resources, especially to ensure adequate financial support.

Using strategies similar to the referral/follow-up intervention, the public health nurse next works with individuals and families to identify helpful resources and to design a detailed plan to access these resources. An effective planning process outlines each step to link the client to services and resources. Because families with multiple needs often require complex resources to meet these needs, the plan should incorporate strategies to form a multidisciplinary team. Early linkages across helping professions facilitate coordination and collaboration to meet individual/family needs. The individual/family remains part of this multidisciplinary team to assist with "troubleshooting" to resolve actual or potential barriers to service acquisition and use. Periodic formative evaluations of service organization, coordination, and case management are conducted with providers and the individual/family target of care (Rippke et al., 2001).

Case management by public health nurses has been found to improve health outcomes among women receiving Temporary Assistance for Needy Families (TANF). Kneipp et al. (2011) provided on-site public health nursing case management for women participating in an existing Welfare Transition Program (WTP), a requirement for those receiving TANF. Based on the development of trust with these women, the public health nurse provided case management interventions of "health access or entry into primary care for newly identified symptoms; care coordination; health education; health and social service referrals; obtaining preventive services, screening, and routine care; and assistance in meeting health goals participants had set for themselves" (p. 1761). In combination with the training provided by the WTP, the case management intervention led to improved health status among these women, including improved healthcare visit rates for mental health, reduced symptoms of depression, and improved functional status (Kneipp et al., 2011).

CASE MANAGEMENT INTERVENTION AT THE SYSTEM AND COMMUNITY PRACTICE LEVELS

Application of the case management intervention at the system and community practice levels is similar to those for the referral/follow-up intervention. The primary goal is "to create needed resources where resources do not exist or are inadequate" (Rippke et al., 2001, p. 97). The public health nurse intervening at the system or community practice level first identifies population subgroups whose quality of life is at risk and then conducts a resource assessment (similar to a community assessment such as the Public Health Nursing Assessment Tool presented in this text) to determine availability, accessibility, acceptability, and cultural competence of existing community resources. Having identified any gaps in community services or in the service system, the nurse collaborates with community organizations and systems to develop a plan to address existing gaps. In collaboration with community partners, the public health nurse also ensures that new resources and services are adequate and equitable. Periodic community assessment seeks to determine this "community's capacity to meet the quality-of-life needs of identified populations-at-risk" (Rippke et al., 2001, p. 97).

Delegated Functions

Delegated functions are direct care tasks that "a registered professional nurse carries out under the authority of a healthcare practitioner as allowed by law. Delegated functions also include any direct care tasks a registered professional nurse entrusts to other appropriate personnel to perform" (Keller et al., 2008, p. 199). In relation to the delegated functions intervention, the public health nurse may initiate **delegation** of functions to others as the delegator or receive delegated function from others as the delegatee. Because the focus of delegated functions is on direct care tasks, this public health nursing intervention occurs primarily at the individual/family level of practice. Consultation, collaboration, coordination, and communication have important impacts on care and services, but these are not delegated functions. No other public health nursing intervention discussed in this book requires another health professional's authority; all other interventions are nursing functions conducted independently under the local state's nurse practice act (Rippke et al., 2001).

A public health nurse might delegate to unlicensed assistive personnel, such as outreach workers conducting home visits in a maternal health program. In this case, the public health nurse delegates, for example, prenatal education to the outreach worker. In situations where a public health nurse trains lay health advisors, the nurse does not delegate nursing functions to them, and the lay health advisors share health information to their peers on an informal, "every mother knowledge" basis (Watkins et al., 1994). A school nurse may, in some states and for some skills, delegate to a school secretary, but the school nurse cannot delegate to parents assisting with vision screenings because they are not operating in an official capacity.

The delegated functions intervention also differs from the referral and follow-up intervention. Neither a referral from a hospital to a public health agency nor a referral from a school nurse to a support group is delegation. A referral given to an individual or family to seek additional services from a community agency does not involve delegation of skilled care tasks. In the same sense, coordination of care with a multidisciplinary team does not include transfer of nursing functions to others. Referrals from a physician or nurse practitioner for maternal–child home visiting or for home healthcare visits are not delegation, because home visiting is an independent nursing function. In this case, the physician or nurse practitioner's orders meet insurance reimbursement requirements rather than the legal requirements of delegation.

PUBLIC HEALTH NURSE AS DELEGATOR

The National Council of State Boards of Nursing (NCSBN) and the American Nurses Association (ANA), as well as nursing specialty areas (Timm, 2003), have demonstrated heightened interest in delegation since the late 1980s (ANA & NCSBN, 2005; NCSBN, 1995, 2005). Because every healthcare worker's contributions are necessary to address "the public's increasing need of accessible, affordable, quality health care" (NCSBN, 1995, para. 1), appropriate delegation of responsibilities and tasks must be ensured. Because NCSBN and ANA have been most concerned with nurse delegation to others (rather than the nurse as delegatee), delegation is defined as "[t]ransferring to a competent individual the authority to perform a selected nursing task in a selected situation. The nurse retains accountability for the delegation" (NCSBN, 1995, para. 5). In this context a nurse cannot delegate the practice functions of assessment, evaluation, and nursing judgment, and this means that a specific task cannot be "routinely and uniformly delegated" (NCSBN, 2005, para. 9); the nurse must determine the individual needs of each patient for each event of delegation.

FIVE RIGHTS OF DELEGATION

When the public health nurse contemplates delegating a function to another licensed professional or to unlicensed assistive personnel (Zimmerman & Kirkpatrick, n.d.), the nurse must consider the five rights of delegation to determine whether delegation can be done. The first right is whether it is the "right task": Is this a task that may be delegated? Nursing assessment, for example, cannot be delegated under most states' nurse practice acts. In school nursing, the appropriateness of delegating medication administration has received increased attention (National Association of School Nurses, 2010, 2011; Resha, 2010). A 2008 California Supreme Court decision concluded that unlicensed school employees may not administer insulin, based on a provision of the California Nurse Practice Act that specifically prevented nurse delegation of insulin administration (Block, 2009).

The second right is whether "the care setting, available resources, and other relevant factors [are] conducive to assuring client safety" (Rippke et al., 2001, p. 115). Especially when there is low potential for harm, low task complexity, minimal problem solving, and predictable task outcomes, a task is more likely to be appropriate to delegate. For example, many school systems do not provide a school nurse for each school, resulting in hours or days when a nurse is unavailable to children requiring health services. One New Jersey nonpublic school system developed and implemented a careful plan to allow delegation of epinephrine administration by unlicensed school personnel when the registered professional nurse was unavailable. Public health nurse consultants and the school system established detailed policies that balanced the risk of epinephrine injection against the benefit of its administration in carefully defined situations with carefully constructed checks and balances (Truglio-Londrigan et al., 2002).

In the third right, the nurse considers the characteristics of the delegatee: Does the potential delegatee have "reasonable knowledge, training, and experience to assure consistent and safe performance of the task" (Rippke et al., 2001, p. 115)? A nurse may delegate any nursing functions to another registered nurse, as long as the second nurse has appropriate knowledge, training, and experience for safe and consistent performance of the delegated task. An advantage of delegating to another registered professional nurse is that the nurse delegator can pass both responsibility and accountability to the second nurse, because both have the same licensure. This third step also requires the delegator to consider whether the patient's condition is sufficiently stable and whether potential patient responses to the delegated task are sufficiently predictable that the delegatee's knowledge and judgment are sufficient.

The fourth right considers whether the task's objectives, directions, and expectations can be clearly communicated (Hansten & Washburn, 1992): What is the right communication? If the task is unfamiliar to the delegatee or requires multiple steps and complex decision making, the task is less likely to be delegated. Maternal outreach workers, who provide antepartal and postpartum health education and support to women at risk for delivering low-birth-weight infants, are selected based on their experiences in working with pregnant and postpartum women and are provided significant additional training. These programs have demonstrated effective and predictable contexts in which to delegate public health nursing functions to unlicensed assistive personnel.

Supervision and surveillance by the public health nurse delegator is the fifth right. The delegator must be available to monitor, provide feedback, and answer questions. In public health nursing, when services are delivered in a variety of locations and delegator and delegatee may be in different places, a plan for ensuring opportunities for supervision and evaluation should be concrete. For example, in home healthcare services, the public health nurse supervises a home health aide at regular intervals and is available for questions by telephone. New or emerging patient or home health aide needs can be addressed with supplemental home visits, if needed.

PUBLIC HEALTH NURSING AS DELEGATEE

The public health nurse must also consider the implications of these principles when the nurse accepts delegation from other healthcare professionals, including physicians and advanced practice nurses. For nurses working in population health and working under independent statutory authority, there may be confusion about whether the public health nurse actions are delegated by a physician under relevant laws. One state supreme court determined that public health nurses were independently liable when they provided long-term medication management of a patient with diagnosed tuberculosis but failed to identify and respond to clear symptoms of a severe medication reaction that required liver transplantation. In this case the court determined that the health department physician was immune from prosecution as a public official and that this physician owed a duty to the public and no particularized duty to the patient (*State ex rel. Howenstine v. Roper*, 155 S.W. 3d 747 [Mo. Sup. Ct. 2005]).

When the public health nurse accepts delegation from a healthcare professional and the delegation is allowed by law, the five rights of delegation should be considered to guide the nurse in determining whether or not to accept the delegation. First, is the task to be delegated within a professional nurse's legal scope of practice? Although a nurse may have the knowledge or skill to complete a task, whether or not it is legal may vary according to state nurse practice acts. Second, a public health nurse must consider whether the circumstances are right to implement a task. A hospital-based physician seeking to delegate the task may be unaware or may not appreciate the complexity of the proposed task if it is implemented in an individual's home. The task must also be consistent with the public health nurse's agency policies and procedures, with which the delegator may be unaware or unfamiliar (Rippke et al., 2001).

The third right focuses on the public health nurse's "knowledge, training, and experience to assure safe performance of the task" (Rippke et al., 2001, p. 116). The nurse should not accept responsibility for a task when the nurse lacks or doubts his or her ability to ensure safe and effective care. The nurse must also consider whether the task is appropriate for this individual client and whether this client is stable enough at this time to attempt the proposed task given the public health nurse's knowledge, training, and experience. Fourth, the public health nurse must consider whether the orders, directions, and communications from the physician or nurse practitioner are clear and accurate. The fifth right is ensuring the right supervision is available: Who is responsible and accountable? The nurse must be clear that the task is within the nurse's legal scope of practice.

Whether public health nurses are the delegator or the delegatee, registered professional nurses retain professional accountability for their decisions. As the delegatee, it is insufficient for a client task to be ordered; it must also be within the scope of nursing practice. As a delegator, the registered professional nurse may delegate responsibility for task completion but retains accountability for the task—unless the nurse is delegating to another registered professional nurse (Rippke et al., 2001). Concerns for ensuring appropriate public health nursing interventions for delegated functions go well beyond exact performance of tasks. The scope of nursing practice, the relevant state nurse practice act, and legal decisions shaping nursing practice must all be considered.

Minnesota Department of Health Population-Based Public Health Nursing Practice Intervention Wheel: Application to Practice

Frequently, the frail, elderly population is at increased risk for neglect and abuse. In this population it is essential to have providers who understand their distinctive needs and clinical presentation of disease. A percentage of the elderly will be found in the nursing home or adult home. Within the walls of these nursing homes is a subpopulation of poor, minority, older adults who present with a complexity of needs.

In caring for the geriatric population, nurse practitioners face numerous challenges, such as clinical presentation of disease, limited access to specialists, and limited access to care. For example, the clinical presentation of a specific disease process in an older adult may be very different from a younger adult, such as in the case of a urinary tract infection. In a younger adult, a urinary tract infection most likely presents with urinary urgency, urinary frequency, and supra pubic tenderness, whereas in an older adult it can present as confusion, delirium, or fever. The American adult population is growing older, yet the specialists in this field have not kept pace with this growth.

The Case for Case Management

The following is a case study that exemplifies one of the intervention wheel's population-based strategies known as case management. After the case study there is a discussion as to the process of the case management and an exploration as to the application of case management in relation to the three levels of practice: individual/family, community, and system. In addition, **Box 10-1** provides questions for further contemplation by the reader after reading the case study.

CASE STUDY

NURSE PRACTITIONERS ENHANCING GERIATRIC MEDICINE

Shirley Franco, MSN, FNP

Gericine, a nurse practitioner primary healthcare group, was created to provide quality care to an underserved population. The nurse practitioners at Gericine care for and manage one of the most vulnerable populations, older adults residing in long-term care. This practice is located in the northeast, outside of New York City. The Gericine model provides accessible health care while facilitating and planning treatment options that meet the resident's needs. Nurse practitioners provide a comprehensive and individualized treatment plan and become the care manager for the population they serve.

Care managers are licensed healthcare providers who combine advanced practice nursing care with case management. The care manager becomes the primary care provider, advocate, and facilitator for the resident. He or she is responsible for providing residents with options and available resources while understanding the resident's status and life-to-death trajectory. Ultimately, the nurse practitioner care manager promotes quality, cost-effective outcomes. A nurse practitioner functioning in the care manager role commonly is faced with providing care for a resident like the situation described below.

An 87-year-old Hispanic man with a history of hypertension, chronic obstructive pulmonary disorder, chronic heart failure, gastric paresis, and recent gastrostomy tube placement for significant weight loss is newly admitted to a long-term care facility. This resident has been seen multiple times by a gastrointestinal specialist who suggested to the family that a gastrostomy tube may stabilize his weight. Despite the gastrostomy tube, the resident is losing weight and has had a 5-pound weight loss in 2 weeks. The resident's weight before the gastrostomy tube placement was 112 pounds, but now he is 107 pounds. The resident's wife is Spanish speaking and does not understand why her husband is still losing weight.

The nurse practitioner is challenged with providing culturally competent care to this resident with multiple comorbid conditions while trying to help the wife understand the disease process and where the patient is in the life-to-death trajectory. The nurse practitioner has carried out a comprehensive assessment, including talking to the resident's family and assessing the community where the resident had lived the past 50 years of his life. The nurse practitioner notes that both the resident and his wife were active in their community church and that the resident has been an active member of the "Green Thumb" club. In fact, the resident has won many awards for the flowers and vegetables that he has successfully tended over the years.

The nurse practitioner decides that she will need a multidisciplinary approach to provide comprehensive care for the resident and his wife. The nurse practitioner seeks out the assistance of a social worker to support her need for advance care planning, and she requested that the gastrointestinal specialist be present along with the dietary and nursing staff. Together, the multidisciplinary team is able to present to the resident and his wife the options and available resources located within the long-term care facility and the local community. They are able to create a plan that changes the current feedings to a higher caloric concentration and a slower infusion rate for easier absorption, and they explain the disease processes of gastroparesis and diabetes so that the resident and his wife understand the current situation and how the diseases progress. The team also establishes a comprehensive advance care plan that encompasses many of the aspects that the resident stated he wanted.

In this case, the nurse practitioner focused on delivering a collaborative, communicative, and comprehensive plan of care to the resident and his wife. As the nurse practitioner care manager, the focus is on the quality of the care that is delivered while balancing the most cost-effective positive outcome for the resident.

Box 10-1 Field Exercise

- Who is the population of interest in this case?
- Why would this population be considered a "vulnerable" population?
- What were the major issues for this particular resident and his wife?
- How would you describe the processes of case management that are taking place in the case study?
- What roles did the nurse practitioner exemplify in this case study?
- Can you think of any other healthcare team members who could have been engaged?
- Would there be a situation in which referral and follow-up was necessary? If yes, explain.
- Would there be a situation when delegation would be beneficial? If yes, explain.
- As the nurse practitioner engaged in the process of case management, what other ways could she be engaged at the community and systems level to enhance the care of the resident and his wife?

In the case study described above, it is the nurse practitioners who are involved in the case management process as they care for their population of older adults and their families. This process begins with the assessment that is beyond the individual assessment but also includes the family members with a look out into the community from where the resident was admitted. It is evident that the nurse practitioner works together with other members of the healthcare team but that this collaboration also includes family members. There is a give and take between all members with the focus being the resident and the resident's wife. The role of the nurse care manager is very evident as an educator, communicator, collaborator, and provider of care.

The nurse practitioner who is working as the care manager in this situation practices at the individual/family level as evidenced by the education taking place with the resident and the resident's wife, as well as the support and counseling. In addition, work at the community level may also be explored as this nurse practitioner care manager can reach out into the community and encourage members of their church and the Green Thumb club to come to visit the resident. In fact, the nurse practitioner may also encourage the community members to do more than just visit but to be engaged. For example, the members of the Green Thumb club may consider planting with the resident in small pots on the resident's unit or if possible work with administration to have a small section of the grounds dedicated to resident gardening. In this way the nurse practitioner is attempting to change attitudes of the community to look at the long-term care organization as a building that people can walk into and engage with the residents rather than walk by the building door. The nurse practitioner may also carry out the intervention of case management on the system level in the following way. From his or her experience, he or she may note that for some individuals in this vulnerable population the complexity of their problems may warrant more than the already established multidisciplinary team meetings as directed by Medicare and Medicaid. The nurse practitioner may request and lobby for a change in the long-term care system. The request may be in the form of a suggestion that, for newly admitted long-term care residents with multiple needs, weekly meetings take place for the first 6 months to ensure a smooth transition.

Conclusion

This chapter addresses three public health interventions in the green wedge of the intervention wheel: referral and follow-up, case management, and delegated functions. Each intervention was discussed in detail along with exploration as to how these interventions may be implemented at the individual/family, community, and systems levels of practice. The argument for case management exemplified a nurse practitioner case management model where the nurse functioned as a care manager for an older adult living in a nursing home. This case presents a real-life experience for the reader where the intervention of case management was explored, as well as how the nurse practitioner practiced at the individual/family, community, and system levels. The field exercise provided the context where the reader was able to reflect on the case and think beyond the field exercise box. In general, the green wedge offers the public health nurse additional strategies for the provision of care to populations.

References

Allender, J. A., & Spradley, B. W. (2005). *Community health nursing: Promoting and protecting the public's health* (6th ed.). Philadelphia, PA: Lippincott Williams & Wilkins.

American Nurses Association (ANA) & the National Council of State Boards of Nursing (NCSBN). (2005). *Joint statement on delegation.* Retrieved from https://www.ncsbn.org/Joint_statement.pdf

American Nurses Credentialing Center. (2008–2009). *Nursing case management.* Retrieved from http://www.nursecredentialing.org/NurseSpecialities/CaseManagement.aspx

Beilman, J. P., Sowell, R. L., Knox, M., & Phillips, K. D. (1998). Case management at what expense? A case study of the emotional costs of case management. *Nursing Case Management, 3*(2), 89–95.

Block, D. (2009). Reflections on school nursing and delegation (Editorial). *Public Health Nursing, 26,* 112–113.

Bokhaut, T., & Mahoney, I. E. (1960). A referral plan that serves babies. *American Journal of Nursing, 60,* 824–827.

Bower, K. A. (1992). *Case management by nurses.* Washington, DC: American Nurses Publishing.

Brooten, D. (1995). Perinatal care across the continuum: Early discharge and nursing home follow-up. *Journal of Perinatal & Neonatal Nursing, 9*(1), 38–44.

Cady, L. L. (1952). Planning referral forms. *American Journal of Nursing, 52,* 175–176.

Cave, L. A. (1989). Follow-up phone calls after discharge. *American Journal of Nursing, 89,* 942–943.

Champion, V. L., & Skinner, C. S. (2008). The health belief model. In K. Glanz, B. K. Rimer, & K. Viswanath (Eds.), *Health behavior and health education: Theory, research, and practice* (4th ed., pp. 45–65). San Francisco, CA: Jossey-Bass.

Clemen-Stone, S., McGuire, S. L., & Eigsti, D. G. (2002). *Comprehensive community health nursing: Family, aggregate, and community practice* (6th ed.). St. Louis, MO: Mosby.

Dieckmann, J. L. (1999). *Caring for the chronically ill: Philadelphia, 1945–1965.* New York, NY: Garland Publishing.

Donaldson, N. E. (1977). Fourth trimester follow-up. *American Journal of Nursing, 77,* 1176–1178.

Flynn, L., Budd, M., & Modelski, J. (2008). Enhancing resource utilization among pregnant adolescents. *Public Health Nursing, 25,* 140–148.

Hansten, R., & Washburn, M. (1992). What do you say when you delegate work to others? *American Journal of Nursing, 92,* 48–49.

Hogben, M., McNally, T., McPheeters, M., & Hutchinson, A. B. (2007). The effectiveness of HIV partner counseling and referral services in increasing identification of HIV-positive individuals. *American Journal of Preventive Medicine, 33*(2S), S89–S100. doi:10.1016/j.amepre.2007.04.015

Katz, M. B. (1996). *In the shadow of the poorhouse: A social history of welfare in America* (rev. ed., 10th anniversary ed.). New York, NY: Basic Books.

Keller, L. O., Strohschein, S., & Briske, L. (2008). Population-based public health nursing practice: The intervention wheel. In M. Stanhope & J. Lancaster (Eds.), *Public health nursing: Population-centered health care in the community* (7th ed., pp. 186–214). St. Louis, MO: Mosby Elsevier.

Kersbergen, A. L. (1996). Case management: A rich history of coordinating care to control costs. *Nursing Outlook, 44,* 169–172.

Kneipp, S. M., Kairalla, J. A., Lutz, B. J., Peneira, D., Hall, A. G., Flocks, H.,... Schwartz, T. (2011). Public health nursing case management for women receiving Temporary Assistance for Needy Families: A randomized controlled trial using community-based participatory research. *American Journal of Public Health, 202,* 1759–1768.

Knollmueller, R. N. (1989). Case management: What's in a name? *Nursing Management, 20*(10), 38–40, 42.

Kraus, B. C. (1944). The patient referral system. *American Journal of Nursing, 44,* 387–391.

Lillibridge, J., & Hanna, B. (2008). Using telehealth to deliver nursing case management services to HIV/AIDS clients. *Online Journal of Issues in Nursing, 14*(1). Retrieved from http://www.nursingworld.org/MainMenuCategories/ANAMarketplace/ANAPeriodicals/OJIN/TableofContents/Vol142009/No1Jan09/ArticlePreviousTopic/TelehealthandHIVAIDSClients.aspx

Manfredi, C., Lacey, L., & Warnecke, R. (1990). Results of an intervention to improve compliance with referrals for evaluation of suspected malignancies at neighborhood public health centers. *American Journal of Public Health, 80,* 85–87.

McGuire, S., Gerber, D. E., & Clemen-Stone, S. (1996). Meeting the diverse needs of clients in the community: Effective use of the referral process. *Nursing Outlook, 44*(5), 218–222.

National Association of School Nurses. (2010). *Position statement: Delegation* (rev.). Retrieved from http://www

.nasn.org/PolicyAdvocacy/PositionPapersandReports /NASNPositionStatementsFullView/tabid/462/Article Id/21/Delegation-Revised-2010

National Association of School Nurses. (2011). *Medication administration in the school setting* (rev.). Retrieved from http://www.nasn.org/PolicyAdvocacy/PositionPapers andReports/NASNPositionStatementsFullView/tabid /462/ArticleId/86/Medication-Administration-in-the -School-Setting-Revised-2011

National Council of State Boards of Nursing (NCSBN). (1995). *Delegation concepts and decision-making process: National Council position paper*. Retrieved from https://www.ncsbn.org/323.htm#

National Council of State Boards of Nursing (NCSBN). (2005). *Working with others: A position paper*. Retrieved from https://www.ncsbn.org/Working_with_Others.pdf

Office of Minority Health, U.S. Department of Health and Human Services. (2001). *National standards for culturally and linguistically appropriate service in health care. Final report*. Retrieved from www.omhrc.gov /assets/pdf/checked/finalreport.pdf

Resha, C. (2010). Delegation in the school setting: Is it a safe practice? *Online Journal of Issues in Nursing, 15*(2). Retrieved from http://www.nursingworld .org/MainMenuCategories/ANAMarketplace /ANAPeriodicals/OJIN/TableofContents/Vol152010 /No2May2010/Delegation-in-the-School-Setting.aspx

Rippke, M., Briske, L., Keller, L. O., Strohschein, S., & Simonetti, J. (2001). Public health interventions: Applications for public health nursing practice. *PublicHealth Nursing Section, Division of Community Health Services, Minnesota Department of Health*. Retrieved from http://www.health.state.mn.us/divs/cfh /ophp/resources/docs/phinterventions_manual2001.pdf

Tahan, H. A. (1998). Case management: A heritage more than a century old. *Nursing Case Management, 3*(2), 55–62.

Timm, S. E. (2003). Effectively delegating nursing. *Home Healthcare Nurse, 21*, 260–265.

Truglio-Londrigan, M., Macali, M. K., Bernstein, M., Kaider, G., Peterson, S., & Tumnio, M. C. (2002). A plan for delegation of epinephrine administration in nonpublic schools to unlicensed assistive personnel. *Public Health Nursing, 19*, 412–422.

U.S. Department of Health and Human Services (U.S. DHHS), Task Force on Community Preventive Services. (2011a). *Community preventive services: Interventions to identify HIV-positive people through partner counseling and referral services*. Retrieved from http://www.thecommunityguide.org/hiv/partner counseling.html

U.S. Department of Health and Human Services (U.S. DHHS). (2011b). *Healthy People 2020: HIV*. Retrieved from http://healthypeople.gov/2020/topicsobjectives2020 /ebr.aspx?topicid=22

Wald, L. D. (1902). The nurses' settlement in New York. *American Journal of Nursing, 2*(8), 567–575.

Watkins, E. L., Harlan, C., Eng, E., Gansky, S.A., Gehan, D., & Larson, K. (1994). Assessing the effectiveness of lay health advisors with migrant workers. *Family & Community Health, 16*, 72–87.

Will, M. B. (1977). Referral: A process, not a form. *Nursing 77, 7*(12), 44–55.

Wingert, W. A., Teberg, A., Bergman, R., & Hodgman, J. (1980). PNPs in follow-up care of high-risk infants. *American Journal of Nursing, 80*, 1485–1488.

Wolfe, I. (1962). Referral—A process and a skill. *Nursing Outlook, 10*, 253–256.

Zimmerman, P. G., & Kirkpatrick, C. (n.d.). *Delegating to unlicensed assistive personnel*. Retrieved from http://ce.nurse .com/ce124-60/delegating-to-unlicensed-assistive -personnel/

For a full suite of assignments and additional learning activities, use the access code located in the front of your book to visit this exclusive website: http://go.jblearning .com/londrigan. If you do not have an access code, you can obtain one at the site.

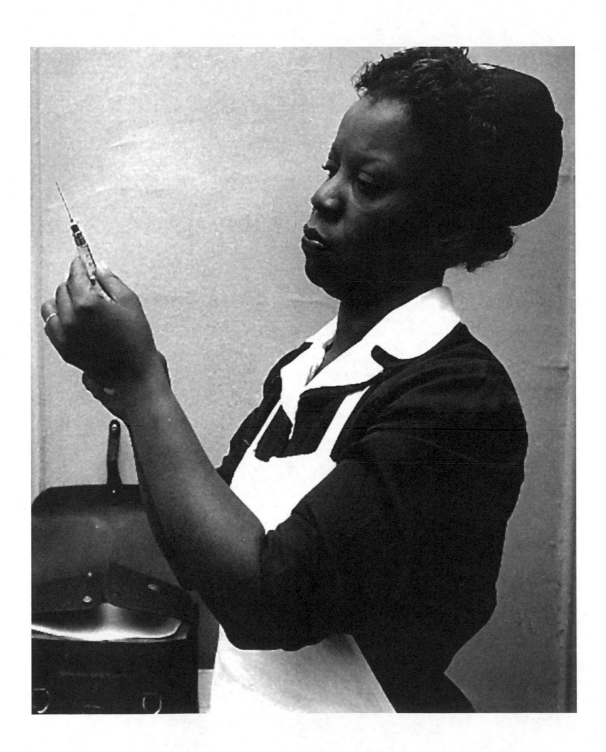

Chapter 11

Working It Out: Consultation, Counseling, and Health Teaching

Lin Drury

One of the most important points of a visiting nurse's work is the instructions she must give in the homes. The people must be taught some of the rules of hygiene and sanitation, and something of how to care for their sick.... Indeed, all of these people are not ignorant of what good nursing is, and I am sure every nurse has learned something from some one of them" (Moore, 1900, pp. 19–20).

www

LEARNING OBJECTIVES

At the completion of this chapter, the reader will be able to

- Describe the Minnesota Department of Health Population-Based Public Health Nursing Practice Intervention Wheel Interventions of counseling, consultation, and health teaching.

- Differentiate between individual/family, community, and system levels of public health practice.
- Analyze the application of the population-based public health nursing interventions of counseling, consultation, and health teaching to the presiding case study.

www

KEY TERMS

❏ Consultation
❏ Counseling

❏ Health teaching
❏ Vulnerable populations

The Minnesota Department of Health Population-Based Public Health Nursing Practice Intervention Wheel Interventions (Keller, Strohschein, & Briske, 2008; Minnesota Department of Health, 2001) exemplifies how public health nurses work with individuals/families and populations in communities to promote health, prevent disease, and limit the impact of illness. The population-based public health nursing practice intervention wheel is used to demonstrate public health nursing practice, to generate evidence on the best practices concerning public health nursing services, and ultimately to promote funding for research and health initiatives that public health nurses develop, initiate, and evaluate. The population-based nursing practice intervention wheel specifies 17 distinct interventions that are initiated through three levels of practice: individual/family, community, and systems that are population-based. In this text, these 17 interventions are grouped into five themes. This chapter focuses on the blue wedge, termed "working it out." Specifically, these interventions are counseling, consultation, and health teaching. The purpose of this chapter is to first define and describe these interventions, then to identify an issue in public health practice, and finally to demonstrate via a case study the "applying" and the "doing" of these interventions.

This intervention wheel also serves as a tool for conceptualizing public health nursing and facilitating a cognitive and practice shift from individual to population-based nursing. Providers and the general public are more than likely to envision the healthcare system as it is depicted on television—high technology interventions delivered to individuals in life-threatening situations. This vision, however, overlooks the health care that is delivered outside of acute care settings to individuals/families, populations, and the communities within which they live.

Throughout the 20th century, diagnosis and treatment of acute illness have driven reimbursement and shaped unsystematic services focused on sickness rather than health (Institute of Medicine, 2011; Partnership for Prevention, 2007; Schoen, Osborn, How, Doty, & Peugh, 2008; Wennberg, Fisher, Goodman, & Skinner, 2008). Consequently, it is much more difficult to envision a system focused on promoting and maintaining health and preventing and/or managing chronic illness. Nursing students and registered nurses who are engaged in hospital-based care may wonder how public health nurses design and deliver preventive services for entire populations because their practice is focused on the provision of care to individuals within a circumscribed inpatient unit (Benner, Sutphen, Leonard, & Day, 2010). The very thought may be overwhelming and sometimes confusing. The public, conditioned by prior experience, may wonder why they should see a nurse if they are not sick. The population-based interventions depicted in the blue wedge of the wheel—counseling, consultation, and health teaching—are critical processes for bridging these gaps and moving providers and the public into preventive care.

Minnesota Department of Health Population-Based Public Health Nursing Practice Intervention Wheel Interventions

Counseling

The public health nursing intervention of **counseling** begins with professional conversations between the nurse and the individual, family, and/or target population within the context of the community. Counseling "establishes an interpersonal relationship with a community, system, family, or individual intended to increase or enhance their capacity for self-care and coping. Counseling engages the community, a system, family or individual at an emotional level" (Keller et al., 2008, p. 199). The counseling relationship helps the population to reflect, clarify views, identify alternatives, examine available resources, and explore options in a supportive context. The public health nurse encourages the individual/family and population to consider the consequences of potential courses of action and to formulate their own decisions.

Counseling relationships evolve as the public health nurse earns trust through continuing contact with the population. Deborah Antai-Otong (2007) notes "Trust is germane to therapeutic and authentic nurse-client relationships.... The client's capacity to trust is governed by early interactions with patients and caregivers.... However, trust evolves through nurse-client relationships that convey acceptance, empathy, caring, and understanding" (p. 29). A study of public health nurses in Canada highlighted the role of trust in client empowerment. Aston, Meagher-Stewart, Edwards, and Young (2009) found that public health nurses fostered trust by shifting the balance of power away from the "nurse as expert" and instead engaging clients in transparent dialogue through active listening, believing in the client's strengths, and creating an atmosphere of safety and accessibility. Truglio-Londrigan (2008) spoke about trust as a process that forms through a connection that unfolds over time, allowing for a working together that further builds the relationship.

Vulnerable populations who have previous negative experiences with "the system" may require extended time to develop even a tenuous level of trust. Cultural norms and current life stressors may also extend the time required to earn trust (deChesny & Anderson, 2012; Drury, 2008a). In addition, as the sphere of communication widens from individuals/family through community and systems, and to populations, the possibility for miscommunication multiplies. Public health nurses as well as other public health practitioners need to be conscious of this as they seek to work "with" individuals/families and populations, always practicing actions that build trust.

Although public health nurses often deal with sensitive issues such as intimate partner violence, addiction, or homelessness, it is important to keep discussions focused on "here and now" problem solving via counseling. Psychotherapy is not within the scope of practice for public health nurses, and referrals to prescreened sources should be facilitated when needed (Browne, Doane, Reimer, MacLeod, & McLellan, 2010; Clark, 2008; Keller et al., 2008). The prescreening process takes place as the public health nurse locates organizations and agencies to serve as partners. These partners may assist the public health nurse in the provision of services such as psychotherapy. The prescreening process clarifies eligibility requirements, fees, and waiting lists, ensuring that those being served will not encounter bureaucratic barriers to treatment. This prescreening process ensures a place where the needs of the individual/family or a population can be addressed. The public health nurse in this situation promotes trust by facilitating access to care and following up on its efficacy.

The literature presents evidence of the importance of counseling as a population-based public health nurse intervention strategy. Edinburgh and Saewyc (2008) studied a home-visiting intervention that helped young (10- to 14-year-old) sexually assaulted adolescent runaways. The authors noted that the teens in this study refused traditional counseling as an intervention, and that traditional counseling was not culturally congruent with the needs of this specific age group. The authors noted "the solution was to offer all teens participation in a therapeutic empowerment group, which met after school weekly under the guidance of a skilled therapist" (p. 45). Other interventions in this home-visiting intervention program included mental health and screening referrals, health education, and daily living skills. Outcomes were positive in terms of reconnecting these young runaways to school and family. Hollenbeck (2008) advocated for universal newborn hearing screening and stressed the importance of providing emotional support, counseling, and education throughout the process, particularly if the screening identified that further examination was needed.

Frank and Grubbs (2008) studied the effectiveness of a faith-based screening and education program focusing on diabetes, cardiovascular disease, and stroke. The study outcomes noted the importance of conducting the programs in small groups that facilitated one-to-one counseling. Huang, Lin, and Li (2008) addressed the vulnerable population of older adults. These authors studied the service needs of residents in community-based long-term care and noted a need for psychological support and counseling pertaining to lifestyle change, role change, and environmental change. The importance of counseling as a population-based intervention is also noted among other public health practitioners. Olshtain-Mann and Auslander (2008) studied parents' stress and perceptions of competence 2 months after their preterm infant was discharged from a neonatal intensive care unit. These authors noted the importance of emotional support and counseling during the first year after discharge. Although this work comes out of the social work literature, many public health nurses work in early childhood programs supporting families during these first few years after discharge. Counseling is an intervention strategy

that public health nurses in all settings "apply" and "do" daily in their practice.

Consultation

The complexity of public health practice may require a wide range of expertise. Public health nurses may therefore find themselves seeking the **consultation** of others in their practice. These consultation services may include health officers, sanitarians, health educators, area professionals, epidemiologists, environmentalists, and media experts. Public health nurses may consult with a media expert if they need assistance on how to reach out into the community and gain the attention of a targeted population. Or, the public health nurse may seek consultation services of many different types of professionals or organizations. In this situation the development of a coalition may be the answer, and the public health nurse may be instrumental in the organization of this coalition and the development of a partnership between and among all involved.

Part of the success of partnerships and coalitions is that every organization involved in the coalition is actively seeking consultation from the other. Working together in these types of partnerships facilitates sharing of ideas and information where everyone's expertise is honored and used in the decision-making process. The public health nurse works within coalitions to mediate power and to ensure that decision making remains within the target population. Consultation "seeks information and generates optimal solutions to perceived problems or issues through interactive problem solving with a community, system, family or individual. The community, system, family or individual selects and acts on the option best meeting the circumstances" (Keller et al., 2008, pp. 199, 204). Just as the public health nurses draw upon multiple sources of information to assist populations to meet their needs, they may in turn be sought for consultation purposes to provide nursing expertise within the community at large. Ideally, the coalition includes members of the targeted population.

Hopson and Steiker (2008) demonstrate consultation in adapting the evidence-based drug abuse prevention program called "Keepin' it REAL" to a variety of schools. The authors noted that schools differ and that each and every school has its own culture and population of students. "Interventions that work well at one school may be a poor fit for others" (p. 116). To address this issue Hopson and Steiker used a participatory action research (PAR) approach to consult with students and staff to improve the program's "fit within a particular school" (p. 118). "PAR is dialogical and proactive typically focusing on empowerment and with researchers' and participants' values both being central to the planning process" (Kidd & Kral, 2005, p. 187). Kidd and Kral noted that collaboration exists in every phase of a PAR project. The collaborative partnership of the students and staff of the schools is critical so that the researchers may not only collaborate but also engage in consultation and learn from these partners about interventions that are most likely to succeed at each school.

Health Teaching

Health teaching focuses on providing information needed by the individual/family or population so they may become more aware of the promotion of health, the prevention of disease and injury, health screenings, available community services, and how to access those services. Health teaching "communicates facts, ideas, and skills that change knowledge, attitudes, values, beliefs, behaviors, and practices of individuals, families, systems, and/or communities" (Keller et al., 2008, p. 199). Health teaching engages participants at an intellectual level, whereas counseling engages participants emotionally. In practice, health teaching proceeds from the counseling relationship. For example, if a public health nurse is developing a mammography program for a particular population residing in a particular community, the nurse may first have to provide counseling services to address barriers to participation such as fear. The public health nurse must carefully assess the population and structure information accordingly. Once this assessment is completed, the public health nurse can develop educational programs tailored to the priorities of the individual/family or population. Information must be provided in a "user friendly" form and offered in measured amounts that can be absorbed easily. The goal for the public health nurse is to facilitate outcomes such as knowledge attainment and behavior change in the individual/family or population.

The public health nurse takes a flexible approach that helps the individual/family or population to progress gradually from non-threatening topics to areas that may be more emotionally or culturally challenging. For example, a public health nurse who offers a support group for battered women may have minimal attendance; however, offering a "mothers' group" instead may bring women who eventually, once trust is established, reveal abuse. These mothers may explain that if their partner caught them attending a group focused on domestic violence, their risk of battering would increase.

If we are to consider that public health is an interdisciplinary science, of which nursing is a critical participant, we may see the entire process of the development of educational programs in the following way. For example, multiple organizations in a particular community may form a coalition to promote health. The members of this coalition together have agreed to a formal partnership and have identified one of the organizations as the lead agency. Methods of communication, formal and informal, have been developed to reduce miscommunication. The coalition decides to collectively conduct an assessment of the community to identify issues and to organize these issues in order of priority. The coalition also has members of the community involved as key participants. All the data from the community assessment are compiled, and an analysis reveals several issues. One of the issues is obesity in elementary school children. Once the key issue is decided, the members of the coalition must collectively determine who the targeted individual/family or population will be, what content will be delivered, how the content will be delivered, where and when the content will be delivered, and by whom. Table 11-1 identifies these areas with examples of some of the key questions that the members of the coalition and the public health nurse must ask in the development, implementation, and evaluation of the educational program.

Many of these areas noted in Table 11-1 correspond with the determinants of health noted in the Graphic Model for *Healthy People 2020* (U.S. Department of Health and Human Services [U.S. DHHS], 2010). The determinants of health depicted in this model include: physical environment, health services, social environment, individual behavior, and biology and genetic. Policymaking, however, although not depicted in the Graphic Model for *Healthy People 2020* is described as a determinant of health in the *Healthy People* website (U. S. DHHS, 2010). Each determinant is considered here as it applies to health teaching and from here forward is referred to as a Systematic Approach to Health Teaching, understanding that there is an overlap of each of these determinants.

Biological/genetic determinants such as age, gender, and ethnicity can influence whether an individual seeks out new information, places relevance on the information, and puts that information to use. For example, Kaye, Crittenden, and Charland (2008) noted that "reaching and properly serving older men can be a challenge for practitioners" (p. 9). Older men may fail to participate in health education programs or to actively seek help because "many older men believe that a stigma is attached to seeking help" (p. 9). Age is associated with learning styles, sensory capacity, and familiarity with technological developments (Knowles, Holton, & Swanson, 2005). For example, the act of producing a pamphlet requires the public health nurse to be conscious of normal aging changes with regard to vision, requiring the production of pamphlets that have larger print and colors that are easily identifiable.

Working with children also brings challenges. The public health nurse must secure the cooperation of school or organizational officials in addition to obtaining each child's parental consent before any information is presented. Teaching about bodily functions, family life, and sexuality are likely to evoke worry and require extensive preliminary work with organizational officials and parent groups. Detailed consent and opt-out procedures must be agreed on before proceeding. Children's developmental levels are also important—for example, the adolescent's sense of invincibility pairs poorly with information structured to startle or scare participants into compliance. Strategies that emphasize active participation and peer group values are more likely to catch the interest of adolescents. Finally, attention to the determinant of genetics suggests that we look at the inherited conditions of particular populations such as sickle-cell anemia, cystic fibrosis, and family history of health disease as a guide to health teaching.

Social environment as a determinant, such as education and culture, are critical considerations in health teaching. Individuals may be reticent to reveal language, educational, or literacy issues

Table 11-1 QUESTIONS TO ASK IN THE DEVELOPMENT OF HEALTH TEACHING PROGRAMS

Who: Individual/Family/Population	What Is the Issue?	How Is the Program Delivered and By Whom?	When and Where?
Who is the targeted individual/family or population? What do we know about the targeted individual/family or population? What is their age? What is the gender? What are their cultural ideas, values, and beliefs? What is their level of education? What is the primary language spoken? What is their income level? What are past health experiences? What are significant past experiences? What behaviors or lifestyle characteristics does the individual/family/population exemplify? Are there any physical barriers to participating in the educational program, such as pain, hunger, or illness? Is the individual/family/population ready to learn or is there an emotional barrier present? Or, does the individual/family/population not see the issue as a priority at the present time? Are there marital issues or concerns? Child care issues or concerns? Transportation issues or safety issues that must be taken into consideration?	What is the content or the message that must be covered? How detailed is the content or message? Can the content or message be divided into sessions? How will the public health nurse know if the educational program is successful? In other words, what will be the evaluation process? What behavioral change is expected? Did the educational program connect with the individual/family/population and get the message across?	What is the best way to deliver the content given the information pertaining to the individual/family/population? What is the best channel that the message will be delivered given individual/family/population age, gender, physical and behavioral characteristics, etc. For example: Will the educational program be delivered via lecture, one-to-one, small group discussion, demonstration, media such as billboards, television, or radio. Will the Internet be used as a channel, including text messaging, Facebook, etc.? What materials will be used to deliver the message? For example: Will there be pamphlets, books, songs, games, or toys? Are the materials appropriate? Is the message clear and to the point? Who is the best person to deliver the message? For example: If the issue involves adolescent boys who are involved in sports, perhaps an athlete is the best person to present the information.	When and where is the best time to conduct the educational program? When and where is the best place to connect with the individual/family/population? For example: if the public health nurse wishes to conduct child car safety seat checks, it may be best to conduct this educational program at parks where young families may bring their children on the weekends.

that can interfere with accurate interpretation of health information. Translating written material into the first language of individuals/family or populations may be ineffective if limited education and health literacy are not also considered or if cultural mores render some topics taboo. When the public health nurse is working with an individual or family, discussion of written materials in private to solicit feedback and confirm comprehension while protecting self-esteem is essential. In other situations, enlisting a culturally appropriate licensed medical translator should also be considered.

Economics overlap heavily with social determinants in terms of educational background, available income, and access to resources (Summers, et al. 2009). Individuals/families and populations with limited income may find it difficult to gain access to health education programs even if they are free. Transportation costs or costs affiliated with babysitting may make participation in these programs impossible. In addition, the implementation of health recommendations such as including fresh fruit and vegetables in the diet may not be an attainable goal. The public health nurse must adapt teaching materials to fit the needs and the economic resources of the target population, providing information on economical substitute sources of fiber, vitamins, and minerals.

Physical environmental determinants such as characteristics of the structural environment may necessitate the tailoring of information or the way in which information is provided. For example, many clinics have environments that are not conducive to teaching given the constant interruptions and the noise, yet many clinic nurses make do with what they have and offer great educational programs. Examples of educational programming in waiting rooms include reading and math corners for young children to enhance literacy while at the same time modeling

behavior for families, food corners with varying boxes and cans from grocery stores that can be used as props to teach clients how to read labels, and healthy menu guides that are culturally congruent for the targeted clinic population. **Box 11-1** illustrates this use of clinic waiting time for educational programming.

Individual behavior as a determinant may be viewed in a wide variety of contexts: for example, whether or not a person chooses to engage in cigarette smoking or an exercise program. Yet another example may be the consideration of the psychological status of the target population to determine readiness for learning and behavioral change. Public health nurses frequently encounter individuals and family members in the community who have been discharged from the hospital after an episode of acute illness. Before hospital discharge, these individuals and family members receive volumes of information, typically diet sheets, medication schedules, activity restrictions, and follow-up instructions—all during the stress of illness and compounded by anxiety related to going home. Short hospital stays make this pattern hard to avoid, but nevertheless the public health nurse must plan accordingly. Expect the newly discharged to be overwhelmed and confused. Allow time during early visits to contact providers, clarify instructions, and adapt the information to fit the client's circumstances (Drury, 2008b). In addition, public health nurses find themselves working with vulnerable populations with complex needs, such as people who are homeless or have mental illnesses compounded by comorbid chronic diseases. These situations must also be accounted for in the development of teaching sessions and/or programs (Drury, 2008c).

Policy as a determinant must also be considered and assessed. In situations where there is a law that has been developed and implemented to protect the public, such as bike helmet laws, the

> ## Box 11-1 What To Do When Waiting: Example of Group Health Teaching Diabetes Education
>
> *Anny M. Eusebio, RN, MSN, FNP-BC*
>
> I practice in an outpatient satellite clinic affiliated to a major hospital in the New York area. The population is about 75% Latino and has limited reading skills in either English or Spanish. There is a high rate of obesity and diabetes in this clinic population. Furthermore, the majority have uncontrolled diabetes despite the best efforts of health care providers.
>
> In 2007 we attended an informational session where RNs and NPs were introduced to and taught how to use the U.S. Diabetes Conversation Map Kits created by Healthy Interactions in collaboration with the American Diabetes Association.
>
> The concept was intriguing. It uses visually stimulating maps (in 5 topics) as teaching aides for individuals in group settings. They are appropriate for all educational levels and are available in English and Spanish. These maps provide the data needed for individuals to improve diabetes self-management in a fun and interactive manner. This easy and engaging method facilitates discussion and is appropriate to populations such as ours with limited formal education.
>
> About a year ago the program was launched in our clinic in an effort to improve education via groups. The education included information such as diet modification and the expected health outcomes included improved fasting glucose and HbAIc levels. We have one English-speaking diabetes educator who supervises the group meetings. A Spanish-speaking nurse was also educated in the use of the Conversation Maps.
>
> Over the past 4 months this forum was extended to include the family members of the individual participants. This creates a further bond between spouses, children/parents, grandchildren/grandparents, and siblings. In particular, the family members that prepare meals for the individual clients are invited, but all family interested in expanding their knowledge of diabetes are welcome.
>
> These Conversation Maps are an interesting way to teach about diabetes, not only to individuals but groups in a culturally sensitive and congruent way.
>
> *Source:* Healthy Interactions, Inc., 2008.

public health nurse must be aware of how the law is implemented and develop health teaching for the population to facilitate compliance. In addition, when developing health teaching, the coalition and its members must constantly ask if the targeted population will be able to access the program they are developing. This question involves discussion pertaining to time of the program, cost of the program, transportation to the program, location of the program, and how the content of the program addresses the targeted populations ideas, values, emotions, and beliefs pertaining to the topic. Similar questions pertain to the determinant of *Health Services* and reflect the "seven A's" of the Public Health Nursing Assessment Tool as presented in Chapter 3 of this text.

Collective Consideration of Counseling, Consultation, and Health Teaching

What is of interest in the above description of counseling, consultation, and health education is how many of the population-based interventions are closely intertwined with one another. For example, public health nurses find they must carry out counseling first to emotionally support individuals through their decision-making process and at the same time provide education and seek consultation from others. Several well-established and extensively evaluated nurse-managed public health programs demonstrate complete integration of counseling, consultation, and health teaching.

The Transitional Care Model (TCM) (Naylor et al., 2009) provides in-hospital planning and home care support for chronically ill older adults. The nurse-led multidisciplinary team uses hospital visits, consultations with inpatient and outpatient providers, patient and family teaching, home visits, telephone support, and coordination of services to ease patient's transitions from hospital to home and to prevent readmissions. A randomized clinical trial of the TCM versus standard care for Medicare patients with congestive heart failure demonstrated a savings of $5,000 per TCM patient (Naylor et al., 2004). Multiple clinical trials over the past 20 years have measured the program's success in improving quality of care, preserving physical function, enhancing quality of life, increasing satisfaction with care, and reducing costs (Coalition for Evidence-Based Policy, 2010).

The Nurse Family Partnership (NFP) (Olds et al., 2010) supports first-time teen and/or unmarried low-income mothers with home visits from public health nurses throughout the pregnancy and for 2 years after birth. The nurses teach the mothers how to care for themselves and their infants; promote maternal growth through family planning, education, and workforce involvement; and facilitate access to community resources for mother and child. Outcomes for the mothers and their children have been tracked for up to 19 years in randomized controlled trials in at least 3 different locations. Overarching outcomes compared to controls that are consistent across at least two of the three locations are as follows: child abuse, neglect, and injuries down by 20–50%; subsequent births during late teens or early twenties down by 10–20%; and child educational attainment up by 6 percentile points in grades 1–6 reading/math. The total cost for the 3 years of monthly visits is approximately $12,500 per family in 2010 (Coalition for Evidence-Based Policy, 2011).

Insite is North America's first medically supervised injection facility, a place where users of illegal drugs can obtain clean supplies and inject their pre-obtained drugs with less risk of bloodborne disease or death by overdose. Public health nurses in Vancouver, British Columbia, Canada operate the multidisciplinary program that oversees 700–1,000 individuals every 18 hours, 7 days a week. The program was opened to address a human immunodeficiency virus prevalence of 17–30% and hepatitis C virus rates greater than 90% among drug users. The nurses do not supply or administer the drugs, but they observe clients at the injection booths from a centrally located nurses' station. They monitor clients for overdose symptoms, anaphylaxis, or unsafe injection practices. The nurses provide nonjudgmental teaching to reduce harm and offer assistance with any issues or concerns, including primary health care. They work with a network of community partners to help Insite's clients obtain access to basics such as food, clothing, and shelter. Addiction counselors and peer workers are on-site. Intense scrutiny by community and governmental stakeholders has led to rigorous data collection and analysis by external evaluators. Outcomes include a 35% decrease in fatal overdoses in the area and a 30% increase in the use of detoxification services. A 2008 decision by the British Columbia Supreme Court ruled that Insite should remain open and gave the Canadian federal government a year to make necessary changes to laws in order to relieve Insite from the burden of seeking continuous exemptions (Lightfoot et al., 2009).

The Case/Issue

In the other intervention chapters of this text, the authors present issues that public health nurses work with every day. Many of these issues and challenges are disease processes that are communicable, noncommunicable, and chronic illnesses. For this chapter, instead, a community is presented as a system under study with its many issues and challenges. These issues and challenges have a profound affect on the individuals/ families and the population that reside within its borders. What follows is a description of this community in need.

Community in Need

The Henry Street Settlement (HSS) is a not-for-profit social service institution located on the Lower East Side of Manhattan in New York City. Since 1893, the settlement has focused on meeting the needs of vulnerable populations and has expanded to include 19 sites serving more than 100,000 clients from around the world and across the life span. Although HSS was founded by the early 20th century nursing leader Lillian Wald to address the health problems of impoverished immigrants, Wald's insights into the determinants of health led to the development of programs encompassing education, recreation, the arts, sociopolitical activism, and economic development in addition to home and agency-based nursing care (Lewenson, Keith, Kelleher, & Polansky, 2001).

Today's HSS programs reach clients in their homes, in day care centers, youth groups, workforce training, homeless shelters, mental health centers, summer camps, senior centers, and in the performing arts. Ironically, nursing did not remain among HSS's core services. As the settlement grew over the decades and professional specialization increased, nurses left HSS and formed the Visiting Nurse Service of New York in 1944. Following this separation, HSS referred clients to outside medical providers (Feld, 2008).

Like their predecessors, current HSS clients are at high risk for a wide range of physical and psychosocial health problems. Substantial populations at HSS today were born in China, Africa, Latin America, or Russia. Disenfranchised by language, culture, and economic barriers, the needs of today's clients are complex and interdependent. Meanwhile, constraints on healthcare spending have reduced providers' incentives to accept such patients. As a result, HSS found its referral sources dwindling and its clients poorly equipped to compete for increasingly scarce public health care.

THE COMMUNITY

In 1893, the lower East side was a neighborhood of impoverished immigrants geographically and socially isolated from the wealthy sections of Manhattan. Lillian Wald found families

The Lower East Side of New York City, 1893.

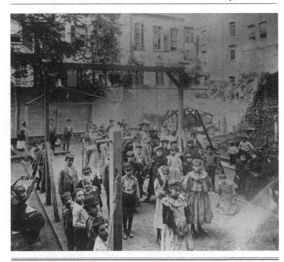

Source: Courtesy of the Visiting Nurse Service of New York.

doubled and tripled up in small, deteriorating apartments. Airless rooms, inadequate plumbing, and vermin joined with malnutrition and overwork to foster disease. Poverty and social isolation enforced by language and cultural differences contributed to despair. Residents in the early 1900s had few options for improvement (Wald, 1915).

Today, the lower East side is gentrifying. Luxury housing and business developments are replacing the tenements and attracting upscale residents (National Trust for Historic Preservation, 2008). The shrinking supply of affordable apartments has concentrated the HSS client population into dense blocks of New York City Housing Authority buildings and deteriorating rent-stabilized units. Immigrants still come to the area, and poor families repeat the pattern of previous centuries, doubling up or taking in boarders to meet rising rents in substandard accommodations. Henry Street Settlement clients share the geography of the Lower East Side but are isolated from their affluent neighbors by an unmarked economic boundary line.

The Lower East Side of New York City today.

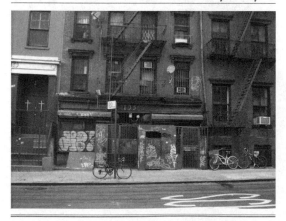

Source: Collection of Lin Drury.

POPULATION AND PROGRAMS

Henry Street Settlement clients range in age from newborns to centenarians. The population is outstandingly diverse, reflecting New York City in terms of race/ethnicity, culture, religion, and education/literacy. Specific programs target selected high-need groups. For example, the Parent Center provides drop-in support, education, and socialization to parents of infants and toddlers. The overwhelming majority of participants are African American or Spanish-speaking women of childbearing age, but there are no restrictions on attendance, and an occasional father or grandparent joins the program. Children in HSS Head Start programs reflect the demographics of families within walking distance of the centers. At one HSS Head Start site, nearly all the children are monolingual Chinese. The Housekeeping program serves more than 2,000 elderly and/or disabled clients throughout the city. On a single day, the caseload of that program includes 62 languages or dialects and an even larger number of cultures.

DETERMINANTS OF HEALTH: ECONOMIC

Clients across HSS programs have one characteristic in common, poverty. In addition, HSS grows its own employees by offering entry-level jobs to successful program participants. Consequently, HSS clients, plus most of the rank and file employees, represent vulnerable populations in terms of socioeconomic level, cognitive status, illness or disability, and life circumstances (Aday, 2001; de Chesnay & Anderson, 2012). City demographic data divide Manhattan into 10 clusters by zip code. The HSS area cluster is combined with two more-affluent zip codes in calculating the median household income, but it still ranks fourth from the bottom (Thompson, 2007).

Economic factors are strong determinants of population health in New York City (Summers et al., 2009). In September 2007, the city comptroller released a report on a 15-year study of the health of city residents. A key finding was the widening gap in illness rates between rich and poor New Yorkers. Since data collection began in 1990, preventable and manageable chronic disease has risen among low-income residents. For example, hospitalization of people with type 2 diabetes has increased 82% citywide, with poor individuals five times more likely to require hospital care than individuals from the city's wealthiest neighborhoods. The diabetes death rate was 125.2 per 100,000 people in the poorest neighborhoods but only 14.8 per 100,000 people in the richest neighborhoods.

The city comptroller summed up the report by stating that New York needs to do a better job of providing primary and preventive care. He acknowledged that low Medicaid reimbursement rates for routine care and wellness visits contribute to providers' preference for emergency department services for their publicly insured clients (Thompson, 2007).

Low-income New Yorkers are at high risk for a wide range of preventable physical and psychological disorders. They are two to six times more likely to experience serious psychological distress than their counterparts with higher incomes, and they are four times more likely to be hospitalized for substance abuse and/or mental health treatment instead of receiving outpatient care (Karpati et al., 2004; Thompson, 2007).

DETERMINANTS OF HEALTH: SOCIAL AND HEALTH SYSTEM

In addition to the economic disparity, many HSS clients are recent immigrants who face documentation issues, language barriers, employment disparity, and cultural distance from healthcare workers. Long-term HSS clients, therefore, not only must deal with poverty but also with social determinants that have an impact on their health. The HHS clients commonly suffer from

congestive heart failure, diabetes, hypertension, arthritis, emphysema, cancer, depression, and alcoholism. These individuals would benefit from case management and/or monitoring by a visiting nurse, but most are not eligible for these services under current Medicare or Medicaid regulations. Limited coverage for hearing, vision, and dental care further restricts many clients' functional capacities.

Working-poor clients and HSS front-line employees often hold jobs that do not provide paid sick days; thus, they cannot afford to miss work while seeking care. If offered, their health insurance is high in cost and low in coverage; many cannot justify this expense amid conflicting budget priorities. Clients and employees alike seek health care only when they are acutely ill.

For both clients and front-line employees at HSS, contact with healthcare providers is often limited to emergency department treatment, and opportunities for preventive care are lacking. Both clients and employees need user-friendly services that are culturally appropriate and available in a context they trust. In response to this burgeoning need for health care, HSS opened an on-site medical office. A multilingual physician and a culturally diverse staff run the office, but appointments during the workday are required. Medicaid and Medicare are accepted, but no free services are available, even for HSS employees. Perhaps as a result, since it opened in 2002 the office has been underutilized (V. Stack, personal communication, 2007). Recent efforts to expand participation in Medicaid managed care plans and community outreach projects are improving awareness and use of the office.

DETERMINANTS OF HEALTH: ENVIRONMENTAL

The unmarked economic boundary line separating low-income and upscale housing on the Lower East Side also determines the accessibility of shops and services for HSS clients. One subway line runs at the periphery of the area, and taxis do not cruise the streets as they do in middle class neighborhoods. The blocks within walking distance of HSS are dominated by retailers who aim for low-income customers: currency exchanges, bodegas (gritty urban convenience stores), 99-cent stores, and "greasy spoon" diners. At the local bodegas, clients on the Supplemental Nutrition Assistance Program (SNAP), commonly referred to as "food stamps," find it impossible to spread their entitlement of approximately $5 per day across the entire month. Food pantries draw long lines, but the fruits, vegetables, and whole grains recommended for a healthy diet are not among the available items.

Retailers and professional offices targeting upscale customers have recently opened several blocks away but are inaccessible to most HSS clients because of economic disparity, distance, language, and culture. Clients seeking a bank, supermarket, department store, gym, or restaurant must speak English, must have the agility to board a bus or have cash for a "gypsy" cab (informal and unregulated car service), and then muster up the energy to transport their purchases (and sometimes several children as well) up multiple flights of stairs or unreliable elevators to their apartment. A common refrain among clients is "It's just all too much. . ."

Minnesota Department of Health Population-Based Public Health Nursing Practice Intervention Wheel: Applying and Doing

The Intervention

The above presents a picture of a community with needs that have a profound health effect on the individual/families and the population who reside in that community. The proposed answer was to develop a university/community partnership to reintegrate public health nursing in a social service setting through a faculty/student public health nursing clinical practice.

The Partnership: Application of Consultation, Counseling, and Health Teaching

In the mid-1990s, HSS administrators were looking for healthcare resources for their clients while faculty from Pace University Lienhard School of Nursing sought community health experiences for their nursing students. They discovered a mutual opportunity. Consultations between the school of nursing and HSS led to an AmeriCorps grant in 1995. Ongoing faculty efforts plus internal funding from the school of nursing provided the groundwork for the current partnership between HSS and the school (Lewenson et al., 2001).

In 2004, a Lienhard School of Nursing faculty member, with a specialty in public health nursing, approached HSS with a proposal to develop a faculty practice and student clinical practicum in public health nursing on-site. Henry Street Settlement administrators recognized an opportunity to integrate preventive care, health teaching, and counseling activities into their social service delivery programs. The faculty member initiated the public health nursing practice and began planning for the current partnership.

The purpose of the partnership was to expand the breadth and depth of public health nursing practice at the HSS. The overall goal was to improve the health of an underserved population, HSS clients and employees, by engaging them in the process of community health planning with public health nursing faculty and students from the Lienhard School of Nursing. Thus the partnership incorporates the public health nursing faculty member, students from the school of nursing, clients and employees from HSS, and community residents and professionals who have interest or expertise on community issues. The partners decide what health issues should be addressed and suggest approaches. All members of the partnership jointly determine what evidence will be collected to assess the outcomes of its work. Members of the partnership continuously discuss where they are going and what process will work best to get them there. This consultation approach is particularly appropriate at HSS, given the facility's history and current pattern of service delivery. The Settlement was founded on the wisdom of listening to its constituency and then acting on the information obtained (Wald, 1915). Most HSS programs go a step further in empowering the population by employing current or former service recipients to mentor new clients: Children are trained as peer counselors, teens run a retail bicycle shop, mental health clients operate a clothing boutique, vocational program graduates gain paid employment within the housekeeping program, formerly homeless people work with shelter residents in preparation for permanent housing, and ambulatory senior citizens visit homebound elderly. The public health nurse faculty member continuously consults with all participants in the partnership to create interventions that provide learning opportunities for the students and positive outcomes for clients and employees. Many of these interventions take the form of health teaching and counseling.

How the Collaborative Partnership Works: Counseling, Consultation, and Education at the Individual/Family, Community, and Systems Levels

Public health nursing practice inclusive of health teaching, counseling, and consultation are often linked, particularly when working with

vulnerable populations whose past experiences with the healthcare and social services systems have inspired mistrust. In an attempt to engage a broad range of clients and employees, information, materials, and professional expertise from the school of nursing faculty and students are available at multiple HSS locations. The cultural diversity and life experiences of the school of nursing students make it possible to match the special skills and interests of students with particular populations at HSS. The public health nursing faculty member and students spend time at each location counseling clients and employees and offering nonthreatening health teaching sessions to build trust. As clients and employees share their interests and concerns, the school of nursing faculty member and students respond with information, hands-on interventions, and individualized counseling as needed. The partnership works collectively and collaboratively to design, implement, and evaluate health promotion, early intervention, and disease management programs for the HSS population-at-large. The nursing students perform community health assessments, conduct group health educational programs, organize activity sessions, provide one-on-one health counseling, make home healthcare visits, and provide referrals and follow-up care. The school of nursing provides loaner and donor equipment and supplies to assist the population in self-monitoring of health or management of chronic illness.

For example, the HSS population is at high risk for a comorbidity pattern of obesity, diabetes, hypertension, and heart disease. A healthy diet is key to interrupting this pattern, but the economic and environmental disparities detailed above foster diets high in carbohydrates, sodium, and fat. Students intervene at the systems level by joining with advocacy groups to increase SNAP allocations, contacting the city council to permit the use of food stamps at farmers' markets, and participating in a neighborhood coalition to obtain city-sponsored "green carts" for the area. At the community level, students canvass local bodegas and more distant grocery stores to counsel managers about the condition and price of perishable foods in an attempt to protect the public. They make reports to the department of health when needed and follow up on results. In addition, students consult with food service administrators on menu planning and provide classes for the cooking staff in the day care and senior centers. They work with the housekeepers and senior companions to select healthy foods when doing grocery shopping and light meal preparation for homebound seniors. On the individual and family level, students offer classes and cooking demonstrations throughout HSS that are focused on healthy eating on a budget.

Each counseling and health teaching activity leads to others, sometimes progressing from the individual or group out to a wider audience. Students discovered that homeless clients in residential shelter program had little experience in meal planning and preparation. They created a series of groups, including grocery shopping field trips, as a way to council and teach this vulnerable population. Shelter clients found they could not stretch their SNAP allotment across the month unless they bought in bulk, but their rooms came with individual-size refrigerators. The students organized their clients to meet with the shelter director and to begin a letter-writing campaign requesting larger refrigerators with freezer space. The building has a complex funding stream, multiple layers of management, and subcontracted program operations. It was a challenge just to determine who should receive the letters, but working through the system has united the clients around a common goal. It may be a long time before the Department of Housing and Urban Development responds to the client's request, but they have developed a "voice" within the shelter program.

Outcomes

The partnership began with eight students during one semester in one HSS program serving one population. After 6 years, 80 to 100 students deliver year-round care to clients and employees in 12 distinct HSS programs at multiple sites that serve populations across the organization. There is increased participation by clients and employees at each site as well as an increase in requests for further public health nursing services. Employees are taking an increasingly active role in urging nonparticipating clients and coworkers to obtain services. Public health nurses were hired for HSS programs that had not previously employed them, and recent graduates from the school of nursing with experience in the partnership were hired to provide professional nursing assessments for clients in the housekeeping program. A director of nursing was hired to launch a home healthcare service at HSS.

LESSONS LEARNED

A partnership between two organizations with multiple "players" is always a work in progress with multiple unknowns. The public health nursing faculty member has made a substantial commitment of time and energy to become a trusted figure within HSS. Changes in clients' circumstances, employee turnover, and school of nursing student rotations are constants that require continuous adjustment and modification. Organizational dynamics, funding issues, and political variables can dramatically alter the climate in which the partnership works. The global economic crisis had an immediate and devastating impact on governmental, corporate, and philanthropic funding to HSS. Budgets have been cut, programs have been trimmed, and some of the new nursing positions have been lost. The number of clients in need of HSS services is rising while staff and other resources are shrinking.

To address this crisis, the partnership between Lienhard School of Nursing (now part of Pace University's new College of Health Professions) and HSS has expanded and widened its scope to include undergraduate students in computer sciences. A small University grant provides clients in senior services programs at HSS with refurbished wireless computers and mentoring into online social networks. Undergraduate students in nursing and computer sciences work in teams making home visits to homebound low-income older adults who need a virtual social network, but who lack the equipment and expertise to gain access. Nursing students assess the client's cognitive and physical capacity to use computers, determining if the client is literate and mentally clear, if a large keyboard is needed because of arthritis, or if an extra large monitor is required because of visual impairment. Computer science students refurbish donated computers and adapt them to meet the senior's needs. They install these customized computers and make a series of home visits to provide one-to-one mentoring on how to use email, video chat, and Web searches. Nursing students make continuing contact with the client online and by home visit to reduce social isolation and to monitor ongoing health needs. Henry Street Settlement staff members get regular updates on each senior and provide referrals for additional services as needed.

Providing seniors with computers and Internet access brings a virtual community into their homes, fostering mental activity and "neighborly" monitoring when assistance is needed. Online seniors can stay connected with family and support services without traveling, often forestalling institutional placement. We envision the gradual progression of a virtual senior center for the growing number of HSS clients who can no longer walk to the physical facility. Teaching clients how to use the computer and counseling them in Internet communication strategies will allow thinly stretched HSS case workers to keep in touch with their expanding caseloads online. Virtual home visits will help caseworkers to prioritize when a costly face-to-face visit is required. Cost benefit data are being collected and funding is being sought to sustain and expand the program.

The partnership is fluid and ever changing. Participation in all activities and programs is voluntary for all clients and employees who choose to be involved. Data collection is limited to what clients and employees are comfortable in providing. Risks to participants are limited to minor discomfort associated with some screening procedures and potential stress associated with discussing personal issues. Participants benefit, however, by obtaining free and convenient attention for health concerns and by having access to nursing students and a faculty member who provide health teaching and counseling within their own home community. Referrals and follow-up are available for any participant who needs additional care, but still some choose not to take advantage of the services offered. The partnership continues to reach out.

Conclusion

The HSS case study highlights the enormous impact of the determinants of health on the individual/family or population and demonstrates that the nursing interventions of counseling, consultation, and health teaching must address health disparities at the systems level while simultaneously providing direct care to people. The *systematic approach to health teaching* and the seven A's assist the public health nurse to synthesize information in a complex environment. The PAR ensures that the population guides public health nurses in collaborative practice with the community.

References

Aday, L. A. (2001). *At risk in America: The health and health care needs of vulnerable populations in the United States*. San Francisco, CA: Jossey-Bass.

Antai-Otong, D. (2007). *Nurse-client communication: A life span approach*. Sudbury, MA: Jones and Bartlett.

Aston, M., Meagher-Stewart, D., Edwards, N., & Young, L. M. (2009). Public health nurses' primary care practice: Strategies for fostering citizen participation. *Journal of Community Health Nursing, 26*, 24–34.

Benner, P., Sutphen, M., Leonard, V., & Day, L. (2010). *Educating nurses: A call for radical transformation*. San Francisco, CA: Jossey-Bass.

Browne, A. J., Doane, G. H., Reimer, J., MacLeod, M. L. P., & McLellan, E. (2010). Public health nursing practice with 'high priority' families: The significance of contextualizing 'risk.' *Nursing Inquiry, 17*(1), 26–37.

Coalition for Evidence-Based Policy. (2010). *Top tier evidence initiative: Evidence summary for the Transitional Care Model*. Washington, DC: Author.

Coalition for Evidence-Based Policy. (2011). *Top tier evidence initiative: Evidence summary for the Nurse-Family Partnership*. Washington, DC: Author.

Clark, M. J. (2008). *Community health nursing: Advocacy for population health*. Upper Saddle River, NJ: Pearson Education.

de Chesnay, M., & Anderson, B. A. (Eds.). (2012). *Caring for the vulnerable: Perspectives in nursing theory, practice, and research*. Sudbury, MA: Jones & Bartlett Learning.

Drury, L. J. (2008a). From homeless to housed: Caring for people in transition. *Journal of Community Health Nursing, 25*(2), 91–105.

Drury, L. J. (2008b). Increasing competency in the care of homeless patients. *Journal of Continuing Education in Nursing, 39*(4), 153–154.

Drury, L. J. (2008c). Transition from hospital to home care: What gets lost between the discharge plan and the real world? *Journal of Continuing Education in Nursing, 39*(5), 198–199.

Edinburgh, L. D., & Saewyc, E. M. (2008). A novel, intensive home-visiting intervention for runaway, sexually exploited girls. *Journal Compilation, 14*(1), 41–48.

Feld, M. N. (2008). *Lillian Wald: A biography*. Chapel Hill, NC: University of North Carolina Press.

Frank, D., & Grubbs, L. (2008). A faith-based screening/education program for diabetes, CVD, and stroke in rural African Americans. *ABNF Journal, 19*(3), 96–101.

Healthy Interactions, Inc. (Healthyi) in collaboration with the American Diabetes Association. (2008).

U.S. D. conversation map program. Retrieved from http://healthyinteractions.com/us/en/diabetes/hcp/about/program

Hollenbeck, L. (2008). Advocating for universal newborn hearing screening. *Creative Nursing, 14*(2), 75–81.

Hopson, L. M., & Steiker, L. K. H. (2008). Methodology for evaluating an adaptation of evidence-based drug abuse prevention in alternative schools. *Children & Schools, 30*(2), 116–127.

Huang, J.-J., Lin, K.-C., & Li, I.-C. (2008). Service needs of residents in community-based long-term care facilities in northern Taiwan. *Journal of Clinical Nursing, 17*(1), 99–108.

Institute of Medicine. (2011). *The future of nursing: Leading change, advancing health*. Washington, DC: National Academies Press.

Karpati, A., Kerker, B., Mostashari, F., Singh, T., Hajat, A., Thorpe, L., . . . Frieden, T. (2004). *Health disparities in New York City*. New York, NY: New York City Department of Health and Mental Hygiene.

Kaye, L. W., Crittenden, J. A., & Charland, J. (2008). Invisible older men: What we know about older men's use of healthcare and social service. *Generations, 32*(1), 9–14.

Keller, L. O., Strohschein, S., & Briske, L. (2008). Population-based public health nursing practice: The intervention wheel. In M. Stanhope & J. Lancaster (Eds.), *Public health nursing: Population-centered health care in the community* (pp. 199–205). St. Louis, MO: Mosby Elsevier

Kidd, S. A., & Kral, M. J. (2005). Practicing participatory research. *Journal of Counseling Psychology, 52*(2) 187–195.

Knowles, M. S., Holton, E. F., & Swanson, R. A. (2005). *The adult learner: The definitive classic in adult education and human resource development* (6th ed.). Boston, MA: Elsevier.

Lewenson, S., Keith, K. A., Kelleher, C., & Polansky, E. (2001). Carrying on the legacy of Lillian Wald: Partnership with the Henry Street Settlement and the Lienhard School of Nursing at Pace University. *Nursing Leadership Forum, 5*(4), 116–121.

Lightfoot, B., Panessa, C., Hayden, S., Thumath, M., Goldstone, I., & Pauly, B. (2009). Gaining insite: Harm reduction in nursing practice. *Canadian Nurse, 105*(4), 16–22.

Minnesota Department of Health/Office of Public Health Practice. (2001). Public health interventions: Applications for public health nursing. Retrieved from www.health.state.mn.us/divs/cfh/ophp/resources/docs/ph-interventions_manual2001.pdf

Moore, E. J. (1900). Visiting nursing. *American Journal of Nursing, 1*(1), 17–21.

National Trust for Historic Preservation. (2008). National trust for historic preservation names: 2008 list of America's 11 most endangered historic places. Retrieved from http://www.nationaltrust.org

Naylor, M. D., Brooten, D. A., Campbell, R. L., Maislin, G., McCauley, K. M., & Schwartz, J. S. (2004). Transitional care of older adults hospitalized with heart failure: A randomized, controlled trial. *Journal of the American Geriatric Society, 52*(7), 675–684.

Naylor, M. D., Feldman, P. H., Keating, S., Koren, M. J., Kurtzman, E. T., Maccoy, M. C., & Krakauer, R. (2009). Translating research into practice: Transitional care for older adults. *Journal of Evaluation in Clinical Practice, 15*(6), 1164–1170.

Olds, D. L., Kitzman, H. J., Cole, R. C., Hanks, C. A., Arcoleo, K. J., Anson, E. A., . . . Stevenson, A. J. (2010). Enduring effects of prenatal and infancy home visiting by nurses on maternal life course and government spending: Follow-up of a randomized trial among children at age 12 years. *Archives of Pediatrics & Adolescent Medicine, 164*(5), 419–424.

Olshtain-Mann, O., & Auslander, G. (2008). Parents of preterm infants two months after discharge from the hospital: Are they still at (parental) risk? *Health & Social Work, 33*(2), 299–308.

Partnership for Prevention. (2007). Preventative care: A national profile on use, disparities, and health benefits. Retrieved from http://www.prevent.org/NCPP

Schoen, C., Osborn, R., How, S. K. H., Doty, M. M., & Peugh, J. (2008). In chronic condition: Experiences of patients with complex health needs in eight countries. Retrieved from http://www.commonwealthfund.org/publications/publications_show.htm?doc_id=726496

Summers, C., Cohen, L., Havusha, A., Slinger, F., & Farley, T. (2009). *Take care New York 2012: A policy for a healthier New York City.* New York, NY: City Department of Health and Mental Hygiene.

Thompson, W. C. (2007). *Health and wealth: Assessing and addressing income disparities in the health of New Yorkers.* New York, NY: Office of the New York City Comptroller.

Truglio-Londrigan, M. (2008). Flattening the field: Group decision-making. In S. B. Lewenson & M. T. Londrigan (Eds.), *Decision-making in nursing: Thoughtful approaches for practice* (pp. 131–144). Sudbury, MA: Jones and Bartlett.

U.S. Department of Health and Human Services (U.S. DHHS). (2010). *Healthy people 2020.* Washington, DC: U.S. Government Printing Office.

Wald, L. D. (1915). *The house on Henry Street.* New York, NY: Henry Holt & Company.

Wennberg, J. E., Fisher, E. S., Goodman, D. C., & Skinner, J. S. (2008). Tracking the care of patients with severe chronic illness. Retrieved from http://www.dartmouthatlas.org

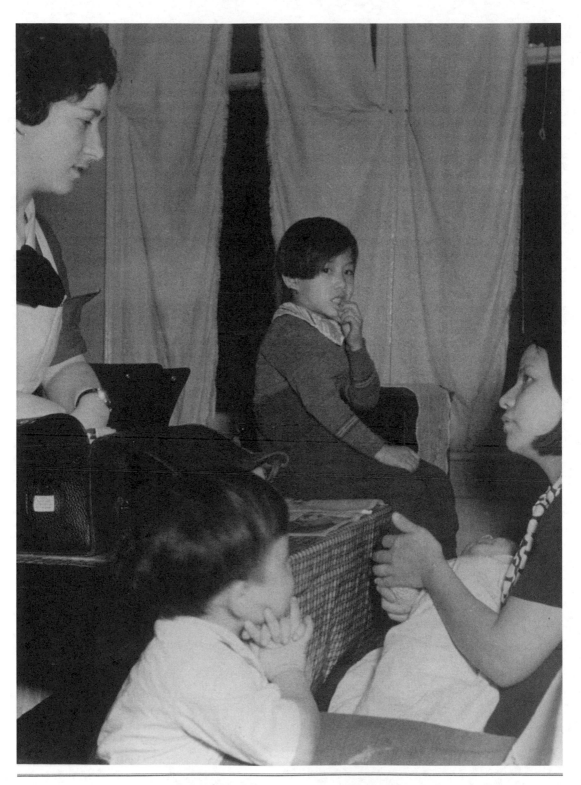

Chapter 12

Working Together: Collaboration, Coalition Building, and Community Organizing

Adrienne Wald

Public health nursing, being closely related to the activities of several other professions and many community organizations, cannot be carried on successfully and productively as an isolated service. The more closely it is coordinated with the interests and activities of other related and cooperating agencies through a constant sharing and interchange of ideas and service, the more soundly and economically will it fulfill its purpose (National Organization for Public Health Nursing, 1939, p. 15).

LEARNING OBJECTIVES

At the completion of this chapter, the reader will be able to

- Define collaboration, coalition building, and community organizing.
- Apply collaboration, coalition building, and community organizing strategies at appropriate levels of practice.

- Explore evidence-based ways that public health nurses practice these strategies to impact public health outcomes.

KEY TERMS

- ❏ Coalition building
- ❏ Collaboration

- ❏ Community organizing

The interventions in the orange section of the Minnesota Department of Health Population-Based Public Health Nursing Practice Intervention Wheel are presented in this chapter. This orange section includes the three interventions of collaboration, coalition building, and community organizing as depicted in the wheel conceptual model (Keller, Strohschein, & Briske, 2008; Minnesota Department of Health, 2001). This chapter devotes a separate section to each of the three interventions. Section one is about collaboration, section two presents coalition building, and section three discusses community organizing. Together, these three interventions are considered types of "collective action" (Keller et al., 2008, p. 193). Each of these three interventions is discussed with examples of how they are applied at the appropriate level of intervention: individual/family, community, and system. Each of the following sections (collaboration, coalition building, and community organizing) describes evidence-based practices used to address the issue examined in depth in this chapter: physical inactivity. The application of these interventions to this important 21st-century public health crisis illustrates aspects of how each intervention strategy works and reinforces key concepts.

Issue: Physical Inactivity Is a Major 21st Century Public Health Concern

Today, leading experts consider physical inactivity to be one of the most critically important public health problems of our times (Blair, 2009; Sallis, 2009). In 2003, physical inactivity was estimated to be responsible for over 200,000 deaths each year in the United States (Pate et al., 2006). Additionally, the World Health Organization (WHO, 2002) estimates that worldwide, 2 million deaths per year can be attributed to

physical inactivity, making it a global health crisis as well. For the second time in history, the United Nations met to focus on a public health issue: the problem of non-communicable diseases (NCDs). At this Summit, organized by the WHO, the critical need to better address the enormous global burden of these diseases was recognized. NCDs include heart attacks and strokes, cancers, diabetes, and chronic respiratory disease, and account for over 63% of deaths in the world (WHO, 2011). Every year, NCDs kill 9 million people under the age of 60. According to the WHO, "NCD's are largely preventable by means of effective interventions that tackle shared risk factors, namely: tobacco use, unhealthy diet, physical inactivity, and harmful use of alcohol" (WHO, 2011, para. 1). Substantial improvements in health and quality of life are possible by including moderate amounts of physical activity in daily life, according to evidence-based findings from a major report updated in 2008 by the Surgeon General on physical activity and health (U.S. Department of Health and Human Services [U.S. DHHS], 1996, 2008). The health benefits of physical activity and its importance in promoting good overall health and in reducing the risk of many chronic diseases, such as heart disease, type 2 diabetes, depression, and some cancers, and obesity are well known (Blair, 2009; Pollard, 2003). Strong evidence is emerging on the role of physical activity in brain health and the delay of cognitive decline (Blair, 2009).

In spite of this evidence that regular physical activity is necessary for health promotion and disease prevention for all populations, individuals in age groups from children to adolescents to older adults are not engaging in sufficient physical activity to achieve these benefits. According to the WHO (2002), 60% of the world's population does not get enough physical activity to achieve even the minimal recommendation of at least 30 minutes of moderate intensity activity per day. For

Figure 12-1 Trend in percent of Americans meeting recommended physical activity (1986–2000).

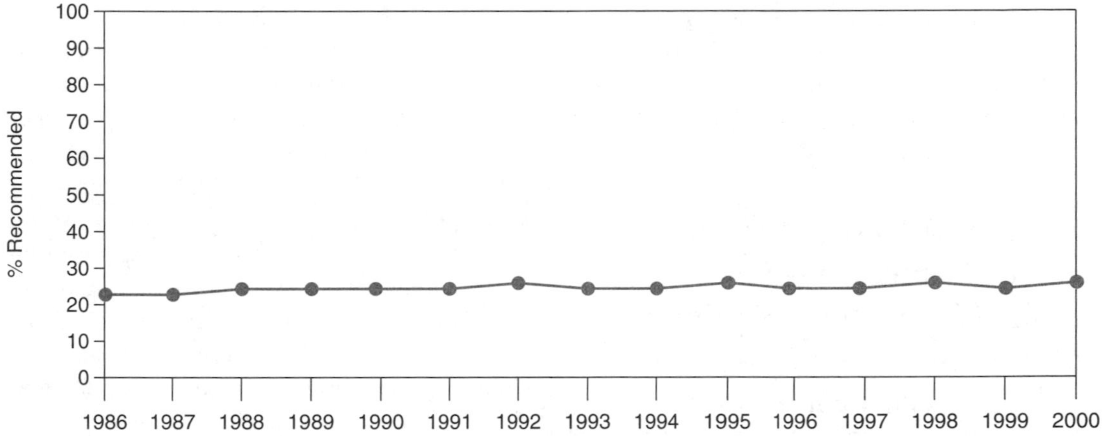

Source: Data from Centers for Disease Control and Prevention, 2000.

those who do not follow the minimum recommendations for physical activity, the risk of getting a cardiovascular disease increases by 1.5 times.

Further, the costs associated with inactivity and obesity accounted for some 9.4% of the national U.S. health expenditure, whereas in Canada physical inactivity accounted for about 6% of total healthcare costs in 1995. Data from 1998 indicate that in the United States, individuals who are physically active save an estimated $500 per year in healthcare costs. It is reported that inactivity alone may have contributed as much as $75 billion to U.S. medical costs in the year 2000 (WHO, 2002). In the United States, there has been no increase in the level of physical activity participation from 1986 through 2000 (**Figure 12-1**), implying that most of the strategies during this time period have been ineffective in increasing physical activity participation in Americans. Indeed, data for deaths from low (cardiorespiratory) fitness indicate that it kills more Americans than smoking, diabetes, and obesity ("smokadiabesity") combined (see **Figure 12-2**) (Khan & Tunaiji, 2011).

Figure 12-2 A comparison of deaths attributable to low fitness (men (m) and women (w)) and the combined effect of smoking (S), diabetes (D) and obesity (O) (men and women). Slide represents the identical data published by Blair (2009).

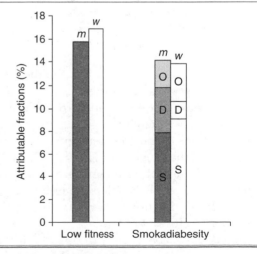

Source: Courtesy of BMJ Publishing Group Ltd and the British Association of Sport and Exercise Medicine.

Experts suggest that new strategies and innovative approaches are needed to impact physical activity participation and health outcomes (Blair, 2009; Pollard, 2003). As discussed, interventions of collaboration, coalition building, and community organizing can be effective in accomplishing this goal.

Minnesota Department of Health Population-Based Public Health Nursing Practice Intervention Wheel Strategies and Levels of Practice

Collaboration

A working definition of **collaboration** has been offered as:

> {A} mutually beneficial and well-defined relationship entered into by 2 or more organizations (individuals) to achieve common goals. The relationship includes a commitment to: a definition of mutual relationships and goals; a jointly developed structure and shared responsibility; mutual authority and accountability for success; and a sharing of resources and rewards. (Mattessich & Monsey, 1992, p. 7)

Collaboration has been defined in the intervention wheel as an approach that "commits 2 or more persons or organizations to achieving a common goal through the enhancement of the ability of one or more of them to promote and protect health" (Keller et al., 2008, p. 204). We know that public health nursing may be practiced by one public health nurse or by a group of public health nurses working together or collaboratively.

Clearly, collaboration with other healthcare professionals or with those in other organizations working toward mutual goals is often part of the work of the public health nurse to promote the health of any population. In fact, the Institute of Medicine (IOM) has called for the integration of interprofessional education into health professions curricula to improve healthcare quality. Six professions, including nursing, collaborated in producing the Interprofessional Education Collaborative report, which states that "policy, curricular, and/or accreditation changes to strengthen teamwork preparation are at various stages of development among the six professions represented in this report" (2011, p. 5). In addition, the American Association of Colleges of Nursing has integrated interprofessional collaboration behavioral expectations into its Essentials for Baccalaureate, Master's and Doctoral Education for Advanced Practice.

Working in collaboration with others to achieve goals requires that public health professionals and practitioners possess or acquire skills that are applied to develop a shared vision and agree on an effective plan of action (Sullivan, 1998). However, although collaboration is often highly effective in increasing the quality of results and offers the potential of many benefits, including the opportunity for a more comprehensive evaluation and assessment of issues, collaborative projects may not always work (Gray, 1998). An understanding of how successful collaborations are formed is important in considering, or undertaking, a collaborative effort.

In 1992, the Wilder Research Center offered a theoretical understanding of what is needed for collaboration to succeed (Mattessich & Monsey, 1992). An initial review of 133 studies identified 18 relevant and valid studies, and the combined findings from these studies resulted in identification of 19 factors reported to influence whether or not a collaboration formed by government agencies and nonprofit organizations will succeed. These factors were grouped into six key categories: (1) environment, (2) membership,

(3) process/structure, (4) communications, (5) purpose, and (6) resources. The 19 factors are listed in the category to which they belong and are described in **Box 12-1**.

This information can be useful in guiding the decision to enter into a partnership with potential collaborators by a careful evaluation of whether the important factors for success exist before undertaking an effort. Not every collaboration, however, is the same, and the exact combination of the factors for success may not always be identical. Consideration of these factors can assist those who work in public health in assessing the potential of a collaborative approach and in maximizing the impact of collaborative projects (Mattessich & Monsey, 1992).

Collaborative approaches to the problem of physical inactivity have taken on a new importance as the evidence base on physical activity has grown. New models of health behavior and health promotion, such as the social–ecological model, have been developed and are being applied to areas such as physical activity participation (Elder et al., 2007). These models offer

---

Box 12-1 Six Categories of Factors That Influence the Success of Collaboration

1. Environment
   A history of collaboration exists in the community.
   The collaborative group is seen as a community leader in the area in which it is focused.
   There is a favorable political/social climate.
2. Membership
   There is mutual respect, understanding, and trust.
   Cross-section of members in the group is appropriate.
   Collaboration is viewed as being in the self-interest of members.
   There is the ability to compromise.
3. Process/structure
   Members share a stake in both the process and groups.
   There are multiple layers of decision making.
   There is flexibility and openness.
   Clear roles and policy guidelines are developed.
   There is adaptability in the face of changing conditions.
4. Communications
   There is open and frequent communication.
   Formal and informal communication links exist.
5. Purpose
   There is a concrete and unique purpose.
   There are clear, realistic, and attainable goals.
   There is a shared vision, with an agreed-on mission, objectives, and strategy.
6. Resources
   Funding is sufficient to support operations.
   The leader, or convener, of the collaborative group is skilled interpersonally and is fair and respected by partners.

Source: Adapted from Mattessich and Monsey, 1992.

new understanding of the many determinants of physical activity and suggest potential interventions at multiple levels of influence on behavior, with a growing emphasis on environmental and policy influences. These models are used to target behavior change beyond the individual level only. As a result, it is increasingly evident to those working in public health and prevention that the decisions and policies in sectors ranging from agriculture to transportation to education may have a huge impact on physical activity participation and health. Yet these groups have not traditionally understood the connections between them nor have they often sought opportunities to collaboratively engage in health promotion efforts.

Important environmental and policy approaches may be implemented by applying collaboration, coalition building, and community organizing interventions. These approaches can effect physical activity participation at the population-based level, complementing the individual-level focus of changing one person's behavior at a time (Heath et al., 2006).

Projects that involve the collaboration of those from multiple sectors are promising approaches to impact physical activity at the population level (Pollard, 2003). The impact of the built environment—the man-made physical structures and infrastructure of communities (Prevention Institute, 2009)—on health and the potential to alter aspects of the built environment to promote health are now being recognized by public health professionals (Pollard, 2003). Offering opportunities for walking and cycling as a regular part of daily life, for example, are important to increasing physical activity and to improving health among a largely sedentary population in the United States. To promote healthier communities, multiple approaches directed at all levels of the government—local, state, and federal—are needed. The creation of communities and transportation systems that promote physical activity require the support of public health professionals working collaboratively with other disciplines such as architects, builders, public officials, bike and pedestrian advocates, and others on common concerns (Pollard, 2003).

The literature shows results of community-led initiatives to improve the built environment. For example, the Prevention Institute (2009) compiled a report that profiled 11 communities around the country to show how they were able to impact the built environment to positively affect the health of community residents. One community, for example, built a jogging path around a cemetery as a way to increase physical activity (Aboelata et al., 2004).

As another example of a collaborative effort to address physical activity, the American Heart Association Council on Nutrition, Physical Activity, and Metabolism (Physical Activity Committee), together with the Councils on Cardiovascular Disease in the Young and Cardiovascular Nursing, issued a scientific statement (Pate et al., 2006) focused on this issue, specifically in youth. Evidence gathered from the 2003 Youth Risk Behavioral Surveillance System indicated that 37% of students (high school-aged youth) did not participate in adequate physical activity (20 minutes or more of vigorous physical activity on 3 or more of the previous 7 days). Also, Black, Hispanic, and female students were less likely to participate in vigorous physical activity at the recommended levels (Pate et al., 2006). Nine key recommendations were made for improving policy and practice to impact physical activity participation at the population level. The statement called for U.S. schools to renew and expand their role in the offering and promotion of physical activity for youth by, for example, delivering evidence-based health-related physical education programs that meet national standards. Also recommended were policies and practices to ensure that all children and youth participate in a minimum of 30 minutes of moderate to vigorous physical activity during the school day as well as other recommendations that, if implemented on a national basis, would better provide U.S. youth with the physical activity needed for health (Pate et al., 2006). This report, the result of a large collaborative approach of bringing together key organizations with a common objective, illustrates how working together to share resources and information can be highly effective. Collaborative efforts such as this, to develop evidence-based guidelines, are an approach to inform practitioners about current best practices.

Another example of a collaborative effort to impact physical activity is the initiative spearheaded by the American College of Sports Medicine, working together with the American Medical Association, to encourage the prescribing of exercise as medicine. Launched in 2007, Exercise is Medicine is a program that calls on U.S. physicians to prescribe exercise and encourage their patients to incorporate physical activity and exercise into their daily routine. It also encourages physicians and primary care providers to assess patients' physical activity level and record it as a vital sign. In addition, this initiative has called for greater collaboration between healthcare professionals and those in the fitness industry, including fitness and athletic trainers, to work together to get clients active and improve health outcomes (Sallis, 2009). Evidence-based guidelines issued by organizations collaboratively may be more comprehensive than would otherwise be possible without the contribution of a range of perspectives brought together in a group effort. For example, as a result of a comprehensive review of the scientific research on physical activity,

in October 2008 the U.S. DHHS released new physical activity guidelines (PAG). These new guidelines, revised from a decade earlier, provide evidence-based recommendations to improve individuals' health through appropriate physical activity and are intended for use primarily by policymakers and health professionals. The PAG were used as the basis for the objectives related to physical activity identified in *Healthy People 2020*, updated from the previous *Healthy People 2010* objectives "to reflect the strong state of the science supporting the health benefits of regular physical activity among youth and adults, as identified in the PAG. Regular physical activity includes participation in moderate and vigorous physical activities and muscle-strengthening activities" (U.S. DHHS, 2010). In addition to the guidelines issued by the federal government, several other government agencies and health organizations also issued guidelines for physical activity based on their own scientific research and made recommendations for the public or for practitioners. These guidelines or recommendations each were written with a somewhat different emphasis or focus (i.e., to prevent chronic disease, to promote health, or to manage weight) and address a specific population (i.e., adults or children). The evidence-based recommendations from some of the major government and health organizations are summarized in **Box 12-2.**

INDIVIDUAL-FOCUSED LEVEL

At the individual level of practice, a public health nurse working in an agency may be caring for an older adult, female, Hispanic client with early heart disease who has received an exercise prescription from her physician or nurse practitioner. The exercise prescription was based on evidence in the literature indicating that writing an exercise prescription has been shown to be more successful than if healthcare professionals

Box 12-2 Overview of Key National Guidelines and Recommendations on Physical Activity

Population: Adults

American College of Sports Medicine/American Heart Association—jointly issued, 2008

- A minimum of 30 minutes of moderate intensity aerobic physical activity 5 days per week (150 minutes) or 20 minutes of vigorous intensity aerobic physical activity 3 days per week—to promote health and prevent chronic disease.

American Cancer Society Guidelines on Nutrition and Physical Activity for Cancer Prevention, 2006

- Balance caloric intake with physical activity—to maintain a healthy weight throughout life.
- Engage in at least 30 minutes of moderate to vigorous physical activity, above usual activities, on 5 or more days of the week; 45 to 60 minutes of intentional physical activity are preferable.

U.S. Department of Health and Human Services: 2008 Physical Activity Guidelines for Americans

- At least 2 hours and 30 minutes (150 minutes) of moderate aerobic exercise per week or 1 hour and 15 minutes of vigorous aerobic exercise per week, or an equivalent combination of moderate- and vigorous-intensity aerobic physical activity, performed in episodes of at least 10 minutes and should be spread throughout the week—to promote health and prevent chronic disease.
- Increase aerobic exercise to 300 minutes (5 hours) of moderate intensity per week or 150 minutes of vigorous aerobic exercise per week, or an equivalent combination of moderate- and vigorous-intensity aerobic physical activity—to achieve additional and more extensive health benefits.
- Do muscle-strengthening activities (that are moderate or high intensity and involve all major muscle groups) on at least 2 nonconsecutive days per week—to achieve additional health benefits.
- Avoid inactivity; some physical activity is better than none—to achieve some health benefits.

Population: Youth (Children and Adolescents)

U.S. Department of Health and Human Services: 2008 Physical Activity Guidelines for Americans

- Aerobic: most of the 60 minutes a day should be either moderate- or vigorous-intensity aerobic physical activity; it should include vigorous-intensity physical activity on at least 3 days a week.
- Muscle-strengthening: as part of their 60 minutes of daily physical activity, muscle-strengthening physical activity should be included at least 3 days of the week.
- Bone-strengthening: as part of their 60 minutes of daily physical activity, bone-strengthening physical activity should be included at least 3 days of the week.

Population: Older Adults

U.S. Department of Health and Human Services: 2008 Physical Activity Guidelines for Americans

- Older adults who cannot do 150 minutes of moderate-intensity aerobic activity a week because of chronic conditions should be as physically active as their abilities and conditions allow.
- Older adults should do exercises that maintain or improve balance if they are at risk of falling.
- Older adults should determine their level of effort for physical activity relative to their level of fitness.
- Older adults with chronic conditions should understand whether and how their conditions affect their ability to do regular physical activity safely.

Sources: Haskell et al. (2007); Lawrence et al. (2006); Nelson et al. (2007); U.S. DHHS (2008).

merely discuss the benefits of physical activity with a patient (Sallis, 2009). The nurse may collaborate with other healthcare professionals, such as the prescribing physician or nurse practitioner or perhaps an exercise physiologist or fitness specialist, to ensure that an appropriate program for this particular client is offered. In this case, the common goal of this collaborative effort is to provide the most effective treatment plan as prescribed for the client.

Further, data from a study on the association of physical activity-related social support in a national U.S. sample of minority women ($N = 2,912$) indicate that social support from family and friends can impact an individual's participation in physical activity (Eyler et al., 1999). Of the determinants of physical activity that were studied, social support is one of the strongest correlates, and providing additional social support may be an important component of interventions that aim to increase physical-activity participation in a population of sedentary women of racially/ethnically diverse backgrounds (Eyler et al., 1999). Knowing this, the public health nurse may collaborate at the individual-focused level by working with a member of a family or a friend of the client who may be able to assist in meeting the care goal for this client by offering social support and encouragement for the client's physical activity program.

COMMUNITY-FOCUSED LEVEL

At the community level, the public health nurse may collaborate with others such as staff in the local parks department or leaders in local fitness businesses to initiate a collaborative effort to identify the available resources in the local area for those at risk of cardiovascular disease seeking information on active lifestyles and physical activity. To help direct these members of the community to safe locations in which to engage in physical activity, they may work together to develop a list or brochure of local resources such as parks and trails as well as gyms and community facilities that are available. They can then disseminate these materials to members of the community, perhaps by using the social marketing intervention, discussed later in this text.

SYSTEM-FOCUSED LEVEL

At the systems level, practice is focused on making a change in organizations, policies, laws, or power structures within a community, according to the assumptions of the intervention wheel (Keller et al., 2008, p. 192). A public health nurse may collaborate with leaders of other organizations that have a mutual interest in or concern with increasing physical activity, for example, in children who are at risk of being physically inactive. They may begin by gathering data on local and other policies that impact the issue of children who are not sufficiently physically active in their community and decide to work together to make a change by lobbying the state for a school-based state policy to increase physical activity by offering after-school programs. The nurse may identify leaders of local organizations such as the Parent-Teacher Association, as well as religious or other community groups, that are concerned about physical inactivity among local school children, or who serve children as part of their mission. This collaboration may lead to coalition building, the next intervention in the intervention wheel that also entails collective action.

Coalition Building

Whereas collaboration can occur at the individual-focused level, the other two interventions in the orange wedge of the intervention wheel, coalition building and community organizing, are not applicable at the individual level. These two interventions most often take place at the community or systems level of practice. For the most part, the interventions in the orange wedge are used by public health nurses who are focused on impacting community- and systems-level practice in their work rather than on individual-level practice (Keller et al., 2008). A coalition can be described as an alliance of individuals, groups, or organizations that come together or join forces for a specific or common purpose.

As defined in descriptions in the intervention wheel model, **coalition building** "promotes and develops alliances among organizations or constituencies for a common purpose. It builds linkages, solves problems, and/or enhances local leadership to address health concerns" (Keller et al., 2008, p. 204). Often, by forming a coalition the new organization or alliance or group becomes more effective in achieving a goal or goals. Usually, by bringing people or organizations together in pursuit of a common goal, resources can be maximized and more can be accomplished than could be by any individual person or organization alone.

Coalitions have been considered to be a foundation for creating successful change within a community. Because a range of local interests is represented and brought together, forming a coalition can build a powerful base of key individuals or organizations that can work to influence social change of a mutual concern. There are a number of types of coalitions that can be formed. Coalitions may be permanent or temporary; they can be formed to address a single issue or multiple issues. Typically, a coalition that is well organized and broad based will be more successful in effecting policy change, increasing knowledge of the public, and creating innovative solutions to complex problems of concern (Wisconsin Clearinghouse for Prevention Resources, 2009).

A mission statement is important to provide direction and purpose for a group of people or organizations brought together in a coalition. In fact, this mission statement provides a common vision for all involved. It is developed collaboratively and typically contains specific components. **Figure 12-3** includes more information about the development of a mission statement.

In addition to the mission statement, eight key steps have also been identified as critically important to coalition building (Butterworth, 2009). These eight steps are listed in **Box 12-3**. Following these steps may help ensure the success of a coalition.

SYSTEM-FOCUSED LEVEL

Coalition building is an intervention used to address the problem of physical inactivity at

---

Figure 12-3 A mission statement should answer the question, "What are we doing here?"

Misson Statement ➡➡➡ **Goals** ➡➡➡ **Objectives**

A mission statement should:
- Include a program overview.
- Include a program aim.
- Incorporate a short narrative that describes the general focus of the program, including the intent and philosophy behind the program.
- Help to guide program planners in the development of program goals and objectives.

Source: Courtesy of the Minnesota Department of Health, Center for Health Promotion (n.d.).

> ### BOX 12-3 STEPS TO COALITION BUILDING
>
> 1. Clarify/reaffirm coalition's vision and mission.
> 2. Create community ownership of the coalition.
> 3. Solidify coalition infrastructure and processes.
> 4. Recruit and retain an active, diverse membership.
> 5. Develop transformational leaders.
> 6. Market your coalition.
> 7. Evaluate your coalition.
> 8. Focus on action and advocacy.
>
> *Source:* Courtesy of CoalitionsWork. Butterworth, 2009.

the policy or system level. For example, there is an initiative underway that has built a coalition of organizations to develop a national physical activity plan to assist Americans in becoming more physically active (National Plan for Physical Activity, 2008). The plan will be developed by a combination of efforts from researchers, educators, healthcare professionals, and mass media experts from across the country.

The coalition that will develop the plan was initially formed under the leadership of the Centers for Disease Control and Prevention and the Prevention Research Center at the University of South Carolina, who are providing the organizational infrastructure. The importance of having a strong organizational structure for a collaboration or coalition to succeed has been previously mentioned, and the strength of these two leading and reputable organizations can help ensure its success. Other organizations who are part of the coalition include the American Academy of Pediatrics; American Alliance for Health, Physical Education, Recreation, and Dance; American Association of Retired Persons; American Cancer Society; American College of Sports Medicine; American Heart Association; Active Living Research, American Association for Cardiovascular and Pulmonary Rehabilitation; and the National Coalition for Promoting Physical Activity, itself a coalition with a clear mission statement (**Box 12-4**).

Community Organizing

Community organizing, as defined in the intervention wheel, "helps community groups to identify common problems or goals, mobilize resources, and develop and implement strategies for reaching the goals they collectively have set" (Minkler, 1997, as cited in Keller et al., 2008, p. 204).

> ### BOX 12-4 EXAMPLE OF A COALITION TO ADDRESS PHYSICAL ACTIVITY IN THE UNITED STATES AND ITS MISSION STATEMENT: NATIONAL COALITION FOR PROMOTING PHYSICAL ACTIVITY (NCPPA)
>
> NCPPA is "an extraordinary group of national organizations that independently address a host of issues pertaining to physical activity including health/science, education, environments, population specific outreach, and activity behavior" (NCPPA, n.d., n.p.).
>
> Mission: to "unite the strengths of public, private, and industry efforts into collaborative partnerships that inspire and empower all Americans to lead more physically active lifestyles" (NCPPA, n.d., n.p.).
>
> *Source:* Courtesy of the National Coalition for Promoting Physical Activity.

COMMUNITY-FOCUSED LEVEL AND SYSTEM-FOCUSED LEVEL

The Safe Routes to School (SRTS) program provides an example, or case study, of a framework for community organizing aimed at providing options that would allow children to walk and bicycle to school safely and thereby increase physical activity opportunities for school children. The program was first started in Denmark in the 1970s and was initiated in the United States in The Bronx and Florida in 1997. It has a grassroots history whereby the success of pilot community projects led to federal interest and funding. The national SRTS program was funded for $612 million from 2005 to 2009 by federal transportation legislation, and its success illustrates how collaboration and coalition building, along with local community organizing around an issue, can expand into further intervention actions such as advocacy and policy implementation (National Center for Safe Routes to School, 2009).

A framework that has been successfully used is available on the SRTS website (http://www .saferoutesinfo.org) to support the development of other programs in local communities and is illustrative of how a community-based approach can begin with a grassroots effort focused on a particular community concern. The framework suggested by SRTS is based on the evidence of what has worked in other communities starting a program. The steps are outlined for others who are interested in starting a program, and they are meant to provide guidance on a process that has worked. However, each community is unique, and using these steps in a different order may work better for some communities, or some communities may require different approaches than outlined in the steps suggested by SRTS. The seven steps are to (1) bring the right people together, (2) hold a kickoff meeting and set a vision, (3) gather information and identify issues, (4) identify solutions, (5) make a plan, (6) get the people and the plan moving, and (7) evaluate, adjust, and keep moving (National Center for Safe Routes to School, 2009).

Another effective community organizing approach to promoting physical activity among underserved older adults is the Southeast Senior Physical Activity Network (SESPAN) in southeast Seattle (Cheadle, Egger, LoGerfo, Walwick, & Schwartz, 2010). SESPAN is based on an organizing strategy that involved networking between several community-based organizations (including senior housing buildings and religious organizations), senior centers, and other organizations to meet two broad objectives. The first objective was to create new senior physical activity programs where there were no programs by making connections between two or more community-based organizations. Networking among organizations led to the creation of a number of potentially sustainable walking and exercise programs that are reaching previously underserved communities within southeast Seattle. A second objective was to build a broader coalition of groups and organizations to assist in making environmental and policy changes on a larger scale. After a health fair event, organizations involved in the event decided to continue to work together. A health coalition was established with the potential to continue to develop new programs and larger scale environmental changes (Cheadle et al., 2010).

Beaglehole and colleagues (2004) suggested that "a suitable definition of public health is collective action for sustained population-wide health improvement" (Beaglehole, Bonita, Horton, Adams, & McKee, 2004, p. 2085). This definition of public health focuses attention on the importance of the interventions of collective action discussed in this text and highlights the key role they play in achieving public health goals.

Minnesota Department of Health Population-Based Public Health Nursing Practice Intervention Wheel: Application to Practice

The following case study illustrates how one nurse practices in a way that exemplified the "doing" of the intervention wheel strategies described in this chapter. Once you have read and discussed the case, collaborate with each other on the field exercise in **Box 12-5**.

WWW

CASE STUDY
UNFIT UNIVERSITY GETS ACTIVE — INTERVENTIONS OF COLLECTIVE ACTION

An Ivy League university in the northeast, Unfit University (UU), is a member of the American College Health Association (ACHA), a national professional organization that serves college health professionals (http://www.acha.org/about_acha/history.cfm). A nurse (Ms. Fit, RN, MPH) who works at the University Health Services Center has a public health background, and part of her role is to work with the UU community and serve as a resource and to develop and implement evidence-based student health programs to meet the needs of the UU student population. Unfit University participates in the ACHA-National College Health Assessment (NCHA) survey to collect data on the health behaviors of their student population, and they use these data to help inform decisions on priority needs and programs and to determine resource needs.

Ms. Fit has seen national data published from the ACHA-NCHA survey on the health behaviors of college students who participate in the assessment and from these data learns that inadequate physical activity participation in college students is a concern nationally (American College Health Association, 2009). Further, she read a review study published in the *Journal of American College Health* that reports high percentages of college students (about 40–50%) who are not sufficiently physically active to achieve health benefits. Of note, it is reported that female students met the guidelines significantly less than male students (Keating, Guan, Pinero, & Bridges, 2005).

In addition, Ms. Fit knows that *Healthy Campus* 2010 has identified lead indicators for health, including physical activity, and has set targets for physical activity in college students by 2010.

(continues)

CASE STUDY (*continued*)

One target, objective 7-3b11, "is to increase the proportion of college students who have received information on physical activity and fitness from the baseline of 33.5% to the 2010 target of 55%" (American College Health Association, 2009). A second objective, 22-2/3, is "to increase the proportion of college students who engage in physical activity at least 3 days/week at moderate intensity for at least 30 minutes, or vigorous physical activity for 20 minutes or more minutes, from the baseline of 40.3% to the 2010 target of 55%" (American College Health Association, 2009, PowerPoint no. 26). (Note: At the writing of this chapter, *Healthy Campus 2020* objectives regarding physical activity are not publically available; however, they are in development and it is suggested that the American College Health Association website (http://www.acha.org) be checked regularly for the release of *Healthy Campus* 2020 objectives). The population of interest is inactive or insufficiently active students (i.e., those not meeting the *Healthy Campus* target at UU in Anytown, USA). The problem is that insufficiently active college students are at risk of chronic illness, including cardiovascular disease, obesity, depression, diabetes, and cancer (Blair, 2009). Unfit University is an all-women's university and is concerned that, based on these national data, their students are at risk of not engaging in sufficient physical activity for acute health benefits and for long-term health outcomes.

Community Level

Ms. Fit of UU's Health Services Department brings together leaders of several key groups at the University, including the leaders of the student environmental committee, the student wellness committee, and student athletes (team captains) to conduct an audit to evaluate the University's environmental facilitators and barriers to physical activity on the UU campus and to make recommendations to the university administration on ways to increase physical activity for all students on campus.

Systems Level

Ms. Fit is invited by Administration to work with the architects and designers who are developing plans for expanding the campus at UU to collaborate on ways to improve environmental factors to encourage physical activity, such as expanding bike paths and adding more recreational facilities.

Individual/Family Level

Ms. Fit meets with the Student Health Services nurses to collaborate on how individual students can be better assessed for physical activity level and counseled on the importance of physical activity for their unique health and activity status. Ms. Fit and the nurses decide that the Health Services nurses will screen for physical inactivity on all students who visit the clinic and offer a Fitness Challenge on a monthly basis, campus-wide, to raise awareness of physical fitness levels.

Conclusion

This chapter presents the interventions of the orange section of intervention wheel aimed at collective action. The intervention wheel model considers that the three interventions in the orange section that were described in this chapter are all part of "collective action" (Keller et al., 2008, p. 193).

Collaboration, coalition building, and community organizing are the interventions aimed at harnessing the collective energy of more than one person or group. Perhaps Margaret Mead said it best when describing the power of collective action: "Never doubt that a small group of thoughtful, committed citizens can change the world: indeed it is the only thing that ever has" (Margaret Mead® used with permission).

As we have discussed in this chapter, when presenting a variety of approaches to the problem of physical inactivity, public health nursing can incorporate best practices and evidence-based interventions when engaging in or supporting collective action to address this concern effectively. The strategies used in public health nursing consist of the development of collaborative efforts that maximize the efforts of each individual or organization for a mutual goal. Further, this chapter shows how public health nursing strategies can be applied on the community, systems, and individual/family levels. Public health professionals are often key players in any community-based effort. They can support important initiatives whether on the issue of physical activity or any other health concern by applying the intervention wheel interventions.

References

Aboelata, M. J., Mikkelsen, L., Cohen, L., Fernandes, S., Silver, M., & Parks, L. F. (2004). *The built environment and health: Eleven profiles of neighborhood transformation.* Oakland, CA: Prevention Institute. Retrieved from http://www.preventioninstitute.org/pdf/BE_full_document_110304.pdf

American College Health Association. (2009). Healthy campus 2010: Making it happen. PowerPoint presentation *Healthy People 2010, Healthy Campus 2020*, slide no. 26, presented at the ACHA Annual 2002 meeting. Retrieved from http://www.acha.org/Info_resources/hc2010.cfm

Beaglehole, R., Bonita, R., Horton, R., Adams, O., & McKee, M. (2004). Public health in the new era: Improving health through collective action. *Lancet, 363*(9426), 2084–2086.

Blair, S. N. (2009). Physical inactivity: The biggest public health problem of the 21st century. *British Journal of Sports Medicine, 43*(1), 1–2.

Butterworth, F. D. (2009, May 9). *Strength in numbers: Building strategic partnerships to advocate for change.* New Orleans, LA: SOPHE State Health Policy Summit.

Centers for Disease Control and Prevention (2000). *Behavioral Risk Factor Surveillance System Survey data.* Atlanta, GA: U.S. Department of Health and Human Services, Centers for Disease Control and Prevention.

Cheadle, A., Egger, R., LoGerfo, J. P., Walwick, J., & Schwartz, S. (2010). A community-organizing approach to promoting physical activity in older adults: The Southeast Senior Physical Activity Network. *Health Promotion and Practice, 11*(2), 197–204.

Elder, J. P., Lytle, L., Sallis, J. F., Young, D. R., Steckler, A., Simons-Morton, D., ... Ribisl, K. (2007). A description of the social-ecological framework used in the trial of activity for adolescent girls (TAAG). *Health Education and Research, 22*(2), 155–165.

Eyler, A. A., Brownson, R. C., Donatelle, R. J., King, A. C., Brown, D., & Sallis, J. F. (1999). Physical activity social support and middle- and older-aged minority women: Results from a US survey. *Social Science & Medicine, 49*(6), 781–789.

Gray, B. (1998). *Collaborating*. San Francisco, CA: Jossey-Bass.

Haskell, W. L., Lee, I. M., Pate, R. R., Powell, K. E., Blair, S. N., Franklin, B. A., ... Bauman, A. (2007). Physical activity and public health: Updated recommendation for adults from the American College of Sports Medicine and the American Heart Association. *Medicine & Science in Sports & Exercise, 39*, 1423–1434.

Heath, G. W., Brownson, R. C., Kruger, J., Miles, R., Powell, K. E., Ramsey, L. T., and the Task Force on Community Preventive Services. (2006). The effectiveness of urban design and land use and transport policies and practices to increase physical activity: A systematic review. *Journal of Physical Activity and Health, 3*(Suppl. 1), S55–S76.

Interprofessional Education Collaborative Expert Panel. (2011). *Core competencies for interprofessional collaborative practice: Report of an expert panel*. Washington, DC: Interprofessional Education Collaborative.

Keating, X. D., Guan, J., Pinero, J. C., & Bridges, D. M. (2005). A meta-analysis of college students' physical activity behaviors. *Journal of American College Health, 54*(2), 116–125.

Keller, L. O., Strohschein, S., & Briske, L. (2008). Population-based public health nursing practice: The intervention wheel. In M. Stanhope & J. Lancaster (Eds.), *Public health nursing: Population-centered health care in the community* (pp. 187–214). St. Louis, MO: Mosby Elsevier.

Khan, K. M., & Tunaiji, H. A. (2011). As different as Venus and Mars: Time to distinguish efficacy (can it work?) from effectiveness (does it work?). *British Journal of Sports Medicine, 45*(10), 759–760.

Lawrence, H., Kushi, L. H., Byers, T., Doyle, C., Bandera, E. V., McCullough, M., ... American Cancer Society 2006 Nutrition and Physical Activity Guidelines Advisory Committee. (2006). American Cancer Society guidelines on nutrition and physical activity for cancer prevention: Reducing the risk of cancer with healthy food choices and physical activity. *Cancer Journal for Clinicians, 56*, 254–281.

Mattessich, P. W., & Monsey, B. R. (1992). *Collaboration: What makes it work*. St. Paul, MN: Amherst H. Wilder Foundation.

Minnesota Department of Health. (2001). *Public health interventions: Applications for public health nursing practice*. St. Paul, MN: Author.

Minnesota Department of Health, Center for Health Promotion. (n.d.). Developing a mission statement.

Retrieved from http://www.health.state.mn.us/divs/hpcd/chp/hpkit/text/tea_mission.htm

National Center for Safe Routes to School. (2009). Retrieved from http://www.saferoutesinfo.org

National Coalition for Promoting Physical Activity. (n.d.). *NCPPA to manage implementation of national physical activity*. Retrieved from http://www.ncppa.org

National Organization for Public Health Nursing. (1939). *Manual of public health nursing* (3rd ed.). New York, NY: MacMillan.

National Plan for Physical Activity. (2008). Retrieved from http://www.physicalactivityplan/org

Nelson, M. E., Rejeski, W. J., Blair, S. N., Duncan, P. W., Judge, J. O., King, A. C., ... Castaneda-Sceppa, C. (2007). Physical activity and public health in older adults: Recommendation from the American College of Sports Medicine and the American Heart Association. *Medicine & Science in Sports & Exercise, 39*, 1435–1445.

Pate, R. R., Davis, M. G., Robinson, T. N., Stone, E. J., McKenzie, T. L., & Young, J. C. (2006). Promoting physical activity in children and youth: A leadership role for schools. A scientific statement from the American Heart Association Council on Nutrition, Physical Activity, and Metabolism (Physical Activity Committee) in collaboration with the Councils on Cardiovascular Disease in the Young and Cardiovascular Nursing. *Circulation, 114*(11), 1214–1224.

Pollard, T. (2003). Policy prescriptions for healthier communities. *American Journal of Health Promotion, 18*(1), 109–113.

Prevention Institute. (2009). *The built environment and health: 11 profiles of neighborhood transformation*. Retrieved from http://www.preventioninstitute.org/builtenv.html

Sallis, R. E. (2009). Exercise is medicine and physicians need to prescribe it! *British Journal of Sports Medicine, 43*(1), 3–4.

Sullivan, T. J. (1998). *Collaboration: A health care imperative*. New York, NY: McGraw-Hill.

U.S. Department of Health and Human Services (U.S. DHHS). (1996). *2008 physical activity guidelines for Americans*. Retrieved from http://www.health.gov/paguidelines

U.S. Department of Health and Human Services (U.S. DHHS). (2008). *2008 Physical activity guidelines for Americans*. Retrieved from http://www.health.gov/paguidelines

U.S. Department of Health and Human Services (U.S. DHHS). (2010). *HealthyPeople 2020. Physical activity.* Retrieved from http://healthypeople.gov/2020/topics objectives2020/overview.aspx?topicid=33

Wisconsin Clearinghouse for Prevention Resources. (2009). *Prevention—Coalition building.* Retrieved from http://wch.uhs.wisc.edu

World Health Organization (WHO). (2002). *The World Health Report 2002—Reducing risks, promoting healthy life.* Geneva, Switzerland: Author.

World Health Organization (WHO) (2011). *10 Facts on non-communicable disease.* Retrieved from http://www .who.int/features/factfiles/noncommunicable_diseases /facts/en/index4.html

For a full suite of assignments and additional learning activities, use the access code located in the front of your book to visit this exclusive website: http://go.jblearning .com/londrigan. If you do not have an access code, you can obtain one at the site.

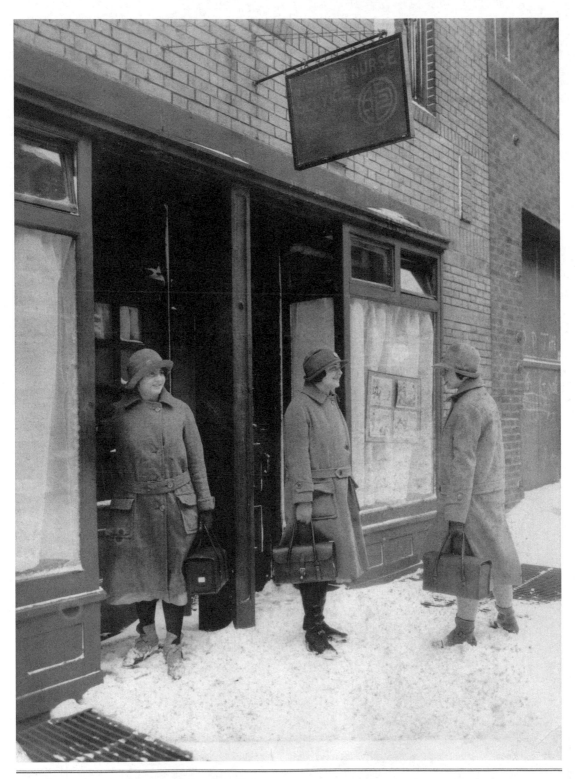

Source: Courtesy of the Visiting Nurse Service of New York.

Chapter 13

Getting the Word Out: Advocacy, Social Marketing, and Policy Development and Enforcement

Susan Moscou

If people knew things—and "things" meant everything implied in the condition of this family—such horrors would cease to exist, and I rejoiced that I had had a training in the care of the sick that in itself would give me an organic relationship to the neighborhood in which this awakening had come (Wald, 1915, pp. 7–8).

LEARNING OBJECTIVES

At the completion of this chapter, the reader will be able to

- Describe social marketing, advocacy, and policy development and enforcement.
- Apply social marketing, advocacy, and policy development and enforcement to the levels of public health practice.

- Explore the ways that public health nursing may apply and do social marketing, advocacy, and policy development and enforcement.

KEY TERMS

- ❑ Advocacy
- ❑ Policy development

- ❑ Policy enforcement
- ❑ Social marketing

The Minnesota Department of Health Population-Based Public Health Nursing Practice Intervention Wheel Strategies describes public health interventions that are applicable to public health nursing. This chapter presents the yellow section of the intervention wheel, otherwise known as advocacy, social marketing, and policy development and enforcement. Advocacy is considered the precursor to policy development, and social marketing is viewed as a strategy for carrying out advocacy (Minnesota Department of Health, 2001).

This chapter is divided into three sections. The first section provides a discussion about overweight and obesity in children. Overweight and obese children are a major public health issue, and this section will focus primarily on overweight and obese children in junior high school. The second section is a case study that highlights this public health issue. Finally, the third section depicts how the public health nurse in the case study engages in the application of three interventions: advocacy, social marketing, and policy development and enforcement through the three levels of public health practice.

This chapter specifically addresses strategies to deal with the growing public health problem of overweight and obese children in the United States. For example, the case study provides a paradigm of how a public health nurse uses the intervention wheel to address the prevalence of overweight and obese junior high school children in a community. The nurse gathers the appropriate facts about the prevalence of overweight and obese children in the school by looking at the present school records pertaining to weight and comparing those data with standards as well as past school records to note trends. Once he or she has these data, the nurse applies the intervention wheel interventions of advocacy and social marketing to develop policy and enforcement strategies around the problem of overweight and obese children attending the school. Advocacy, social marketing, and policy development and enforcement strategies are applied at the community level, systems level, and individual/family levels.

Issue: Overweight and Obesity Are Major 21st Century Public Health Concerns

Overweight and obesity are considered emerging public health problems in the United States. The number of overweight adults, children, and adolescents has increased since the 1970s (Blair & Nichaman, 2002; Ogden et al., 2009). The 2007–2008 National Health and Nutrition Examination Survey found that 10.4% of children aged 2–5 years, 19.6% of children aged 6–11 years, and 18.1% of adolescents aged 12–19 years were obese (Ogden & Carroll, 2010a). Additionally, 34% of adults aged 20 and over were obese and 34% were overweight (Ogden & Carroll, 2010b). The prevalence of obesity in adult men was 32.2% and 35.5% in women (Flegal, Carroll, Ogden, & Curtin, 2010). About 80% of obese adolescents will become obese adults (Jordan & Robinson, 2008). The incidence of weight gain in children has become alarming to the public health community (Harbaugh, Jordan-Welch, Bounds, Blom, & Fisher, 2007). Furthermore, overweight and obesity contribute to various health complaints and chronic diseases (Patterson, Frank, Kristal, & White, 2004) such as diabetes (Yanovski & Yanovski, 2002), cardiovascular diseases such as high blood pressure (Kumanyika et al., 2008), and asthma (Chen, Dales, & Jiang, 2006). In addition, elevated body weights are also correlated with higher death rates.

Body mass index (BMI) determines if a person is underweight, normal weight, overweight, or obese. BMI is a number calculated from a person's weight and height and is a reliable indicator of body fatness for people (Centers for Disease Control and Prevention [CDC], 2009). BMI-defined categories for adults (CDC, 2009) are as follows:

- Underweight = <18.5
- Normal weight = 18.5–24.9
- Overweight = 25–29.9
- Obesity = >30

For children and adolescents, the BMI is calculated the same way as adults, but the criteria to interpret meaning are different. For example, for children and teens BMI age- and sex-specific percentiles are used because the amount of fat changes with age and is also different between girls and boys (CDC, 2009). The prevalence of overweight female children and adolescents from 1999 to 2004 increased from approximately 13% to 16%, while male children and adolescents increased from 14% to 18%; the prevalence of obesity in male adults went from 28% to 31%, and in women the prevalence remained the same, at about 33% (Ogden et al., 2009).

During 2003–2004, 32% of adults were considered obese, and about 17% of children and adolescents in the United States were thought to be overweight. Adults were obese if they had a BMI of 30 or higher, and children were considered overweight if they were at or above the 95th percentile of their BMI specific to age and gender (Ogden et al., 2009).

The prevalence of overweight American children in age groups 6 to 11 and 12 to 19 tripled between 1980 and 2002. Furthermore, overweight and obesity in childhood often persist into adolescence and adulthood (Nader et al., 2006). Although the consequences of overweight children tend to be social rather than medical, many of these children become overweight or obese adults and develop health problems such as type 2 diabetes, high blood pressure, and asthma (de Onis & Blossner, 2000). As a result of this growing trend, many healthcare professionals are now seeing adult-onset diseases in children.

Globally, the prevalence of overweight children has also increased. Flynn et al. (2006) noted the following:

> Available estimates for the period between the 1980s and 1990s show the prevalence of overweight and obesity in children increased by a magnitude of two to five times in developed countries (e.g. from 11% to over 30% in boys in Canada), and up to almost four times in developing countries (e.g. from 4% to 14% in Brazil). (p. 7)

The World Health Organization (WHO) found that childhood obesity is such a problem that obesity warrants consideration along with the continued attention to malnutrition. The WHO ("Childhood Obesity," 2001) is developing population strategies that promote healthy diets and increase physical activity to reduce or reverse the alarming obesity trend.

Related Health Conditions of Overweight and Obesity

Chronic health conditions such as type 2 diabetes, hypertension, coronary heart disease (Kumanyika et al., 2008; Patterson et al., 2004), respiratory illnesses (Chen et al., 2006; Murugan & Sharma, 2008), and osteoarthritis (Yanovski & Yanovski, 2002) are related to overweight and obesity. Since 1960, the percent prevalence of diabetes for all ages has increased by more than 400%. Major risk factors for diabetes are obesity, high-fat diet, and physical inactivity (CDC, 2001). Additionally, diabetes is the fifth-leading cause of death and is responsible for new-onset blindness, kidney failure, and lower limb amputations (Hogan, Dall, Nikolov, & American Diabetes Association, 2003).

Diabetes has reached epidemic levels, and the prevalence of diabetes in the United States continues to increase. The National Health and Nutrition Survey found that 9.3% of Americans 20 years and older (approximately 19 million people) had diabetes; two-thirds had an actual diagnosis and one-third were not diagnosed (Sheehy, Coursin, & Gabbay, 2008). Further, it has been estimated that by 2050, about 43 million people will be diagnosed with diabetes (Narayan, Boyle, Geiss, Saaddine, & Thompson, 2006).

Coronary heart disease, used interchangeably with cardiovascular disease, occurs because the body builds plaque that clogs the inner walls of the arteries. Coronary heart disease is responsible for heart attacks, strokes, and chest pain and is the principal cause of death in the United States (Wallace, Fulwood, & Alvarado, 2008). Cardiovascular disease is associated with poor dietary practices, physical inactivity, overweight, obesity, and cigarette smoking (Lee & Cubbin, 2002).

Obesity is now recognized as a risk factor for developing respiratory diseases such as asthma, pneumonia, and sleep apnea, a condition in which a person will stop breathing several times during the sleep cycle. Weight reduction has been shown to reduce the possibility of developing these conditions or improving the episodes of these conditions (Murugan & Sharma, 2008).

Arthritis is responsible for physical disabilities in elders. Arthritis affects about 70 million Americans. Osteoarthritis is the most common form of arthritis and leads to muscle weakness, which in turn results in decreased physical activity and problems with balance. When this occurs, people are at increased risk for physical disability. Weight reduction and moderate exercise have been shown to improve mobility in overweight and obese adults diagnosed with knee osteoarthritis (Messier et al., 2004). Considering the increasing prevalence of overweight children and adolescents in America, one questions what the future holds for these young individuals as they move into adulthood with regard to these chronic illnesses as well as the corresponding morbidity and mortality rates.

Mental Health and Overweight and Obesity

Individuals diagnosed with such mental illnesses as schizophrenia, depression, and bipolar disorder may be at a higher risk for becoming overweight and obese because of psychotropic medications, decreased physical activity, and inadequate attention paid to nutrition. The prevalence of obesity among people with diagnosed mental health disorders is more than the general population. Women schizophrenics had higher BMIs than nonschizophrenic women, whereas male schizophrenics and nonschizophrenics had comparable BMIs. Experiencing a depressed mood during adolescence may have a role in the prevalence of obesity in this group, but being obese in adolescence does not necessarily cause depression. Young women, however, who were overweight or obese were more likely to experience a depressed mood, which is defined as "feeling sad, blue, or depressed for at least 7 days during the previous month" (Allison et al., 2009).

The prevalence of metabolic syndrome is higher among individuals diagnosed with a mental health disorder than in the general population. Metabolic syndrome is a group of risk factors such as high blood pressure, obesity in the abdominal area, elevated blood sugar levels, elevated bad cholesterol, and lower levels of the good cholesterol (high-density-lipoprotein cholesterol). These conditions often occur together and increase one's risk of developing heart disease, stroke, and diabetes (Newcomer, 2007).

Reasons for the Increase in Overweight and Obese Individuals

The fattening of America is a result of worsening diets, higher carbohydrate intakes, physical inactivity, genetics, sedentary lifestyles, food overproduction because of subsidies, increased portion sizes, and aggressive food marketing of snacks and fast foods (Seiders & Petty, 2004). Aggressive food marketing strategies have also resulted in Americans eating more fast foods, and the "supersizing" trend has resulted in larger portion sizes. Another example of this excessive eating is noted as follows. U.S. food companies produce about 3,800 calories/day per person, whereas food production in 1970 was 3,300 calories/day per person. Further, Americans have vast amounts of food choices in supermarkets, and approximately 12,000 new food products are developed yearly (Blair & Nichaman, 2002). Family-prepared meals have become less frequent because of work schedules, and this has contributed to poorer dietary habits (CDC, 2000). As family-prepared meals have decreased, eating outside the home has increased, resulting in meals that are 20% higher in fat (Ward & Martens, 2000).

Urban sprawl has also contributed to increased rates of overweight and obesity in Americans. Urban sprawl is defined as patterns of housing development that are considered low-density residential areas; therefore, people residing in these areas live in larger houses and commute longer distances to their jobs, often relying on automobiles because of inadequate public transportation (Lopez, 2004). Because these areas lack pedestrian amenities such as walking to school, shopping locally, and socializing with friends within walking distances, urban sprawl is considered a risk factor of overweight and obesity for those residing in those communities.

The composition of a neighborhood can contribute to the overweight and obesity of the residents. Lower BMIs have been associated with neighborhoods that have higher population density, access to public transportation, and mixed land uses that includes houses, apartments, parks, green spaces, access to healthy foods, and private and public resources that encourage healthier lifestyles (Lovasi, Neckerman, Quinn, Weiss, & Rundle, 2009).

Contribution of Schools to Overweight and Obese Children

Children spend a large portion of their day in educational institutions. In 2000, approximately 53 million children attended public and private schools in the United States. Further, schools serve as the location for preschool, after-school, and child-care programs (Koplan, Liverman, & Kraak, 2005). Additionally, many children receive their meals at their schools. Schools, because of loss of monies, may sell foods that are not part of federally reimbursable lunches. Additionally, many schools have become distributors of vending machines that carry candy, beverages, and chips. Vending machines are found in about 43% of elementary schools, 74% of middle schools, and most high schools. These vending machines provide schools with about 50% of the profits from the machines (Seiders & Petty, 2004). On the surface, these profits may appear very attractive to financially struggling schools.

Foods sold outside of federally reimbursed school meals are widely available in educational institutions. These food items sold to students are high in saturated fats and calories, higher in salt content, contain higher levels of sugar, and are of little nutritional value. Additionally, the meals served at these schools often do not meet the lower standards for total fat and saturated fat, 42% do not provide fresh foods and vegetables in their reimbursable lunches, and whole grain breads and rolls accounted for only 5% of meals (Story, Nanney, & Schwartz, 2009).

Fast-food consumption in 2- to 18-year-olds has increased fivefold from 1977 to 1995. Further, fast food was eaten in 9% of all eating situations, and 12% of the required caloric intake came from fast food. Because most fast-food places are located within walking distances from schools, it is thought there is a correlation between the poorer quality diets and weight status (Davis & Carpenter, 2009).

Physical Activity Improves Health

Regular physical activity during childhood and adolescence is related to physical and psychological benefits. Further, it has been found that for youths to start physical activity and maintain regular levels of physical activity, success occurs more often when friends are involved (Salvy et al., 2009).

Moderate physical activity has been shown to reduce or delay chronic health conditions. The Diabetes Prevention Program clinical trial found that walking 2.5 hours a week and eating a low-fat diet resulted in a 58% reduction in the development of type 2 diabetes, and seniors age 60 and older saw a 71% reduction in type 2 diabetes. Participants entered the clinical trial with BMIs of 34 and a medical diagnosis of impaired glucose intolerance, a precursor to diabetes. Individuals who were randomized to modest physical activity saw greater reductions in disease prevention than participants randomized to drug therapy alone (Diabetes Prevention Program Research Group, 2002).

Healthy People 2020 has physical activity as a major topic area along with a series of objectives that speak to this topic (U.S. Department of Health and Human Services [U.S. DHHS, 2010). Lifestyle modifications such as diet and exercise offer enormous benefits to the individual and play a role in the prevention and reduction of many diseases associated with overweight and obesity (Peterson, 2007; Reiser & Schlenk, 2009).

So important is physical activity that in 2008, the federal government issued the first comprehensive guidelines on physical activity (U.S. DHHS, 2008):

> *We clearly know enough now to recommend that all Americans should engage in regular physical activity to improve overall health and to reduce risk of many health problems. Physical activity is a leading example of how lifestyle choices have a profound effect on health. The choices we make about other lifestyle factors, such as diet, smoking, and alcohol use, also have important and independent effects on our health. (p. 1)*

Additionally, First Lady Michelle Obama, in 2009, launched the *Let's Move* campaign to reduce or eliminate childhood obesity (http://www.letsmove.gov/). **Box 13-1** provides information on the Physical Activity Guidelines for Americans and describes the major research findings.

People, however, need assistance in developing routines to maximize adherence to their desired goals. Getting children and adolescents to increase physical activity levels requires multiple approaches, specific community interventions, advocacy strategies, social marketing, and social policy and enforcement.

Minnesota Department of Health Population-Based Public Health Nursing Practice Intervention Wheel Strategies and Levels of Practice

Advocacy

What is **advocacy** and why is it important to the public health nurse? Advocacy can be defined in several ways, depending on one's perspective. Cohen, de la Vega, and Watson (2001) presented a value-neutral view of advocacy

BOX 13-1 PHYSICAL ACTIVITY GUIDELINES FOR AMERICANS MAJOR RESEARCH FINDINGS

1. Regular physical activity reduces the risk of many adverse health outcomes.
2. Some physical activity is better than none.
3. For most health outcomes, additional benefits occur as the amount of physical activity increases through higher intensity, greater frequency, and/or longer duration.
4. Most health benefits occur with at least 150 minutes (2 hours and 30 minutes) a week of moderate intensity physical activity.
5. Both aerobic (endurance) and muscle-strengthening (resistance) physical activity are beneficial.
6. Health benefits occur for children and adolescents, young and middle-aged adults, older adults, and those in every studied racial and ethnic group.
7. The health benefits of physical activity occur for people with disabilities.
8. The benefits of physical activity far outweigh the possibility of adverse outcomes.

Source: U.S. Department of Health and Human Services (2008, pp. vi–vii).

CASE STUDY

Ms. Jones, a public health nurse, has worked at Greene Junior High School's (GJHS) school-based clinic for 10 years. Children come to the healthcare clinic for acute medical problems such as colds and sore throats and chronic medical problems such as asthma and diabetes. In the last several years, Ms. Jones has noticed that children coming to the school-based clinic seem to be more overweight and obese.

During her time at this school, Ms. Jones has seen gym classes reduced and children participate in very little physical activity. Ms. Jones also noted that the school cafeteria offers processed foods that are high in saturated fats, such as fries and chicken nuggets, and the range of nutritious healthy foods is limited. Further, the cafeteria contains several soda and snack machines.

Ms. Jones recently obtained a Master's in Public Health. Armed with knowledge about public health, epidemiology, social epidemiology, and health policy, Ms. Jones decided to examine the prevalence of overweight and obese children at GJHS and determine the average calories of the typical lunch served and if the soda and snack machines contributed to children becoming overweight and obese. Ms. Jones recognizes that obesity is considered an emerging public health problem not only in the United States, but worldwide, and that children are not immune from the overweight and obesity epidemic.

The following sections (advocacy, social marketing, and social policy and enforcement) describe the strategies Ms. Jones can use to address the issue of overweight and obese children at GJHS.

and spoke to this concept as action oriented. They noted how advocacy influenced decisions on the political, economic, and social system front that affects people. For example, Schorr Saxe (2011) demonstrated the importance of advocacy and influence in relation to childhood obesity. This author noted how the solution to childhood obesity goes beyond assisting the patient with lifestyle choices to include community and environmental approaches. These approaches may have the healthcare provider advocating at the local, state, and federal levels to change systems, policies, and laws by participating in writing or speaking campaigns. Here we can see the interrelationship between advocacy as a public health intervention and policy development and enforcement.

Nursing advocacy has been a central role of all nurses and public health nurses specifically. Ballou (2000) discussed the three ideologies present in the contemporary nursing literature. These ideologies included: 1) professional nursing as a moral endeavor, 2) advocacy, and 3) caring. The American Nurses Association Code of Ethics for Nurses with Interpretive Statements (2001) delineates that "The nurse promotes, advocates for, and strives to protect the health, safety, and rights of the patient" (p. 4). Furthermore, the ANA's *Public Health Nursing: Scope & Standards of Practice* (2007) addresses the responsibility of public health nurses to serve and protect the public who cannot address their own concerns.

The public health nurse is participating in advocacy when he or she ". . . pleads someone's cause or acts on someone's behalf, with a focus on developing the capacity of the community, system, individual, or family to plead their own cause or act on their own behalf" (Keller, Strohschein, & Briske, 2008, p. 204). This advocacy is not only an intervention or strategy but a process as well. Bu and Jezewski (2007) noted that this advocacy process consists

of ". . . a series of specific actions for preserving, representing and/or safeguarding patients' rights, best interest and values in the healthcare system" (p. 104). These authors carried out a concept analysis on patient advocacy. Their findings revealed three core attributes: 1) safeguarding patients' autonomy, 2) acting on behalf of patients, and 3) championing social justice in the provision of health care (Bu & Jezewski, 2007). Reflecting upon their findings informs the reader that a nurse is and can be an advocate not only for an individual or family unit but for a group or population as well.

Advocates support a particular cause or issue to get individuals and communities involved in influencing the public and policymakers about their particular issue. Using the above case study, Ms. Jones has identified the presiding problem to be overweight and obesity in a particular population of interest: GJHS children.

The first step in advocacy is to introduce the problem to those who can assist Ms. Jones in reducing the prevalence of overweight and obesity at GJHS. Ms. Jones knows that successful advocacy requires that people are informed and well educated about the issue she wants to address (overweight and obesity at GJHS). Ms. Jones requests to speak at the next Parent-Teacher Association (PTA) meeting. Ms. Jones prepared fact sheets about the emerging problem of overweight and obesity in the United States and in particular the growing problem of children who are overweight and obese. Ms. Jones also prepares a fact sheet about the estimated number of overweight and obese children at GJHS as well as the number of physical education teachers and classes offered for each grade. On the community-focused level, Ms. Jones will conduct research about the actual number of overweight and obese children at GJHS and the contributing social factors such as lack of gym classes, little green space in the

---

BOX 13-2 ADVOCACY INTERVENTION APPLIED AT THE COMMUNITY, SYSTEM, AND INDIVIDUAL/FAMILY LEVELS

Advocacy

- Population of interest: overweight and obese children at GJHS.
- Problem: Overweight and obese children.
- Community example: Ms. Jones, RN, MPH, works with the GJHS Parent-Teacher Association to increase physical activity and to build a walking trail around the school.
- System examples: Ms. Jones works with the Board of Education and local farmers to modify cafeteria offerings and bring healthy and nutritious foods to the children at GJHS. In addition, Ms. Jones works with the Board of Education to remove snack and vending machines from the school that serve only candy, chips, and sodas.
- Individual/family example: Ms. Jones meets with individual parents of overweight and obese children enrolled in the school-based clinic to discuss the importance of weight reduction, healthy foods, and physical activity.

---

community, and few options for fresh food markets. Ms. Jones knows that when parents and teachers have information about the problem, they will be more likely to participate in advocacy activities that can influence decision makers to make changes at GJHS that could lead to lower rates of overweight and obesity. **Box 13-2** provides examples of how Ms. Jones uses advocacy interventions at community level, systems level, and individual or family level. Of note, there is quite a bit of strategic overlap in each of these levels. Ms. Jones can utilize many of the same strategies at the other levels. Reflecting upon the examples provided in Box 13-2 also demonstrates that not only is Ms. Jones being an advocate for these children and their families but also her work with this population is delivered from the perspective of empowering the population. She is providing them with the necessary information that they need to know so that they may use their own voices and speak both individually and collectively.

COMMUNITY-FOCUSED LEVEL

The community-focused level is important to getting the message out about overweight and obese children at GJHS. At the community-focused level, Ms. Jones must identify the dif-

ferent community groups that can play an advocacy role in dealing with this problem. Before Ms. Jones meets with the PTA, Board of Education, and Community School Board, she must have the information needed to educate these groups about the problem. Ms. Jones uses epidemiological and social epidemiological approaches to gather information about children who are overweight and obese. As discussed above, Ms. Jones will gather this information by chart reviews, observation (looking at the level of physical activity at the GJHS), and health statistics about the neighborhoods of the students.

Ms. Jones examined the environmental, social, and personal factors that have contributed to the phenomenon of overweight and obese children. Examples of environmental factors are the cafeteria meals, an overabundance of vending machines in the school, and the decrease in gym classes. Examples of social factors are poverty (within the family and neighborhood of the children), socioeconomic status (family and neighborhood), and discrimination experienced by children growing up in their particular neighborhood. When Ms. Jones completed her study, she then prepared fact sheets for the PTA and an Issue Brief about the rates of overweight and obese children at GJHS, community rates of overweight and obese children, and contributing factors for the Board of Education and Community School Board.

Ms. Jones approached the PTA to advocate for a healthier dietary intake and an increase in physical activity levels for the children at GJHS by building walking trails around the school. When Ms. Jones received a commitment to her cause, Ms. Jones and the PTA advocated their cause to the Board of Education and the local Community School Board. An outcome of the meeting was that the Board of Education agreed to review the nutritional standards for food and beverages served in GJHS. Additionally, the Board of Education and the local Community School Board agreed that the school-based clinic should develop strategies and interventions that would play a role in preventing as well as reducing the number of overweight and obese students at GJHS.

SYSTEM-FOCUSED LEVEL

The systems-focused level is important in setting up partnerships to ensure they buy-in (or have a stake in the process) to strategies to address the problem. At the systems level, Ms. Jones works with the Board of Education, the local Community School Boards, and local farmers to bring healthy and nutritious foods to GJHS. Further, the local Community School Board decides to investigate if setting up a farmer's market in the communities they serve is doable as well as sustainable. Ms. Jones contacts a culinary college located in a nearby community to discuss the possibility of partnering with them to teach school cooks and parents how to prepare healthy meals with local farm produce and to establish student internships at GJHS. (Note that while this appears to be a community level approach there are system level applications present as well.) In addition,

Ms. Jones knows that developing policies that both facilitate and sustain the integration of healthy meals and local produce into the school system meals needs specific mandates to ensure system-level changes.

INDIVIDUAL/FAMILY-FOCUSED LEVEL

The individual/family-focused level is important to ensure that individuals or families have a stake in the process of reducing the incidence of overweight and obesity in children at GJHS. On the individual/family level, Ms. Jones makes arrangements for educational workshops for parents to be held at the school-based clinic. The workshops will address understanding and preventing obesity, nutritional information, and promoting healthy lifestyles. These workshops also provide a venue where Ms. Jones may work with families and individuals.

Ms. Jones identified a problem at GJHS and then developed and implemented advocacy strategies to reduce the prevalence of overweight and obese students at GJHS. Problem identification and developing strategic interventions required an understanding of the role of advocacy as outlined in the intervention wheel.

Social Marketing

Social marketing is defined as the utilization of ". . . commercial marketing principles and technologies for programs designed to influence the knowledge, attitudes, values, beliefs, behaviors, and practices of the population-of-interest" (Keller et al., 2008, p. 204). Social marketing makes use of "commercial marketing strategies to promote public health" (Evans, 2006, p. 1207) on the population level. It is a process that is developed and implemented with a focus on a targeted audience (Grier & Bryant, 2005). The key, in this intervention, is in the answer to the following question. How do public health nurses apply the principles of social marketing to practice? In order to do this, public health nurses need to have the knowledge, competencies, and skills to develop these marketing approaches to a population for the purpose of executing a population based behavioral change. One way to begin is to understand the social marketing mix. According to Daniel, Bernhardt, and Eroglu (2009) there are many activities that a public health professional may develop and implement to influence behavior change; but to ensure maximum effect the best approach is one that comprehensive. The "Four Ps" is a model that depicts this comprehensive marketing mix. The Four Ps is representative of Product, Price, Place, and Promotion (Daniel et al., 2009; Grier & Bryant, 2005; & Storey, Saffitz, & Rimon, 2008).

In social marketing the *product* is the benefit associated with the behavioral change. This, however, may not be easy to determine, and it is for this reason that those responsible for the development of the social marketing initiative must know their targeted audience. "The marketing objective is to discover which benefits have the greatest appeal to the target audience and design a product that provides those benefits" (Grier & Bryant, 2005, p. 323). In the development of a social marketing strategy for children/adolescents who are obese, presenting the product as decreasing one's risk for chronic illness may not be as appealing as being able to participate in sports on a more active and social level. *Price* refers to the cost, from the targeted audience's perspective, in order to receive or achieve the benefit. The targeted audience will weigh the cost and barriers to the benefits when making decisions to engage in behavior change or not to engage in behavior change. *Place* refers to where the targeted audience may be reached or the point of contact for the delivery of the information. As noted above, research may be necessary to identify these locations or the ". . . . life

path points—places people visit routinely, times of day, week, or year of visits, and points in the life cycle—where people are likely to act so that products and supportive services or information can be placed there" (Grier & Bryant, 2005, p. 323). An example of place is when public health nursing students who wish to deliver messages about child safety car seats may stand in front of a food store during morning hours to teach family members as they are placing their young children into their car seats. Finally, *promotion* is the fourth component of the marketing mix. Promotion refers to the communication and the messages that are being delivered. Components of this communication include: type of content; extensiveness of content; language used in the delivery of content and literacy level; ways the content will be delivered (such as pamphlets, flyers, radio announcements, billboards, television, texting, tweeting, songs, and blogs); and who will deliver the message. As previously noted, the component of promotion must also be designed with the specific audience in mind. Ultimately, social marketing is used to influence health behavior. What follows is Ms. Jones' strategy for social marketing at the various practice levels.

Ms. Jones recognizes that using social marketing has the potential to bring about an understanding of problems such as childhood obesity and getting people involved to make changes necessary to prevent and/or reduce overweight and obesity in children. Ms. Jones must use a myriad of communication strategies to ensure that the message is developed, delivered, and received in a way that is targeted to the intended audience so that behavioral change is possible. Before Ms. Jones begins to engage in aspects of social marketing, she must approach the situation with a working knowledge of the 4 Ps and also of behavioral theory. An example of behavioral theory is the health promotion model developed by nurse theorist Pender in 1987 (Sakraida, 2005). The health promotion model is widely used by nursing to identify how well an individual may adhere to preventive health recommendations such as exercise, smoking cessation, and diet modifications. Making changes to existing health behaviors is largely based on how the person perceives his or her risk or susceptibility to a particular disease (Sakraida, 2005). Ms. Jones knows that mass media campaigns will have an effect if the person believes he or she is at risk for becoming overweight or obese. However, because the population in question is children, the families and community must also buy into the notion that overweight and obese children are being seen in epidemic proportions in their communities. The application of the health promotion model, along with the 4 Ps model earlier discussed, may assist Ms. Jones as she makes decisions pertaining to the intervention of social marketing.

To help guide her with the intervention of social marketing, Ms. Jones creates a social marketing wheel to visualize what needs to be accomplished for a public health education campaign around the problem of overweight and obese children in GJHS (**Figure 13-1**). Social marketing is similar to health teaching because they both call for social campaigns to change public attitudes and behavior to solve a particular problem (Kotler & Roberto, 1989). Social marketing overlaps with advocacy as well as policy development and enforcement.

Effective social marketing begins with research about the targeted audience. The information gathered will assist Ms. Jones in the planning, development, and implementation of the social marketing initiative so that it is carefully targeted and tailored to the intended audience. During this beginning research phase, Ms. Jones uses focus groups to assess the level of knowledge of each targeted group (e.g., the family, the teachers, the children in Junior High School) and to gain their input. The focus groups also serve to elicit suggestions about crafting a health promotion campaign to increase physical activity in GJHS as well as out of school and developing healthy eating strategies in school, home, and the neighborhood. Additionally, Ms. Jones works with each of the focus groups to create a health promotion slogan. Slogans may be different depending on the targeted audience. These strategies are needed to ensure that an effective social marketing message will be understood by students, parents, teachers, members of the Board of Education, and the Community School Board. Further, Ms. Jones recognizes that by holding several focus groups, she is able to reach out to many different constituents, which is needed to understand each group's unique perspective about how to approach and address this problem.

Based on the focus groups, Ms. Jones develops a plan on what the health message will be or the content, how the health message will be presented and distributed, and by whom. Specifically, Ms. Jones works with teachers in the art department and media services to create posters, brochures, and a public service announcement. The teachers decide that this will be a school-wide project so that all students will participate. The Board of Education decides to present awards for the most innovative and creative poster, brochure, and public service announcement. The Community School Board works with the local businesses and community centers to appropriately place the media materials.

The implementation phase sees the social marketing being realized followed by evaluation. Part of the evaluation is the determination of whether the social marketing has been successful. For Ms. Jones this may mean tracking the intended targeted audience of children to

Figure 13-1 Obesity campaign social marketing wheel.

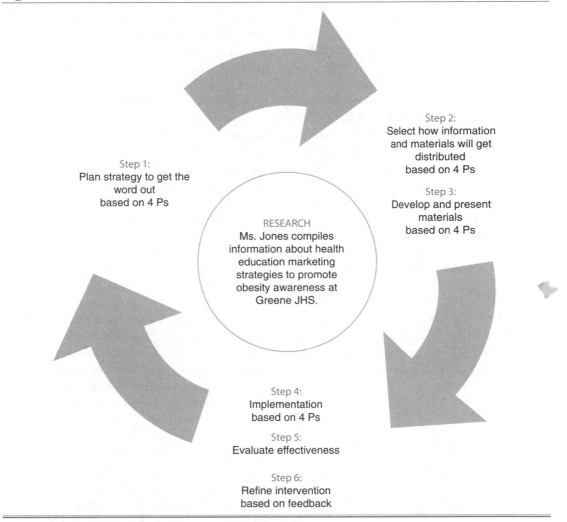

Step 1:
Plan strategy to get the
word out
based on 4 Ps

Step 2:
Select how information
and materials will get
distributed
based on 4 Ps

Step 3:
Develop and present
materials
based on 4 Ps

RESEARCH
Ms. Jones compiles
information about health
education marketing
strategies to promote
obesity awareness at
Greene JHS.

Step 4:
Implementation
based on 4 Ps

Step 5:
Evaluate effectiveness

Step 6:
Refine intervention
based on feedback

Source: Adapted from Evans, 2006.

see if there are changes in eating habits, physical activity or weights. Ms. Jones will accomplish this by tracking data; therefore, she must decide the type of data she is going to collect and track. In addition, Ms. Jones may also consider the actual social marketing and whether or not the program was delivered in the way that it was intended. Based on this type of evaluation, Ms. Jones must determine whether the program continues, continues with minor revisions, continues with major revisions, or if it is discontinued. It is important to note that evaluation really takes place throughout the implementation phase as Ms. Jones continually engages in an ongoing evaluation process by assessing knowledge, attitudes, and beliefs of the participants. Other examples of evaluations on the systems-focused level are the Board of Education removing vending machines from school cafeterias or replacing juice and soda drinks with water. Further, the Board of Education hires more physical education teachers and mandates daily gym classes for all students. Examples of successful outcomes on the community-focused level are the Community School Board working in concert with the local community center's work with local farmers to set up a weekly farmers' market. Examples demonstrating individuals/families-focused level outcomes are behavioral change as evidenced by attendance of families at the weekly shopping and cooking classes at the local churches and community centers.

Policy Development and Enforcement

Policy development is the final resolution of what comes out of advocacy and social marketing. **Policy development**, in fact, is often unsuccessful unless it is carried out in conjunction with advocacy.

> *Policy development places health issues on decision makers' agendas, acquires a plan of resolution, and determines needed resources. Policy development results in laws, rules and regulations, ordinances, and policies.* **Policy enforcement** *compels others to comply with the laws, rules, regulations, ordinances, and policies created in conjunction with policy development."* (Keller et al., 2008, p. 204)

Earlier in this text the chapter *Healthcare Policy and Politics: The Risk and Rewards for Public Health Nurses* gives a detailed accounting of this population-based intervention along with particular strategies. The application of these strategies to the various levels of Ms. Jones' practice is highlighted below.

Ms. Jones has been successful in bringing together all the stakeholders in the school and the surrounding communities to deal with the problem of overweight and obese children. Ms. Jones has seen that the programs addressing healthy eating in schools were developed and that partnerships with local farmers, the culinary school in the nearby community, and the school-based clinic were formed to ensure that the community has access to healthy and nutritious foods as well as learning about the nutritional value of food. Additionally, the local Community School Board established walking programs within the neighborhood, and the Board of Education was committed to increasing physical activity in GJHS.

Ms. Jones knows that she wants the programs started at GJHS and within the community to be sustainable and thus needs to ensure that the interested parties, such as students, teachers, parents, community partners, and the Board of Education, continue their involvement. Ms. Jones is charged with making sure that decision makers are informed about the problem of overweight and obese children so that laws, rules, regulations, ordinances, and policies can be enacted to address this issue. Further, Ms. Jones needs to make certain that the programs and interventions developed are effective, funding is available, surveillance systems are set in place to monitor health statistics, and school-based clinics become a model for addressing overweight and obesity at the community-focused, systems-focused, and individual/family-focused levels. The basic steps needed for policy development and enforcement are illustrated in **Figure 13-2**.

Step 1 requires that Ms. Jones identify the issue (increased numbers of overweight and obese children at GJHS) and the relevance of the issue locally and nationally. By identifying the problem and the target population, Ms. Jones decides what can be done about this issue. During this phase Ms. Jones set a policy agenda

Figure 13-2 Policy development process and enforcement.

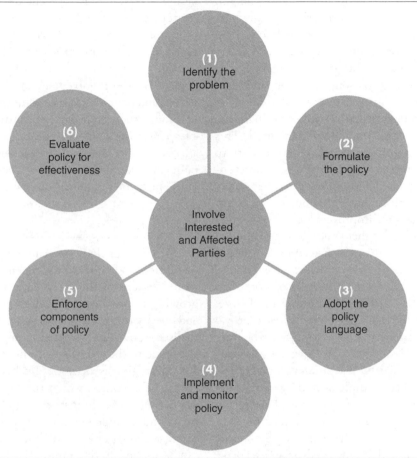

Source: Adapted from Minnesota Department of Health Division of Community Health Services Public Health Nursing Section, 2001.

and identified the local, state, and federal policy-makers who would have authority to develop and mandate policies.

Step 2 requires that Ms. Jones begin to formulate policy and establish goals and objectives to resolve this problem. Because Ms. Jones had already started the advocacy and social marketing process earlier, many of the key stakeholders have already been identified and involved in resolving the problem.

Step 3 requires that Ms. Jones draft a policy to address the issue. The policy should consist of a budget and funding and arrange for public hearings as necessary to bring this problem to the attention of additional stakeholders.

Step 4 requires that Ms. Jones develop rules and guidelines needed to sustain the suggested programs, such as mandating daily gym classes, changing the food choices at the school cafeteria, and setting up local farmers' markets in the community. Ms. Jones has to also decide how these programs will be monitored and who will be responsible for monitoring these programs.

Step 5 requires that Ms. Jones knows how the enforcement of any policy will take place. Strategies for policy enforcement can take many forms such as negotiation, education, and legal repercussions.

Step 6 requires that Ms. Jones evaluate the effectiveness of all policies implemented. This phase is an ongoing process and is necessary to assess the effectiveness of a strategy, intervention, or program. This phase provides policy developers with knowledge about the program and is the basis for improvement.

Ms. Jones knows that policy development and enforcement can also be achieved by legislation or regulation. Legislation provides a legal framework that embodies the principles of a program and the policy basics are unlikely to change. Enacting policy legislatively requires approval by a governing body such as Congress, the state assembly, and so forth. The laws are promulgated and passed by a legislative branch and then, after passage, implemented by local, state, or federal administrative agencies. Legislation provides the basis for the regulatory process; therefore, regulations have the force and the effect of the law that are issued by an executive authority of the government (Milstead, 2008).

Even though Ms. Jones' advocacy, social marketing, and policy development and enforcement strategies were mostly developed on the local level, many of the interventions put into place can lead to government action. The success of enacting legislation and regulations will largely depend on the involvement of the interested parties and ongoing evaluation of the programs. Ms. Jones knows that public health nurses have a responsibility to identify health problems that affect the larger community/population and that policy development and enforcement come out of the principles of public health nursing.

Conclusion

This chapter discusses the advocacy, social marketing, and policy development and enforcement sections of the intervention wheel. The growing public health problem of overweight and obesity in children and adolescents was used to discuss how public health nursing could bring this issue to the attention of interested parties. The strategies used by public health nursing consist of advocacy, which then leads to social marketing, and culminate with policy development and enforcement. Further, this chapter discusses how public health nursing strategies can be applied on the community level, systems level, and individual/family level.

References

Allison, D. B., Newcomer, J. W., Dunn, A. L., Blumenthal, J. A., Fabricatore, A. N., Daudmit, G. L., . . . Alpert, J. E. (2009). Obesity among those with mental disorders: A National Institute of Mental Health Meeting Report. *American Journal of Preventive Medicine, 36*(4), 341–350.

American Nurses Association. (2001). *Code of ethics for nurses with interpretive statements.* Washington, DC: Author.

American Nurses Association. (2007). *Public health nursing: Scope & standards of practice.* Maryland, Author.

Ballou, K. (2000). A historical-philosophical analysis of the professional nurse obligation to participate in sociopolitical activities. *Policy, Politics, & Nursing Practice, 1*(3), 172–184.

Blair, S. N., & Nichaman, M. Z. (2002). The public health problem of increasing prevalence rates of obesity and what should be done about it. *Mayo Clinical Procedures, 77*(2), 109–113.

Bu, X., & Jezewski, M. A. (2007). Developing a mid-range theory of patient advocacy through concept analysis. *Journal of Advanced Nursing, 57*(1), 101–110.

Centers for Disease Control and Prevention (CDC). (2000). *Prevalence of overweight and obesity among adults: United States, 1999.* Retrieved from http:/www.cdc.gov/nchs/nhanes.htm

Centers for Disease Control and Prevention (CDC). (2001). Diabetes. *CDC {Online}.* Retrieved from http://www.cdc.gov/diabetes/statistics

Centers for Disease Control and Prevention (CDC). (2009). *Health weight.* Retrieved from http://www.cdc.gov/healthyweight/assessing/bmi/adult_BMI/index.html

Chen, Y., Dales, R., & Jiang, Y. (2006). The association between obesity and asthma is stronger in nonallergic than allergic adults. *Chest, 130,* 890–895.

Childhood obesity: An emerging public-health problem. (2001). (Editorial). *Lancet, 357*(9273), 1989.

Cohen, D., de la Vega, R., & Watson, G. (2001). *Advocacy for social justice: A global action and reflection guide.* Sterling, VA: Kumarian Press.

Daniel, K. L., Bernhardt, J. M., & Eroglu, D. (2009). Social marketing and health communication: From people to places. *American Journal of Public Health, 99*(12), 2120–2122.

Davis, B., & Carpenter, C. (2009). Proximity of fast-food restaurants to schools and adolescent obesity. *American Journal of Public Health, 99*(3), 505–510.

de Onis, M., & Blossner, M. (2000). Prevalence and trends of overweight among preschool children in developing countries. *American Journal of Clinical Nutrition, 72,* 1032–1039.

Diabetes Prevention Program Research Group. (2002). Reduction in the incidence of type 2 diabetes with lifestyle intervention or metformin. *New England Journal of Medicine, 346*(6), 393–403.

Evans, W. D. (2006). How social marketing works in health care. *British Medical Journal, 332,* 1207–1210.

Flegal, K. M., Carroll, M. D., Ogden, C. L., & Curtin, L. R. (2010). Prevalence and trends in obesity among US adults, 1999–2008. *Journal of the American Medical Association, 303*(3), 235–241.

Flynn, M. A., McNeil, D. A., Maloff, B., Mutasingwa, D., Wu, M., Ford, C., & Tough, S. C. (2006). Reducing obesity and related chronic disease risk in children and youth: A synthesis of evidence with "best practice" recommendations. *Obesity Reviews, 7*(Suppl. 1), 7–66.

Grier, S., & Bryant, C. A. (2005). Social marketing in public health. *Annual Review of Public Health, 26*(1), 319–339.

Harbaugh, B. L., Jordan-Welch, M., Bounds, W., Blom, L., & Fisher, W. (2007). Nurses and families rising to the challenge of overweight children. *Nurse Practitioner, 32*(3), 30–35.

Hogan, P., Dall, T., Nikolov, P., & the American Diabetes Association. (2003). Economic costs of diabetes in the US in 2002. *Diabetes Care, 26*(3), 917–932.

Jordan, A. B., & Robinson, T. N. (2008). Children, television viewing, and weight status: Summary and recommendations from an expert panel meeting. *Annals of the American Academy, 615,* 119–132.

Keller, L. O., Strohschein, S., & Briske, L. (2008). Population-based public health nursing practice: The intervention wheel. In M. Stanhope & J. Lancaster (Eds.), *Public health nursing: Population-centered health care in the community* (pp. 199–205). St. Louis, MO: Mosby Elsevier.

Koplan, J. P., Liverman, C. T., & Kraak, V. A. (Eds.). (2005). *Preventing childhood obesity: Health in the balance.* Washington, DC: National Academies Press.

Kotler, P., & Roberto, E. L. (1989). *Social marketing: Strategies for changing public behavior.* New York, NY: New York Free Press.

Kumanyika, S. K., Obarzanek, E., Stettler, N., Bell, R., Field, A. E., Fortmann, S. P., & American Heart Association Council on Epidemiology. (2008). Population-based prevention of obesity: The need for comprehensive promotion of healthful eating, physical activity, and energy balance. *Circulation, 118,* 428–464.

Lee, R. E., & Cubbin, C. (2002). Neighborhood context and youth cardiovascular health behaviors. *American Journal of Public Health, 92,* 428–436.

Lopez, R. (2004). Urban sprawl and risk for being overweight and obese. *American Journal of Public Health, 94*(9), 1574–1579.

Lovasi, G. S., Neckerman, K. M., Quinn, J. W., Weiss, C. C., & Rundle, A. (2009). Effects of individual neighborhood disadvantage on the association between neighborhood walkability and body mass index. *American Journal of Public Health, 99*(2), 279–284.

Messier, S. P., Loeser, R. F., Miller, G. D., Morgan, T. M., Rejeski, W. J., Sevick, M. A., & Williamson, J. D. (2004). Exercise and dietary weight loss in overweight and obese adults with knee osteoarthritis: The arthritis, diet, and activity promotion trial. *Arthritis & Rheumatism, 50*(5), 1501–1510.

Milstead, J. A. (2008). *Health policy and politics: A nurse's guide* (3rd ed.). Sudbury, MA: Jones and Bartlett.

Minnesota Department of Health Division of Community Health Services Public Health Nursing Section. (2001). *Public health interventions: Application for public health nursing practice.* St. Paul, MN: Minnesota Department of Health.

Murugan, A. T., & Sharma, G. (2008). Obesity and respiratory diseases. *Chronic Respiratory Disease, 5,* 233–242.

Nader, P. R., O'Brien, M., Houts, R., Bradley, R., Belsky, J., Crosnoe, R., & National Institute of Child Health and Human Development. (2006). Identifying risk for obesity in early childhood. *Pediatrics, 118*(3), e594–e601.

Narayan, K. M., Boyle, J. P., Geiss, L. S., Saaddine, J. B., & Thompson, T. L. (2006). Impact of recent increase in incidence on future diabetes burden: U.S., 2005–2050. *Diabetes Care, 29*(9), 2114–2116.

Newcomer, J. W. (2007). Metabolic syndrome and mental illness. *American Journal of Managed Care, 13,* S170–S177.

Ogden, C. L., & Carroll, M. D. (2010a). Prevalence of obesity among children and adolescents: United States, Trends 1963–1965 through 2007–2008. *Health E-Stats.* Retrieved from http://www.cdc.gov/nchs/data/hestat/obesity_child_07_08/obesity_child_07_08.htm

Ogden, C. L., & Carroll, M. D. (2010b). Prevalence of overweight, obesity, and extreme obesity among adults: United States, Trends 1963–1965 through 2007–2008. *Health E-Stats.* Retrieved from http://www.cdc.gov/nchs/data/hestat/obesity_adult_07_08/obesity_adult_07_08.htm

Ogden, C. L., & Carroll, M. D., Curtin, L. R., McDowell, M. A., Tabak, C. J., & Flegal, K. M. (2009). Prevalence of overweight and obesity in the United States, 1999–2004. *Journal of the American Medical Association, 295*(13), 1549–1555.

Patterson, R. E., Frank, L. L., Kristal, A. R., & White, E. (2004). A comprehensive examination of health conditions associated with obesity in older adults. *American Journal of Preventive Medicine, 27*(5), 385–390.

Peterson, J. A. (2007). Get moving! Physical activity counseling in primary care. *Journal of the American Academy of Nurse Practitioners, 19,* 349–357.

Reiser, L. M., & Schlenk, E. A. (2009). Clinical use of physical activity measures. *Journal of the American Academy of Nurse Practitioners, 21,* 87–94.

Sakraida, T. (2005). Nola J. Pender: The health promotion model. In T. A. Marriner-Tomey & A. M. Raile-Aligood (Eds.), *Nursing theorists and their work* (5th ed., pp. 624–639). St. Louis, MO: Mosby.

Salvy, S. J., Roemmich, J. N., Bowker, J. C., Romero, N. D., Stadler, P. J., & Epstein, L. H. (2009). Effects of peers and friends on youth physical activity and motivation to be physically active. *Journal of Pediatric Psychology, 34*(2), 217–225.

Schorr Saxe, J. (2011). Promoting healthy lifestyles and decreasing childhood obesity: Increasing physician effectiveness through advocacy. *Annals of Family Medicine, 9*(6), 546–548.

Seiders, K., & Petty, R. D. (2004). Obesity and the role of food marketing: A policy analysis of issues and remedies. *Journal of Public Policy & Marketing, 23*(2), 153–169.

Sheehy, A. M., Coursin, D. B., & Gabbay, R. A. (2008). Back to Wilson and Jungner: 10 good reasons to screen for type 2 diabetes mellitus. *Mayo Clinic Procedures, 84*(1), 38–42.

Storey, J. D., Saffitz, G. B. & Rimon, J. G. (2008). Social marketing. In K. Glanz, B. K. Rimer., & K. Viswanath (Eds.), *Health behavior and health education: Theory, research, and practice* (4th ed., pp. 435–464). CA: Jossey-Bass.

Story, M., Nanney, M. S., & Schwartz, M. B. (2009). Schools and obesity prevention: Creating school environments and policies to promote healthy eating and physical activity. *Milbank Quarterly, 87*(1), 71–100.

U.S. Department of Health and Human Services (U.S. DHHS). (2008). 2008 Physical activity guidelines for Americans. Washington, DC: Author.

U.S. Department of Health and Human Services (U.S. DHHS). (2010). *Topics and objectives.* Retrieved from http://www.healthypeople.gov/2020/topics objectives2020/default.aspx

Wald, L. (1915). *The house on Henry Street.* New York, NY: Henry Holt & Company.

Wallace, M. F., Fulwood, R., & Alvarado, M. (2008). NHLBI step-by-step approach to adapting cardiovascular training and education curricula for diverse audiences. *Preventing Chronic Disease, 5*(2), 1–7.

Ward, A., & Martens, L. (2000). *Eating out: Social differentiation, consumption, and pleasure.* London, UK: Cambridge University Press.

Yanovski, S. Z., & Yanovski, J. A. (2002). Drug therapy: Obesity. *New England Journal of Medicine, 346*(8), 591–602.

For a full suite of assignments and additional learning activities, use the access code located in the front of your book to visit this exclusive website: http://go.jblearning.com/londrigan. If you do not have an access code, you can obtain one at the site.

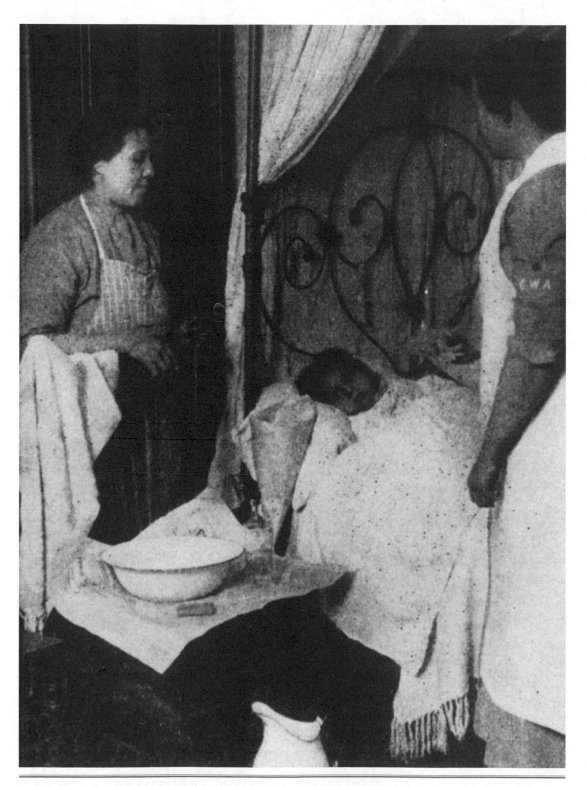

Chapter 14

Protecting, Sustaining, and Empowering: A Historical Perspective on the Control of Epidemics

Christine E. Hallett

Does not the popular idea of "infection" involve that people should take greater care of themselves than of the patient? That, for instance, it is safer not to be too much with the patient, not to attend too much to his wants? Perhaps the best illustration of the utter absurdity of this view of duty in attending on "infectious" diseases is afforded by what was very recently the practice, if it is not so even now, in some of the European lazarets—in which the plague-patient used to be condemned to the horrors of filth, overcrowding, and want of ventilation, while the medical attendant was ordered to examine the patient's tongue through an opera-glass and to toss him a lancet to open his abscess with! True nursing ignores infection, except to prevent it. Cleanliness and fresh air from open windows, with unremitting attention to the patient, are the only defense a true nurse either asks or needs. Wise and humane management of the patient is the best safeguard against infection (Nightingale, 1860/1980, pp. 23–24).

LEARNING OBJECTIVES

At the completion of this chapter, the reader will be able to

- Explore the ways in which human societies have attempted to combat global epidemics.
- Appreciate the role of the nurse, working alongside governments, doctors, and scientists, in the prevention of epidemic diseases.
- Explore the role of the nurse in the treatment and care of patients with life-threatening infectious diseases at different historical moments and in different places.

WWW

KEY TERMS

❏ Epidemic disease   ❏ Pandemic
❏ Infection control

From its beginnings, the human race has shared its habitats with infective microparasites. Harmless—even beneficial—microbes inhabited our planet long before we emerged as a species. They began the long evolutionary process that would enable them to live alongside—often in parasitic or symbiotic relationships with—their neighbors before the antecedents of the human species had even emerged from the primeval ocean. Catalyzing vital processes, such as the decomposition of the planet's toxic organic waste, microbes have long existed in a precarious, yet often positive, relationship with other organic life. Yet human beings notice their presence only when they fail to adapt quietly and harmlessly to the changing patterns of human life.

Of the many microparasites that inhabit our environment, it is the most inefficient—the least well adapted—that cause recognized infections. A "bug" that fails to live symbiotically with its host may expect to limit its own lifespan. If it kills its host, it will die. If it keeps the host alive yet in a weakened state, it can expect that its host will eventually find a way to eradicate it. The purpose of this chapter is to trace the means by which humans have attempted to eradicate certain of those "bugs" they consider harmful: the bacteria and viruses that cause epidemic and endemic infections. The chapter focuses on three case studies of specific diseases appearing at specific historical moments: bubonic plague, as it appeared in the early modern Italian city-states during the 16th and 17th centuries; "Spanish influenza" as it appeared in the cities of the United States in

1918 and 1919; and AIDS as it appeared in the United Kingdom during the 1980s.

The bubonic plague bacillus and the influenza virus caused **epidemic diseases** that affected such large sections of the world's population that they came to be seen as "global epidemics" or, more correctly, as **pandemics**. HIV exists on the cusp between endemic and epidemic disease, affecting large numbers of people worldwide; it is often spoken of as an epidemic because of its capacity to spread rapidly in certain populations and geographical areas of the world at certain times.

Humans have taken a range of measures to protect themselves against or to destroy pathogenic microorganisms. Through its case studies, this chapter considers four different approaches to disease: state-sanctioned control measures, medical interventions, nursing care and support, and individual empowerment. It traces the means by which human societies, more or less effectively, learned to protect themselves against, overcome, and survive severe life-threatening infection on a large scale. It focuses, in particular, on how societies mobilized and used nurses as "front-line" agents in combating infection.

Protecting the People Against God's Wrath: Bubonic Plague in Early Modern Italy

The Black Death—the second recorded pandemic of the disease known as "bubonic plague"—swept across Europe from Central

Asia between 1348 and 1353, causing millions of deaths and devastating entire villages (Alexander, 1980; Hirst, 1953; Preto, 1978; Slack, 1985; Zinsser, 1935). Caused by the bacterium later to be named *Yersinia pestis*, the disease was carried in the body of a particular species of flea known as *Xenopsylla cheopis*, which in turn inhabited a particular species of rat, *Rattus rattus*, also known as the black rat. It may seem extraordinary that a disease carried by one species of microbe in the bloodstream of one species of flea on the back of one species of rat could destroy so many communities, yet the lifestyle of the Middle Ages created an ideal ecological niche for these species. The black rat could live easily in the thatched roofs and grain stores of the largely agrarian communities of the 14th century, and the frequent overcrowding and lack of opportunities for good hygiene practices meant that flea and lice infestations were commonplace. Once the opening-up of trade routes to the East transported the plague to Western Europe, it rapidly gained a foothold there.

The first case study considers one small corner of the world two centuries after the plague caused its first great wave of devastation. The case-fatality rate of bubonic plague was probably around 30%, and its associated form, pneumonic plague, was even more lethal, with an 80% case-fatality rate. Having burned itself out by killing a large proportion of its host population, the Black Death remained endemic in the European rodent population, literally hovering at the gates of the towns and cities of early modern Europe. At particular risk were the inhabitants of the Italian city-states such as Venice, Florence, Naples, and Rome that traded with the East, bringing within their borders goods likely to be infested with the black rat. Although they did not realize the disease was carried by rat fleas, the populations of these cities nevertheless recognized that it was somehow "imported" from outside. These states were the first to introduce systematic measures to protect their populations from plague (Christensen, 2003).

When confronted by plague, the magistrates of the city-states had three aims: to avoid allowing the disease to arise in or to enter the city; to prevent its spread; and to maintain social order while, as much as possible, caring for the sick. Health magistrates, known as "Provveditori alla Sanita," appeared to have thought in terms of a complex relationship between plague and disorder. Plague was itself a form of physical disorder that could most easily arise in a disorderly environment that exuded disease-forming "miasmas" (or "pestilential" states of the air). Once plague had taken hold of a community, the relationship between the disease and social disorder was mutually reinforcing. The effect was perceived to be a spiral one in which the health—both physical and moral—of the community grew increasingly out of control. The work of the magistrates was to arrest this process. To properly coordinate their efforts during epidemics, the governments of Italian city-states appointed specialist Health Boards, known as "Sanita," with wide-reaching powers, which became permanent in many Italian city-states during the course of the 1400s (Campbell, 1931; Carmichael, 1983, 1986; Palmer, 1978).

Arising from a disorder within nature, plague threatened to create chaos within the community. Italian sanitary legislation aimed to prevent such chaos. Many of the measures in force during the Renaissance were introduced by legislation of the early 13th century, which preceded even experience of the Black Death (Carmichael, 1986). There were numerous attempts to legislate for cleanliness within city-states. Unpleasant smells were believed to be particularly dangerous, because they were associated with noxious harmful vapors that composed the miasma. By the end of the

14th century, there was already legislation against the keeping of animals such as pigs and ducks in Florence and against the selling of manure inside the city (Carmichael, 1986). The health authorities came to regard it as their responsibility to control the release of offensive smells associated with industrial activities such as tanning, butchery, and the retting of hemp (Cipolla, 1992; Palmer, 1978).

In taking responsibility for the eradication of plague, the patriciates (nobilities) of early modern cities fulfilled their roles as guardians of order and protectors of the state. King (1986) has identified the main preoccupations of Venetian patricians as evident in their humanistic writings. Noblemen such as Gasparo Contarini, Daniele Barbaro, Paolo Paruta, and Nicolo Contarini promoted the myth of a Venetian republic that was ordered and harmonious and in which the nobility conformed to the principle of "unanimitas." The Venetian patriciate presented itself as the personification of order within the state. Furthermore, its members also saw themselves as the state's defense—as "moenia civitatis," or the "walls of the city" (King, 1986; Pastore, 1988; Ulvioni, 1989). The Italian Health Boards were the most effective and efficient organizations for controlling plague in Western Europe, and their measures became models for the establishment of health controls in other states (Cipolla, 1979, 1992).

Calvi (1989) examined the efforts of magistrates to maintain stability in Florence during the epidemic of 1630–1631. Through a close examination of the criminal trial records of the Health Magistracy and a reading of Francesco Rondinelli's contemporary account of the plague, she discovered that the regulations imposed during the "virtual dictatorship" of the public health officials reflected the desire for order and uniformity. Most of the 300 trials she examined dealt with violations against property, crimes committed by public health workers, and the unlawful hiding of the ill (Calvi, 1989).

It had been recognized since the Black Death that some diseases could be transmitted between individuals (Biraben, 1975; Campbell, 1931). An idea of contagion was part of the general stock of knowledge in early modern Europe. In Thomas More's *Utopia* (1516), the hospitals were situated outside the town so that people with diseases "such as be wont by infection to creep from one to another" (p. 35) might be separated from the rest of the population (Ficino, 1989). However, a theory of contagion was not articulated effectively until the mid-16th century, when it formed the basis of a work by Girolamo Fracastoro (1930). His *De Contagione et Contagiosis Morbis et Eorum Curatione, Libri III*, first published in Venice in 1546, has interested historians because its theories bear some superficial resemblance to a germ theory of disease (Fracastoro, 1930; Nutton, 1990).

Fracastoro emphasized that where plague was concerned, the most frequent means of transmission was contagion between individuals. He distinguished between diseases that were merely common to communities and those that were also contagious (Fracastoro, 1930). The dominant theme in his work was the idea that plague was caused by invasion. It could be passed on from person to person rather than simply arising spontaneously from a disordered environment. It could also be carried in fomites—porous objects such as cloth and wood—and thus be transported between one community and the next. These ideas had immense influence in the Italian city-states, where plague came to be seen as an invading force against which siege measures must be adopted.

During the early modern period, as plague came to be identified more as an invasion from outside the state, measures taken by city-state magistrates to preserve order were increasingly reinforced by a range of defensive strategies; many of these plans were already quite old, dating from the time of the Black Death, but all appear to have been imposed with increasing rigor and determination during the 16th and 17th centuries. In the late 1500s, Gasparo Contarini (1599) commented on the work of the Provveditore alla Sanita, the city's health magistrate:

> *His chiefest office is to forsee that there come not into the citie an contagious infection, which if at any time it happen to creepe in (as sometimes it chanceth) then to take such diligent and carefull order that in as much as maybe the same come not to spread any further. (np)*

Throughout the early modern period, when it became known to its neighbors that a state was affected by plague, it was usual for commerce with that state to be banned. This meant the cessation of all forms of communication, including trade, with the plague-infested region, against whose inhabitants the frontiers were closely guarded (Carmichael, 1983). Banning was controlled by means of a system of health passes that permitted only those who were well or who came from healthy areas to enter a territory. Passes were introduced by Milan during the 15th century and were then used by other states in the first half of the 16th century (Brozzi, 1982; Cipolla, 1973, 1979; Modena, 1988; Palmer, 1978; Petraccone, 1978). Centorio degli Hortensii (1631) described a series of measures introduced by the health deputies of Modena during the plague of 1575–1577: "Besides unpaid officials at the gates, paid officials will be posted at the pass of the Fossa Alta, at the pass of the Marzoia at the high bridge and the low bridge. . . at Buon Porto, on the bank of the River Secchia, at San Marino, on the border with Mirandola" (p. 17). They added that guards at these posts must be able to read and write and must be in possession of an official seal to stamp the passes of those allowed through (Hortensii, 1631). The defensive nature of these measures is striking: They illustrate the extent to which plague came to be associated with invasion.

All ships coming to the early modern state from any area suspected of plague were made to undergo quarantine. Crew members were not permitted to enter the city or unload goods during the quarantine period, which usually lasted 40 days. This measure was originally designed to provide an early warning system for diseases on ships but became one of the most enduring measures against contagion (Campbell, 1931; Carmichael, 1983; Palmer, 1978). It also became a measure for isolating entire communities of people: During a general quarantine, only doctors and members of the government were allowed to leave their homes (Petraccone, 1978; Ulvioni, 1989).

When plague was diagnosed in an Italian city-state, the victims were quickly segregated from the rest of the population. The sick were examined, and persons discovered to be suffering from the plague were taken to the "lazzaretto," or "pest house." The Lazzaretto Vecchio of Venice, founded by decree of the Senate on August 28, 1423, was the first permanent pest house in Europe (Campbell, 1931; Palmer, 1978). It was situated about two miles from the city on a small island off the Lido that had previously been the home of the Eremite Monastery of Santa Maria di Nazareth (Chambers & Pullan, 1992). A decree of the Venetian Senate on April 17, 1464, provided for "two suitable and competent citizens not of noble rank" (Chambers & Pullan, 1992, p. 114) to be appointed for each sestiere of the city to ensure that all infected persons were taken to the Lazzaretto Vecchio and all infected houses evacuated. The notary, Rocco Benedetti, described the horrors of the Venetian

Lazzaretto Vecchio, which seemed to him like "Hell itself" (Chambers & Pullan, 1992):

> From every side their came foul odors, indeed a stench that none could endure; groans and sighs were heard without ceasing; and at all hours, clouds of smoke from the burning of corpses was seen to rise far into the air. Some who miraculously returned from that place alive reported, among other things, that at the height of that great influx of infected people there were three or four of them to a bed. Since a great number of servants had died and there was no one to take care of them, they had to get themselves up to take food and attend to other things. Nobody did anything but lift the dead from the beds and throw them into the pits. . . . And many, driven to frenzy by the disease, especially at night, leapt from their beds, and, shouting with fearful voices of damned souls, went here and there, colliding with one another, and suddenly falling to the ground dead. Some who rushed in frenzy out of the wards threw themselves into the water, or ran madly through the gardens, and were then found dead among the thornbushes, all covered with blood. (pp. 118–119)

A sufferer who died at the pest house was buried there or in a cemetery apart from the city. Survivors were usually sent to a convalescent hospital to undergo a 40-day quarantine before being returned home (Chambers & Pullan, 1992). The lazzaretti were also centers for the disinfection of fomites. In the Venetian lazzaretti, goods from infected homes and ships were aired for 40 days and, during that time, were constantly turned and moved to release any infection they might have absorbed (Brozzi, 1982; Castellacci, 1897; Pastore, 1988).

The monitoring and control of the poor were closely associated with the prevention of plague: It was a means of propitiating God, a measure for promoting order, and a defensive strategy.

Indeed, the development of organized systems of poor relief was probably stimulated by the experience of plague, a disease associated with poverty at an early stage in its history (Preto, 1978; Pullan, 1971, 1992). Governments and physicians observed that the poor were affected in greater numbers than the rich. Theorists devised explanations for this pattern: The poor lived disorderly lives, their inadequate diets were a source of corruption that could spread through the community, and they did not dispose of waste properly and hence lived among filth that might create a poisonous miasma (Anselment, 1989; Biraben, 1975; Carmichael, 1986; Grell, 1990).

During the plague of 1575–1577, physicians expressed the view that the poor were a threat to the health of the community. Nicolo Massa and Girolamo Mercuriale both went so far as to argue that the poor should be removed from towns when there was a threat of plague. Mercuriale referred to them as "fomes" for the disease (Palmer, 1978, p. 144). In August 1576 the state, perhaps acting on such advice, decided that the link between poverty and plague was related to poor housing conditions and chose a site at Zaffusina at which to relocate the poor from plague-affected areas. It was said that the site could have accommodated over 10,000 people, and provision was made for the supply of tents and huts, but the plan was never put into effect (Preto, 1978).

Hospitals originated as hostels for the poor rather than as specialist centers for the cure of disease, and as such they were centers for the isolation of those likely to disrupt the social order (Cartwright, 1977; Pullan, 1992). The poor could be seen as plague in microcosm. The Mendicanti hospitals established in many Italian states from the 1560s onward were designated to remove beggars from public places (Park & Henderson, 1991). By building hospitals, magistrates responded to plague in three ways. First, by caring for its poor, the state obeyed God's commands and might thereby deflect his anger and prevent disease. Second, by housing beggars, the state avoided the problems associated with squalor, dirt, filth, and bad smells that could give rise to miasma. Third, if the poor were seen as carriers of plague in a contagious sense, the state, by isolating them in hospitals, protected healthy citizens from the disease they carried.

Measures adopted by states from the second half of the 1400s illustrate their recognition that plague could easily be brought into cities by immigrants whose origins were uncertain (Carmichael, 1983). In 1498 in Venice, it was decreed that all lodging housekeepers must have licenses (Pullan, 1971). The tendency to associate plague with invasion through theories of contagion is apparent in the way in which particular individuals were blamed for bringing plague into a city. It was believed, for example, that during October 1629 a soldier from Lecco brought the disease into Milan in a bundle of clothing obtained from German troops (Calvi, 1989; Cipolla, 1973; Galassi, 1966–1970).

A decree of the Venetian Council of Ten and Zonta of September 12, 1539, described how orders had been given to the Provveditori alla Sanita (Chambers & Pullan, 1992):

> *To bar from this city many poor persons suspected of carrying the plague, who, as we had heard by letters from Milan, had been expelled from the Milanese state and from Piedmont, and it was thought that they were certain to come here. Not only did the Provveditori carry out these orders both wisely and thoroughly, but they also expelled from Venice some 4000–5000 beggars and other kinds of persons who had recently come to live in this city. (p. 126)*

The approaches of the Italian city-states to the prevention and control of bubonic plague were thus a mixture of the pragmatic and the ideological. By closing their gates to anyone who might carry the disease and removing from their homes all those who were believed to be infected, states protected their healthy citizens. In holding masses and processions and in establishing hospitals for the poor, they worked to propitiate divine wrath. Most did not, however, have the capacity to provide adequate care and attention to those who succumbed to the disease. Early modern pest houses were places of dread—from which one had a poor chance of emerging alive.

Serving and Sustaining a Desperate Population: Influenza in the Modern United States

Modern sensibilities may identify a degree of ruthlessness in the approaches to plague prevention of the early modern Italian city-states. If the beleaguered "Provveditori alla Sanita" took harsh and desperate measures, this can have been only because of their fundamental sense of helplessness when confronted by infectious disease. They had no cure. Keeping their options open, they worked hard to propitiate God; epidemics might, after all, as the Bible suggested, be visitations of divine wrath. Yet, they also directed their energies toward protecting the healthy in their communities. The sick they condemned to the overcrowded pest houses, where desperate and overwhelmed nursing attendants struggled to offer rudimentary support.

Perhaps no greater contrast can therefore be imagined than between the frantic efforts of the early modern pest house attendants and the home care offered by the confident district nurses of modern cities in the early 20th century. The influenza pandemic of 1918–1919 threatened to overwhelm much of Europe, the European colonies, and North America, yet one of the most striking findings of historians is that although medical science stood by helpless before this deadly disease, nursing care seemed effective in reducing death rates. Although no efforts have ever been made to quantify the successes of early-20th-century district nurses (it is impossible to prove definitively that they actually saved lives), the writings of contemporaries indicate that there was a strong belief that good nursing care had made a real difference to survival rates.

This phenomenon of "good nursing care" appears frequently in the writings of physicians and nurses in the late 1800s, but is rarely accompanied by a definition. It appears to refer to those nursing actions that enabled the patient's physiological system to survive best while his or her immune system fought the infectious disease. Thus, the maintenance of a steady temperature by the judicious use of blankets and the warming of "sick rooms"; the provision of copious fluids and nourishing food (usually in the form of nutritious soup); and the maintenance of patient hygiene, rest, and sleep acted both to stabilize the system and to prevent the development of new complications. Providing these prerequisites for recovery seems deceptively simple. In reality, providing core nursing care for a very ill individual required great artistry, skill, and patience, whereas going into a home to care for a person with a known deadly—and incurable—disease required more than a little courage.

The so-called Spanish influenza epidemic of 1918–1919 (caused by the virus H_1N_1) is estimated to have caused a global mortality of between 50 and 100 million (Johnson & Mueller, 2002; Quinn, 2008). It developed toward the end of the World War I and probably killed at least twice as many people as the war itself (Crosby, 1989; Johnson, 2006; Patterson & Pyle, 1991; Phillips & Killingray, 2003). Reid (2005) observed that accurate figures are

difficult to obtain, partly because influenza was not made a notifiable disease until 1918 and partly because early cases were often labeled as bronchitic pneumonia or just pneumonia. It appears to have originated in China and then may have been spread throughout the United States via the mobilization and movement of troops who were housed in overcrowded barracks. From the American military camps it spread rapidly to Europe, where war-weary populations succumbed rapidly (Byerly, 2005; Quinn, 2008). Its most puzzling and unusual feature was its tendency to attack young, apparently healthy adults: Its mortality rate was very high within this group and was lower among the elderly (possibly because of acquired immunity) and the very young (Barry, 2005; Reid, 2005).

A devastating disease, Spanish influenza caused severe headache, cough, breathing difficulties, nosebleeds, aching joints, and intense fatigue. A characteristic symptom was the severe cyanosis that could rapidly turn the faces of sufferers blue or even black. The disease was often extremely rapid in its onset. An apparently healthy individual might suddenly collapse in the street, with blood pouring from his nose, and then die before there was time to get him to a hospital. Already severe in its respiratory symptoms, the disease was frequently complicated by acute and severe bronchopneumonic symptoms, and death was frequently from these complications rather than from the more systemic effects of the virus. Victims of this terrifying disease became feverish to the point of delirium, cyanosed until their skin was black, and weak to the point of utter helplessness (Quinn, 2008).

Joyce Sapwell, a British volunteer-nurse, wrote the following in her diary:

The terrible flu pneumonia epidemic broke out. About one-third of the staff were down with it, and the hospital was full. We had had

*one hundred and eight deaths in eight weeks.
I was put on night duty in charge of four huts
at the bottom of the hospital, the main part
was full, each hut had 20 beds. Three of them
flu pneumonia and one with convalescent colo-
nials. I had not even one orderly to help. Several
patients became delirious, and if they got out of
bed they usually died. (n.d., n.p.)*

Quinn (2008) argued that political leaders were slow to respond to the threat of the
influenza outbreak, prioritizing the war effort
over the fight against the disease. American
President Woodrow Wilson, for example, at
first ignored the advice of doctors to publicize
details of the outbreak and to halt troop movements (Quinn, 2008). Doctors themselves were
helpless against the disease. Just as in the Italian
city-states there had been no cure for bubonic
plague, similarly, 20th-century medical science was unable to discover a "magic bullet"
that would kill the influenza virus. And yet
the perspective on disease of North Americans
in the 1900s was very different from that of
16th century Italians. The emergence of germ
theory in the late 1800s, prompted largely by
the research of scientists such as Louis Pasteur
and Robert Koch, had revolutionized medicine and given both physicians and the societies they served a sense of mastery over disease
(Gradmann, 2001; Latour, 1988). If cures could
not be found immediately, they would, nevertheless, eventually become available. The early
20th century's faith in science gave its people a
belief that they could, collectively, control their
own destiny. In the meantime, a range of remedies was attempted, from the use of opium and
quinine to traditional herbal cures and bloodlet-
ting. "Heroic" remedies such as strychnine and
steam baths, along with smallpox, diphtheria,
and antitetanus serum, were also tried without
success (Quinn, 2008).

The nurses of the United States were also very
different from the largely untrained sick-room
attendants or "servants" of the Early Modern
period. The rapid development of medical science
in the second half of the 19th century meant that
the character of nursing had changed beyond recognition. Retaining their core functions of the care
and nurturing of the sick, nurses were now also
carefully trained technicians who administered the
new, scientific, and often heroic remedies devised
by medical science with dexterity and intelligence.
It was their fundamental nursing skills, however,
that came to the fore when they nursed thousands
of influenza patients from 1918 to 1919. Many of
those who died did so from exhaustion and star-
vation. Nurses could prevent these deaths. They
took soup and hot drinks to the houses of sufferers and offered care and comfort that enabled
the absolute rest that might help the body more
effectively fight the disease (Keen-Payne, 2000).
Quinn (2008) cites the Australian nurse in the
outback town of Byrock, Australia, who delivered
food and medicines "single-handedly" to a town
of 27 families.

Keeling (2009), using New York as a case
study, showed that community-based nursing organizations could have a profound effect
on both the well-being and probably the survival rates of whole communities of individuals. Keeling focused on the efforts of the Henry
Street Settlement, a group of public health
nurses founded in 1893 and working under
the directorship of Lillian Wald. These nurses
had, for decades, been working with the poorest
communities in the city, basing most of their
activities in the Lower East Side, where immigrant families lived in destitution. They were
no strangers to epidemic disease and had at their
disposal an armory of measures to improve the
health, hygiene, and nutritional status and to
promote the comfort of their severely ill patients
(Buhler-Wilkerson, 2001; Keeling, 2007).

Wald and her nurses worked in cooperation with the American Red Cross, the U.S. Public Health Service, volunteer organizations, and city health officials. They used warm blankets, baths, and fresh air to both comfort patients and promote their capacities to fight the infection. Perhaps most importantly, they enabled their patients to obtain complete rest, so enabling their immune systems the best chance of destroying the virus without also overwhelming the body itself. City authorities provided automobiles for their use, and they were able to transport pneumonia jackets and quarts of soup to the homes of the sick, offering warmth and nourishment to patients. They were able to keep large numbers of sufferers at home, thus relieving the desperately overcrowded hospitals, preventing unnecessary journeys for already severely weakened patients, and containing the spread of the disease (Keeling, 2009).

The influenza epidemic of the early 1900s was poorly controlled and contained. It is possible to argue that the governments of Western developed nations had learned nothing from the stringent isolation and quarantine regulations of their forebears in the Early Modern city-states. Yet it can also be argued that the nursing services of the early 20th century were able to ensure that influenza—although just as horrific as bubonic plague in its effects—was not a disease that left its victims totally helpless. Nursing care offered hope, not just to sufferers themselves but to entire societies.

Empowering the Vulnerable: AIDS in Contemporary Britain

The AIDS virus, it can be argued, is a much more efficient microparasite than that which caused Spanish influenza. The reaction of the human body to influenza was rapid and devastating. Death or recovery followed infection within days; both outcomes ultimately destroyed the virus. HIV has a much more hidden effect on the body and can live within its host's cells for several years before the destruction of body systems begins, symptoms emerge, and treatment is sought. This subtle infection has demanded a subtle response—and one, again, in which nurses have been among the active agents in the fight against the spread of the disease.

The third case study focuses on the responses to AIDS within the large cities of the United Kingdom in the 1980s. London, Manchester, Liverpool, Edinburgh, Dundee, and Glasgow were the epicenters of HIV's spread within Britain. It quickly became well known that the AIDS virus thrived within body fluids and was spread by direct contact with those fluids. It was recognized that the virus could live outside the human body only for short periods of time and that it could not survive desiccation or extremes of temperature. Soon after the development of the first cases of HIV, it was recognized that its three main methods of transmission from host to host were via sexual intercourse, through blood transfusion, and through the sharing of hypodermic needles. It was, furthermore, fairly rapidly realized that the virus was spreading through the homosexual communities of large cities throughout the world.

The disease appears to have originated in Africa, where its prevalence was—and still remains—very high. Speculation as to the origin of the disease in medical experimentation soon gave way to efforts to combat it and to find a cure. Scientists achieved some success in developing therapies for **infection control** within a human host and transformed the condition from a rapidly fatal disease to one that can be survived as a long-term chronic condition. This moderate success of medical science has, however, been more than matched by the efforts of public health professionals, including nurses, to educate and empower populations to collectively control the disease.

The first cases of AIDS probably developed in the mid to late 1970s. The disease, however, was not recognized as a distinct entity until large numbers of cases of its associated conditions, Kaposi's sarcoma and *Pneumocystis carinii* pneumonia, began to appear in large U.S. cities in 1981 (AVERT, 2009; Hymes, Green & Mann, 1989). Centers for the control of communicable diseases throughout the developed world began to study what was being recognized as a new disease. The first case of AIDS to be documented in the United Kingdom appeared in December 1981 (Dubois, Braitwaite, Mikhail, & Batten, 1981). Because the earliest recorded symptoms affected gay men and because the disease was, at first, so closely associated with the gay community, some believed it could be transmitted only through homosexual contact. The disease was even, for a time, referred to as "gay compromise syndrome" (Brennan & Durak, 1981). Then a rapid increase in cases among hemophiliacs (who acquired the virus through blood transfusions) led to a dawning recognition that the disease could be transmitted in body fluids through both sexual contact and transfusion (Bateman, 1994). The recording of the first cases of the disease in women in January 1983 along with a rapid rise in the incidence among hemophiliacs also drew more public attention to a disease that could no longer be dismissed. Amid widespread fear and uncertainty, the name "acquired immune deficiency syndrome" was coined and the disease clearly defined in September 1982 (Connor & Kingman, 1988). In May 1983, the AIDS virus (at first referred to as the lymphadenopathy-associated virus) was first isolated by scientists at the Pasteur Institute in Paris (Barre-Sinoussi et al., 1983; Harden, 1992).

One of the earliest voluntary organizations for the prevention and control of AIDS was formed in the United Kingdom in 1982 and came to be known as the Terence Higgins Trust, named after one of the disease's earliest victims (Berridge, 1996). Similar organizations developed in other western European countries and in the United States, and it was through these independent, well-organized, and proactive voluntary organizations that AIDS first became a disease that was controlled through individual education and empowerment. By conveying clear messages about how to protect oneself through safe sex, activists within the gay community probably prevented many potential cases of the disease.

By 1985, messages about AIDS prevention were spreading beyond the gay community. Clear statements were being made about which groups were most at risk. These included heroin addicts who shared needles, and the first needle exchanges were established in the Netherlands, soon to be followed by large numbers of other similar projects. In the United Kingdom the first needle exchange was established in Dundee in February 1986 (Robertson, Bucknall, & Welsby, 1986). Later that year, the Kaleidoscope needle exchange in London and the Maryland Street needle exchange in Liverpool were established and a national campaign was launched, based on the message "don't inject AIDS" (AVERT, 2009).

As data became available from parts of Africa where AIDS was a much more established disease, it became clear that heterosexuals were at serious risk. The disease was clearly spreading through the heterosexual community, and vaginal transmission came to be recognized as an important cause of this spread. The first international conference on AIDS, held in Atlanta, Georgia, in April 1985, recognized that the disease was now a global pandemic

(Mann, 1989). Irresponsible media reporting fueled public panic during the mid-1980s. Widespread fear led initially to widespread homophobia and created a scenario of moral panic that damaged the earliest health education campaigns by distorting their message. It also isolated sufferers, limiting the support they obtained (Fowler, 1991; Gronfors & Stalstrom, 1987; Tester, 1994; Wolf & Kielwasswe, 1991). Nevertheless, even amid the mass media–fueled panic of the mid-1980s, clear messages were beginning to reach those at risk and deliberate actions such as safer sex, the use of clean hypodermic needles, and the abstention of those at risk from blood donation were already beginning to have an effect (Arno & Feiden, 1992).

The history of the containment and control of HIV can be interpreted in part as a history of successful self-help. Voluntary organizations, often established by individuals whose friends or family members had died of AIDS, often led the way in developing campaigns that would both raise awareness of the disease and its transmission and overcome prejudice, thus promoting respect and compassion for sufferers. The Cardiff AIDS helpline grew out of an existing telephone service for gay men, and "body positive" groups throughout the country developed centers and helplines to support sufferers and those anxious about the disease. "Body Positive London" was established in 1985 and provided vital help and support for what was really the epicenter of the AIDS epidemic in the United Kingdom (Berridge, 1996). The charity AVERT was founded in 1986 to campaign against AIDS-related prejudice and injustice, and the National Union of Journalists issued a leaflet advising journalists to offer more positive and respectful reporting of those with HIV (Berridge, 1996). In the same year the London Lighthouse, a care center for AIDS sufferers, was planned in the face

of opposition from a small faction of hostile local residents and won widespread support (Cantacuzino, 1993).

In September 1986, the recognition that the drug azidothymidine could slow the progress of the disease led to the development of the first successful drug therapies for AIDS sufferers. Eventually, highly active antiretroviral therapy came to be widely used and dramatically lengthened the lifespans of those who obtained treatment early. Yet it was still successful health education that had the greatest impact on bringing the disease under control and preventing the escalation of the pandemic.

In 1987, the British government developed its prevention campaign through the newly formed Health Education Authority, using mass media to promulgate the message "don't die of ignorance." Advertising on prime-time television and using hard-hitting slogans and visually arresting images, such as an iceberg and a tombstone, the Authority reached millions of viewers. A televised "AIDS week" was held from February 27 to March 8 in which rival television stations simultaneously showed a film entitled "AIDS—The Facts" and advertised an AIDS helpline number. In the same year, the National AIDS Trust was established to coordinate the activities of self-help and voluntary organizations (Berridge, 1996). Also in 1987, Princess Diana opened the first specialist ward for AIDS at the Middlesex Hospital, making the point, by shaking hands with HIV-positive patients, that the virus could not be transmitted by skin contact. In 1988, health education campaigns gained ground throughout the world, and in that year the first annual World AIDS Day was organized by the World Health Organization (1988).

From the discovery of the first cases of AIDS in 1981 to the launch of successful awareness campaigns in the mid-1980s, rapid progress was made in developing projects that would combat the spread of the disease. Health education campaigns are difficult to evaluate, and some of the early attempts to measure the effectiveness of government campaigns in the mid-1980s produced inconclusive or disappointing results (Baggaley, 1988; Sherr, 1987). Nevertheless, it was possible, by the early 21st century, to demonstrate that reductions in the incidence of a range of sexually transmitted infections (among them HIV) had followed and were probably the result of these campaigns (Nicholl et al., 2001). Nicholl and Hamers (2002) showed that incidences of a range of sexually transmitted diseases (not just AIDS) reduced significantly after the campaigns of the mid-1980s. They further argued that, as memory of those campaigns faded, there was a resurgence of HIV, gonorrhea, and syphilis throughout Europe (Nicholl & Hamers, 2002).

Furthermore, awareness-raising campaigns have, at times, had beneficial and unforeseen knock-on effects. The AIDS-awareness campaigns carried benefits on a global scale. Laurie Garrett argued that donations of public and private funds to third world countries increased dramatically because of the awareness-raising campaigns of HIV activists. Though the effects of this philanthropy have been patchy because of the poor coordination of health promotion programs, the tendency of awareness-raising campaigns to arouse the compassion of individuals in the developed world can be seen as a positive development (Garrett, 2007; Leclerc-Madlala, 2005). These developments should not, however, give rise to complacency. African nations in particular have struggled to obtain the drug therapies they require and to develop effective health-promotion strategies in line with the World Health Organization's global program on AIDS (Friedman and Mottiar, 2005; VanderVliet, 2001).

Conclusion

The study of past epidemics offers us perspective on the ways we tackle the threats posed by our own era. It also teaches us that although new threats arise constantly and present new challenges, these threats and challenges are not so different from those faced by our ancestors. What does differ over time are the resources at our disposal to tackle new epidemic diseases. Among the most vital resources at the disposal of modern governments are the skilled workforces that combat epidemics, and among the largest— but least well recognized—of these are the nurses who care for the sick, empower the vulnerable, and undertake much of the work (in terms of data collection and treatment implementation) that makes it possible for medical science to destroy the causative organisms of disease.

The three case studies presented here were chosen because each demonstrates a distinct response—or more often, reaction—to an epidemic. All three of the diseases presented— bubonic plague, influenza, and AIDS—took their host populations by surprise. A study of the collective responses of some of those populations can offer insight into how humans perceive and combat disease. In the early modern Italian city-states, magistrates adopted a "protective" approach to outbreaks of bubonic plague. They quarantined their cities, they moved the sick and their belongings to pest houses, and they imposed controls aimed at both preventing the spread of disease within their walls and propitiating "divine wrath." Their approach was a classic containment strategy.

In New York and other U.S. cities during the early 1900s, the movement of the sick was not controlled (in fact, troop movements probably exacerbated the epidemic), quarantines were not strictly imposed, and, although antisocial and obviously dangerous behaviors like spitting in public were outlawed, controls on public behavior were relatively mild. The American (and European) approach to Spanish influenza was one in which compassion overrode protectionism and enlightened self-interest ensured both negative consequences (the spread of the disease throughout the world) and, ultimately, positive outcomes (the support of individual sufferers).

The response to the AIDS epidemic in the United Kingdom was one in which self-help groups, often supported by local health professionals, led the way in offering information and support to vulnerable groups and demonstrating how clear messages could be conveyed to those at risk. The awareness and education campaigns of the mid-1980s in the United Kingdom were interesting and valuable because of their audacity (in the context of their time) and because of the commitment they demonstrated. Against a backdrop of mass media-induced fear and negative, stereotypical attitudes to sufferers, self-help groups were able to develop awareness programs that probably saved lives. The government followed swiftly, launching some of the most effective mass media campaigns ever devised for health education purposes. One of the problems with such campaigns was the difficulty of evaluating their effectiveness. It was only in retrospect that researchers were able to demonstrate epidemiological patterns that pointed to their success.

These differences in approach to disease highlight the differences between societies and their cultural norms. In early modern Italy, even though some city-states were nominally republics, the power of state and church was paramount; by contrast, the modern, liberal society of early-20th century New York was one in which every individual life was considered more important than the power of the state. In the United Kingdom during the 1980s, an open society with a free press and a highly active National Health Service at first distorted and

later promoted a health promotion strategy that depended on the conveying of clear messages to vulnerable and often ostracized communities.

In each of these scenarios, nurses, however independently they defined their roles and however determinedly they pursued their health-promoting strategies, were highly dependent on states and local authorities to sanction and enable their work. The pest-house attendants of Early Modern cities struggled in the face of hopelessness and lack of resources. The nurses of early-20th century New York, by contrast, supported as they were by local authorities, the Red Cross, and numerous voluntary agencies, were able to move rapidly into effective action. In the British cities of the 1980s, nursing personnel in a range of scenarios, such as genitourinary medicine clinics, specialist AIDS units, community health centers, and public health departments, were, after some initial delay, assisted by effective mass media campaigns to offer clear health-promoting messages to their client groups.

It would be all too easy to present this story as one of progress, one in which governments and societies became increasingly compassionate and effective. Such a perspective would be both complacent and distorting. States and societies have never been capable of doing more than the virulence of disease and the limitations of resources have permitted. As our own societies confront the advent of new and terrifying diseases, such as severe acute respiratory syndrome and Ebola, we can learn from the struggles of those past societies that confronted similar terrors and stood and fought then with all the means they had at their disposal. But the lessons are not simple ones. We should also be heartened by the knowledge that states and societies—with nurses among their vanguards—have survived epidemic diseases.

Perhaps, ultimately, societies will completely escape the ravages of epidemics only when they have learned to fully understand the nature of their cohabitants on this planet: the vast range of microorganisms that cause both harm and good to human populations. All too often it seems that the spread of disease can be traced to human behavior: the opening up of trade routes, troop movements, lifestyle changes, and possibly even the direct scientific manipulation of exist-

ing microorganisms. Perhaps only when human societies have learned to recognize quickly the consequences of their collective actions and have gained the skills required to launch concerted efforts that override vested interest will they cease to encounter the devastation caused by epidemic disease.

References

Alexander, J. T. (1980). *Bubonic plague in early modern Russia*. Baltimore, MD: Johns Hopkins University Press.

Anselment, R. A. (1989). Smallpox in seventeenth-century English literature: Reality and the metamorphosis of wit. *Medical History, 33*, 72–95.

Arno, P. S., & Feiden, K. L. (1992). *Against the odds: The story of AIDS development, politics and profits*. London, UK: HarperCollins.

AVERT. (2009). Retrieved from http://www.avert.org

Baggaley, J. P. (1988). Perceived effectiveness of international AIDS campaigns. *Health Education Research, 3*(1), 7–17.

Barre-Sinoussi, F., Chermann, J., Rey, F., Nugeyre, M. T., Chamaret, S., Gruest, J., . . . Montagnier, L. (1983). Isolation of a T-lymphotrophic retrovirus from a patient at risk for acquired immune deficiency syndrome (AIDS). *Science, 220*(4599), 868–871.

Barry, J. (2005). *The great influenza: The epic story of the deadliest plague in history*. New York, NY: Viking Press.

Bateman, D. (1994). The good bleed guide: A patient's story. *Social History of Medicine, 7*(1), 115–133.

Berridge, V. (1996). *AIDS in the UK. The making of a policy, 1981–1994*. Oxford, UK: Oxford University Press.

Biraben, J. (1975). *Les hommes et la peste en France dans les pays europeens et mediterraneens*. Two volumes. Paris, France: Mouton.

Brennan, R. O., & Durak, D. T. (1981). Gay compromise syndrome. *Lancet, 2*, 1338–1339.

Brozzi, M. (Ed.). (1982). *Peste Fede e Sanita in una Cronaca Cividalese del 1598*. Milan, Italy: Giuffre.

Buhler-Wilkerson, K. (2001). *No place like home: A history of nursing and home care in the United States*. Baltimore, MD: Johns Hopkins University Press.

Byerly, C. (2005). *Fever of war: The influenza epidemic in the US Army during World War I*. New York, NY: New York University Press.

Calvi, G. (1989). *Histories of a plague year. The social and the imaginary in baroque Florence*. (D. Biocca & B. T. Ragan, trans.). Berkeley, CA: California University Press, Berkeley.

Campbell, A. (1931). *The Black Death and men of learning*. New York, NY: Columbia University Press.

Cantacuzino, M. (1993). *Till break of day*. London, UK: Heinemann.

Carmichael, A. G. (1983). Legislation in the Italian Renaissance. *Bulletin of the History of Medicine, 57*, 516–536.

Carmichael, A. G. (1986). *Plague and the poor in renaissance Florence*. Cambridge, UK: Cambridge University Press.

Cartwright, F. F. (1977). *A social history of medicine*. London, UK: Longman.

Castellacci, D. (Ed.). (1897). *Curiosi ricordi del Contagio Di Firenze nel 1630. Archivio Storico Italiano* (5th series). Anno XX.

Chambers, D., & Pullan, B. (1992). *Venice. A documentary history*. Oxford, UK: Blackwell.

Christensen, P. (2003). "In these perilous times": Plague and plague policies in early modern Denmark. *Medical History, 47*, 413–450.

Cipolla, C. M. (1973). *Cristofano and the plague*. London, UK: Collins.

Cipolla, C. M. (1979). *Faith, reason and the plague*. Brighton, UK: Harvester Press.

Cipolla, C. M. (1992). *Miasmas and disease*. (E. Potter, trans.). New Haven, CT: Yale University Press.

Connor, S., & Kingman, S. (1988). *The search for the virus. The scientific discovery of AIDS and the quest for a cure*. London, UK: Penguin Books.

Contarini, G. (1599). *The commonwealth and government of Venice*. (L. Lewkenor, trans.). London, UK: John Windet.

Crosby, A. W. (1989). *America's forgotten pandemic: The influenza of 1918*. Cambridge, UK: Cambridge University Press.

Dubois, R. M., Braitwaite, M. A., Mikhail, J. R., & Batten, J. C. (1981). Primary Pneumocystis carinii and cytomegalovirus infections. *Lancet, ii*, 1339.

Ficino, M. (1989). *Three books on life*. (C. V. Kaske & J. R. Clark, trans.). Binghamton, NY: Medieval and Renaissance Text and Studies.

Fowler, R. (1991). *Language in the news: Discourse and ideology in the press*. London, UK: Routledge.

Fracastoro, H. (1930). *De Contagione et Contagiosis Morbis et Eorum Curatione, Libri III*. (W. C. Wright, ed. & trans.). New York, NY: G. P. Putnam and Sons.

Friedman, S., & Mottiar, S. (2005). A rewarding engagement? The treatment action campaign and the politics of HIV/AIDS. *Politics and Society, 33*(4), 511–565.

Galassi, N. (1966–1970). *Dieci Secoli di Storia Ospedaleria a Imola*. Vol. II. Imola, Italy: Galeati.

Garrett, L. (2007). The challenge of global health. *Foreign Affairs, 86*(1), 14–38.

Gradmann, C. (2001). Robert Koch and the pressures of scientific research: Tuberculosis and tuberculin. *Medical History, 45*, 1–32.

Grell, O. P. (1990). Plague in Elizabethan and Stuart London: The Dutch response. *Medical History, 34*(4), 424–439.

Gronfors, M., & Stalstrom, O. (1987). Power, prestige, profit: AIDS and the oppression of homosexual people. *Acta Sociological, 30*(1), 53–66.

Harden, V. A. (1992). Koch's postulates and the etiology of AIDS: An historical perspective. *History and Philosophy of the Life Sciences, 14*(2), 249–269.

Hirst, L. F. (1953). *The conquest of plague*. Oxford, UK: Clarendon Press.

Hortensii, Centorio degli. (1631). *I cinque libri de gli avvertimenti, ordini, gride et editti: fatti et osservati in Milano, ne'tempi sospetosi della peste de gli anni MDLXXVI & LXXVII*. Milano, Italy: Bidelli.

Hymes, K. B., Green, J. B., & Mann, J. M. (1989). AIDS: A worldwide pandemic. In M. S. Gottlieb, D. J. Jeffries, D. Mildvan, A. J. Pinching, & T. C. Quinn (Eds.), *Current topics in AIDS* (Vol. 2). London, UK: John Wiley & Sons.

Johnson, N. (2006). *Britain and the 1918–19 influenza pandemic*. London, UK: Routledge.

Johnson, N. P. A. S., & Mueller, J. (2002). Updating the accounts: Global mortality of the 1918–1920 "Spanish influenza" pandemic. *Bulletin of the History of Medicine, 76*, 105–115.

Keeling, A. (2007). *Nursing and the privilege of prescription, 1893–2000*. Columbus, OH: Ohio State University Press.

Keeling, A. (2009). "When the city is a great field hospital": The influenza pandemic of 1918 and the New York City nursing response. *Journal of Clinical Nursing, 18*(19), 2732–2738.

Keen-Payne, R. (2000). "We must have nurses": Spanish influenza in America, 1918–1919. *Nursing History Review, 8*, 143–156.

King, M. L. (1986). *Venetian humanism in an age of patrician dominance*. Princeton, NJ: Princeton University Press.

Latour, B. (1988). *The pasteurization of France*. (A. Sheridan & J. Law, trans.). Cambridge, MA and London, UK: Harvard University Press.

Leclerc-Madlala, S. (2005). Popular responses to HIV/AIDS and policy. *Journal of Southern African Studies, 31*(4), 845–856.

Mann, J. M. (1989). AIDS: A worldwide pandemic. In M. S. Gottlieb, D. J. Jeffries, D. Mildvan, A. J. Pinching, & T. C. Quinn (Eds.), *Current topics in AIDS* (Vol. 2). London, UK: John Wiley & Sons.

Modena, L. (1988). *Life of Judah*. (M. R. Cohen, ed. & trans.). Princeton, NJ: Princeton University Press.

More, T. (first published 1516). *Utopia*. (R. Robinson, trans.). Ashgate Publishing.

Nicholl, A., & Hamers, F. (2002). Are trends in HIV, gonorrhoea, and syphilis worsening in western Europe? *British Medical Journal, 324*, 1324–1327.

Nicholl, A., Hughes, G., Donnelly, M., Livingstone, S., De Angelis, D., Fenton, K.,. . . Catchpole, M. (2001). Assessing the impact of national anti-HIV sexual health campaigns: Trends in the transmission of HIV and other sexually transmitted infections in England. *Sexually Transmitted Infections, 77*, 242–247.

Nightingale, F. (1860/1980). *Notes on nursing. What it is and what it is not*. Edinburgh, UK: Churchill Livingstone.

Nutton, V. (1990). The reception of Fracastoro's theory of contagion. *Osiris. Second Series, 6*.

Palmer, R. J. (1978). The *control of plague in Venice and Northern Italy, 1348–1600*. Unpublished PhD thesis, The University of Kent at Canterbury.

Park, K., & Henderson, J. (1991). The first hospital among christians: The Ospedale di Santa Maria Nuova in early sixteenth century Florence. *Medical History, 35*, 164–188.

Pastore, A. (1988). Tra Giustizia e Politico: Il Governo della Peste a Genova e Roma nel 1656/7. *Rivista Storica Italiana. Anno 100*, 126–154.

Patterson, D. K., & Pyle, G. F. (1991). The geography and mortality of the 1918 influenza pandemic. *Bulletin of the History of Medicine, 65*, 4–21.

Petraccone, C. (1978). La Difesa Contro la Peste. *Archivio Storico per le Province Napoletane. Third Series, Anno XVI*, 253–280.

Phillips, H., & Killingray, D. (2003). *The Spanish influenza pandemic of 1918–19. New perspectives*. London, UK: Routledge.

Preto, P. (1978). *Peste e Societa a Venezia nel 1576*. Vicenza, Italy: Neri Pozza.

Pullan, B. (1971). *Rich and poor in renaissance Venice*. Oxford, UK: Basil Blackwood.

Pullan, B. (1992). Plague and perceptions of the poor in early modern Italy. In T. Ranger & P. Slack (Eds.),

Epidemics and ideas (pp. 101–123). Cambridge, UK: Cambridge University Press.

Quinn, T. (2008). *Flu: A social history of influenza*. London, UK: New Holland.

Reid, A. (2005). The effects of the 1918–1919 influenza pandemic on infant and child health in Derbyshire. *Medical History, 49*(1), 29–54.

Robertson, J. R., Bucknall, A. B. V., & Welsby, P. D. (1986). An epidemic of AIDS-related virus (HTLV III/LAV) infection among intravenous drug abusers in Scottish General practice. *British Medical Journal, 292*, 527–530.

Sapwell, J. (n.d.). *The reminiscences of a VAD in two world wars*. London, UK: The Red Cross Archives.

Sherr, L. (1987). An evaluation of the UK government health education campaign on AIDS. *Psychology and Health, 1*, 61–72.

Slack, P. (1985). *The impact of plague in Tudor and Stuart England*. London, UK: Clarendon Press.

Tester, K. (1994). *Media, culture and morality*. London, UK: Routledge.

Ulvioni, P. (1989). *Il Gran Castigo di Dio*. Milan, Italy: F. Angeli.

VanderVliet, V. (2001). AIDS: Losing "the new struggle"? *Daedalus, 130*(1), 151–184.

Wolf, M. A., & Kielwasswe, A. P. (Eds.). (1991). *Gay people, sex and the media*. London, UK: Haworth Press.

World Health Organization. (1988). *AIDS prevention and control: Invited presentations and papers from the World Summit of ministers of health on programmes for AIDS prevention*. London, UK: World Health Organization.

Zinsser, H. (1935). *Rats, lice and history*. Boston, MA: Little, Brown.

For a full suite of assignments and additional learning activities, use the access code located in the front of your book to visit this exclusive website: http://go.jblearning .com/londrigan. If you do not have an access code, you can obtain one at the site.

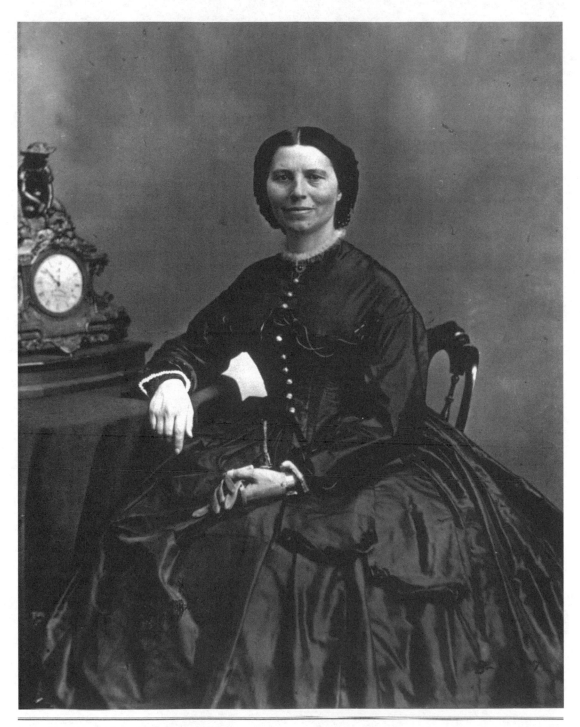

Source: Clara Barton. National Library of Medicine.

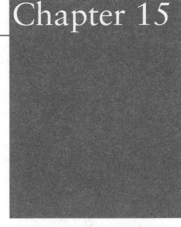

Chapter 15

Historical Highlights in Disaster Nursing

Barbara Mann Wall
Arlene Keeling

Out into pitchy darkness, leaped three men and seven women from a puffing, unsteady train, no physician with them, and no instructions save the charge of their leader as the last leap was made, and the train pushed on. "Nurses, you know what to do, go and do your best. . .(Barton, 1904, p. 150).

LEARNING OBJECTIVES

At the completion of this chapter, the reader will be able to

- Explore historical roots of disaster nursing through the lens of past disasters in the late 19th and 20th centuries.

- Describe the activities of public health nurses as they responded to past disasters.
- Relate past experiences of disaster nursing to present-day problems.

KEY TERMS

- ❏ American Red Cross
- ❏ Disasters

- ❏ Emergency preparedness
- ❏ Nursing history

This chapter examines specific instances of disaster nursing through the lens of **nursing history** to illustrate the important role nurses have had in providing prompt, efficient care to the ill or injured. In her classic text, *Disaster Nursing and Emergency Preparedness for Chemical, Biological* *and Radiological Terrorism and Other Hazards,* Tener Veenema (2007) argues for the importance of disaster responses that are evidence-based. Evidence for practice for disaster management logically comes from history—understanding what worked and did not work in the past.

Although others have recorded the Red Cross and medical responses to disasters, the nursing response and **emergency preparedness** is often overlooked, accepted as "routine" or merely as following doctor's orders.

Nurses' work is highlighted during three late 19th century **disasters**: the yellow fever epidemic of 1888, the Johnstown flood of 1889, and the 1900 Galveston hurricane. These disasters are historically significant because they mark the first **American Red Cross** response, resulting in the federal government giving it a formal charter to provide disaster relief. In addition, the chapter focuses on three 20th century disasters: the 1918 influenza pandemic, the 1947 Texas City ship explosion, and the 1964 Alaska earthquake.

The causes of each disaster varied, and the response was tailored for the problem. In 1888, for example, mosquitoes caused the yellow fever epidemic in Jacksonville, Florida, and in 1889, catastrophic rains caused the Johnstown flood in Pennsylvania. As in Johnstown, the devastation from the 1900 Galveston hurricane—the most deadly hurricane of the 20th century—resulted from a largely uncontrollable force of nature. Death came from drowning or injury, as buildings collapsed and the unexpected and vicious storm surge devastated the coastal city. By contrast, the flu was a biological event—the rapid and overwhelming spread of a deadly virus. The Texas City disaster related to the consequences of increasing industrialization and the growth of the oil industry in the state and demonstrates what happens when hazardous materials are not properly contained. At that time it was the worst industrial accident in the country's history, killing over 500 people. The Alaska earthquake demonstrated the problems that can occur from seismic risks. In 1964, it was the second largest earthquake ever recorded, after the 1960 earthquake in Chile.

Although the disasters resulted from different causes, some related to weather, others to industrialization, and others to the spread of disease, in other ways these disasters reveal similarities. They occurred suddenly and without warning, they devastated communities, and they demanded a nursing and medical response. After each disaster, nurses organized and provided care in both hospitals and the community.

Yellow Fever and the Johnstown Flood

Before World War II there was no permanent program of federal disaster relief in the United States, and private voluntary agencies such as the American National Red Cross and the Salvation Army took primary responsibility for disaster response (Kreps, 1990; Rubin, 2007). The International Committee of the Red Cross was founded in Geneva, Switzerland, in 1863 by Henry Dunant; today, national Red Cross societies exist in nearly every country in the world, with the American National Red Cross, organized in large part by Clara Barton, founded in 1881 (Moorehead, 1998).

During the 1888 yellow fever epidemic in Jacksonville, Florida, the Red Cross recruited nurses to the danger zone. Barton turned to New Orleans for help; there, many people had already had the disease and thus were immune. She recruited 30 nurses, both white and black, to travel with her by train to Jacksonville. On arrival in Jacksonville, however, the train's engineer refused to stop in the epidemic area. Thus, in the midst of a torrential rain, 10 nurses jumped off the moving train so they could assist the sick. Earning $3.00 a day, they worked 72-hour shifts for 79 days. A scandal developed, however, when several men and women refused to work for the $3.00 a day wage in hospitals and instead went into private nursing where they could make more money. Other nurses were accused of immoral conduct (Kernodle, 1949). Barton provided an explanation. She admitted that many of the volunteers she recruited were untrained, and clashes developed between them and the local boards of health, which employed federal and municipal health officers who used newer scientific methods. In addition, many adventurers responded and called themselves Red Cross nurses even though they were not. Consequently, the local health board deported them (Barton, 1904; Dock & Pickett, 1922). Barton believed it was unfair to judge the status of Red Cross nurses by these latter individuals (Barton, 1904).

Consequently, the director of Sandhills Fever Hospital did not rely on Red Cross nurses. Rather, he recruited trained nurses and students, a new type of nurse that he had witnessed as an intern at the Bellevue Hospital in New York City. At Sandhills his chief nurse was Jane Delano, a graduate of Bellevue who later became president of the American Nurses Association and director of the Red Cross Nursing Service (D'Antonio & Whelan, 2004; Kernodle, 1949). One of Delano's classmates, Lavinia Dock, followed her there. As a trained public health nurse, Dock and the other nurses brought improved care to patients through their emphasis on order, cleanliness, ventilation, and nutrition, and they demonstrated the critical importance of what this new nursing profession could offer (D'Antonio & Whelan, 2004; Dock & Pickett, 1922).

A year later, the Red Cross was called on to help at the site of the Johnstown Flood. On the afternoon of May 31, 1889, heavy rains had been pouring down on central Pennsylvania when the decaying South Fork Dam broke. Millions of tons of water and debris came crushing down into the valley in what became the worst flood

in the nation's history. Within 10 minutes, over 2,200 people were killed and tens of thousands more were injured or made homeless. Nurses and physicians from Mercy Hospital in Pittsburgh were among the first to respond, both at the scene and in their hospital (Rafferty, 1974). Clara Barton and her relief team arrived 5 days later, on June 5. They distributed supplies to thousands of survivors and provided warm meals, medical care, and shelter to many in buildings that became known as "Red Cross Hotels" (Kernodle, 1949; National Park Service, 2006). Most of the nursing, however, was handled by a branch of the American Red Cross from Philadelphia not associated with Barton. Led by Lavinia Dock, graduate nurses trained in hospitals and public health worked in tent hospitals set up for the ill and injured. Their nursing proved invaluable as they worked with Barton and other Red Cross relief workers to carry out sanitation measures to prevent disease (Barton, 1904; Dock & Pickett, 1922).

The Galveston Hurricane, 1900

On September 10, 1900, meteorologist and eyewitness John D. Blagden wrote the following to his family (2000):

> *There is not a building in town that is uninjured. Hundreds are busy day and night clearing away the debris and recovering the dead. It is awful. Every few minutes a wagon load of corpses passes by on the street...The more fortunate are doing all they can to aid the sufferers but it is impossible to care for all. (pp. 17–18)*

Two days before, on September 8, a hurricane had hit Galveston, Texas, leaving approximately 8,000 people dead. The image of death pervaded the accounts of the Galveston storm, and by September 12 newspapers were filled with stories about recovering the dead. Eventually, the bodies had to be burned en masse in bonfires throughout the city. During the storm, both blacks and whites took refuge in two local hospitals, John Sealy and St. Mary's Infirmary. Both suffered damage but were able to take patients again within a few days (Bixel & Turner, 2000).

Clara Barton and her staff arrived on September 17 and found an impromptu local relief committee that was tending to disaster recovery needs and collecting supplies. Barton was 78 years old at the time, and this would be her last trip to the scene of a disaster. She had presided over many disasters, and with each one her fame grew (Barton, 1900; Moorehead, 1998). Her arrival in Galveston was met with great fanfare, as one assistant recalled, "When Miss Barton's train got in the guards were ready, soldiers at present arms, everything in very martial style, in fact it was the only spice of the theatrical that there was in the whole business" (Fayling, 2000, p. 91).

Although the Red Cross had recruited nurses during the yellow fever epidemic and the Johnstown Flood in the 1880s, in Galveston it was primarily responsible for obtaining supplies. Rather than assuming total control, Barton and her staff worked with the local relief committee, supplying food, clothing, and shelter. Galveston women had formed a new Red Cross Auxiliary, and Barton ensured they would provide greater leadership at the distribution stations. The Red Cross also worked with volunteers from various charitable and patriotic societies, including the Women's Relief Corps, the Women's Christian Temperance Union, and the Grand Army of the Republic. Blacks had formed their own relief committees, and Barton also set up a special fund for them (Barton, 1900). Barton stayed in Texas for 2 months. In addition to providing help in Galveston, she and her staff distributed supplies to people in towns and villages over a thousand-square-mile area that had suffered

severe damage. Barton had a policy of restarting local work. When the hurricane washed away strawberry plants of farmers in six storm-swept counties and no money was available to buy more, she helped secure over a million plants.

After Barton's retirement, the Red Cross reorganized in 1905 and created state and territorial branches. One of the organization's newly assigned responsibilities included nursing during peacetime emergencies such as fire, floods, pestilence, and other national disasters. The state and local committees of enrolled Red Cross nurses served as volunteer recruiters of other nurses when the need arose. The new structure would be critical to the nursing response to the influenza pandemic when it hit the United States in the autumn of 1918.

The Flu Pandemic, 1918–1919

The influenza epidemic of 1918, killing over 40 million people worldwide and causing over 675,000 deaths in the United States (Hilleman, 2002; Johnson & Mueller, 2002), challenged the nation's public health service, the American Red Cross, the medical and nursing professions, and the U.S. federal government in much the same way it challenged other nations around the world. In 1918, the extremely high death rate—particularly among young adults—from a rare and highly contagious form of influenza was mysterious and frightening. According to one historian (Byerly, 2005):

The influenza and pneumonia of 1918 shocked medical officers and soldiers alike. It rendered strong, healthy men powerless and struggling for breath; it distorted and saturated the lungs of those it killed; it rendered helpless professional physicians of great skill and knowledge; it consumed an enormous amount of army resources; and it killed in such great numbers that images of sick and dead bodies and coffins stayed with the survivors for the rest of their lives. (p. 87)

When the flu hit the cities of the United States and killed citizens, not soldiers, the country was unprepared for the magnitude of the crisis. Reflecting on the events of that year, nurse leader Janet Geister (1957) later wrote: "We weren't ready in plans and resources, nor were we ready in our thinking. A country-wide epidemic was utterly inconceivable" (p. 583). To complicate the situation, the United States had only recently entered the war in Europe and thousands of physicians and nurses had just been deployed. Few were left to cope with a major epidemic at home.

In the United States, influenza first broke out in Kansas at a crowded military recruit camp. It then traveled with the soldiers to the cities of the East Coast, notably Boston, Philadelphia, and New York, where it also arrived on ships from Europe. Within a matter of days it raced south and westward across the country along transportation lines (Crosby, 2003; Markel et al., 2007).

On September 6, 1918, *The Boston Globe* reported an outbreak of "old fashioned grippe" among the sailors on the Commonwealth Pier (Fayling, 2000). By September 17, influenza reports were front page news. Within the next 24 hours health authorities recorded 41 more deaths, and the Boston health commissioner issued a warning against public hysteria. On September 18, only 12 days after the explosion of the epidemic in Boston, the flu spread through Philadelphia, the center of the war industry. Within days hundreds of sailors were ill; civilians were also succumbing to flu. Almost simultaneously, the epidemic erupted in New York City.

Meanwhile, in Boston, where they had been dealing with the flu for over 2 weeks, health officials were alarmed enough to send a tele-gram to the American Red Cross headquarters in Washington, DC, to ask for nurses. In Washington, it was becoming increasingly clear that this was no ordinary flu epidemic. Reports were coming to the Red Cross from cities up and down the East Coast. The new strain had devastated Boston and was now sweeping through New York, Philadelphia, and Washington. It was also racing south and west. The Red Cross had to take action. As a result, on September 24 members of the American Red Cross National Committee assembled in Washington to discuss the federal response. Their plan was to implement the decentralized response they had adopted for home defense a year earlier. The U.S. Public Health Service would manage the medical response and distribute posters and pamphlets educating the public about the illness. The Red Cross National Committee would communicate with its local organizations and direct the nursing response. The major response would have to be done at the local level (Fieser, 1941). Thus, immediately after the meeting, Director of the Red Cross Bureau of Nursing Services Clara Noyes telegraphed all Red Cross Divisions with a directive: "Suggest you organize Home Defense nurses . . . to meet present epidemic . . . Provide nurses with masks" (Noyes, 1918, p. 2).

In New York City, Lillian Wald, director of the Henry Street Settlement, did not need to be told to organize the nurses. In fact, she was all too aware of the alarming rapidity with which the flu was affecting the city's residents; her staff had already been working around the clock. In the slums of the Lower East Side, epidemics of infectious diseases were commonplace, and in September 1918 it seemed this was just another bad flu epidemic—only this time the intensity of the disease and the devastation it caused were remarkable. Finally, on October 10, the Atlantic Division of the Red Cross assembled New York

City nursing leaders to plan their response. At that meeting the nurses created the Nurses' Emergency Council to organize a city-wide response. The Red Cross also inserted a "quarter page advertisement in all the Sunday papers, calling for service from the women of the city" (Doty, 1919, p. 951).

In Philadelphia the situation was becoming increasingly serious, in part because on September 28, despite the fact that 123 civilians had been admitted to hospitals with flu just the day before, the city proceeded with its scheduled Liberty Loan parade to raise money for the war effort. Pandemic then exploded. By October 3, a doctor estimated that the city had seen 75,000 cases since September 11. Finally, the city government allocated $100,000 from its emergency war defense fund "to combat the disease" (Visiting Nurse Society, 1918, n.p.). It also coordinated all relief organizations under the direction of a central office and notified citizens struck with flu to call "Filbert 100" to obtain "a nurse, a doctor, an ambulance or an automobile" (Visiting Nurse Society, 1918, n.p.).

Under the direction of Katherine Tucker, RN, the Philadelphia Visiting Nurse Society handled thousands of influenza cases. In many of the families more than one member was ill; when both parents succumbed, the nurses had to supply food for the entire family. Soup kitchens were set up where the nurses could obtain soup, bread, and milk for such cases. And, as family after family was affected, the city's social infrastructure crumbled. Thousands of city workers were out sick, including streetcar drivers, telephone receptionists, shopkeepers, and garbage collectors. When the few nurses there also became sick, the situation became critical. There were simply not enough nurses. According to Health Director Kreusen (Visiting Nurse Society, 1918), "If you would ask me the three things Philadelphia most needs to conquer the epidemic, I would tell you "Nurses, more nurses, and yet more nurses." (n.p.)

The flu then spread south and west, affecting cities and towns across the nation. Many of the cities suffered extremely high mortality rates, and as the dead piled up, health boards and emergency councils closed theaters, schools, and churches (Barry, 2005). By late November 1918, the virus had made its way around the world. The second wave was over. However, the virus mutated again and a third wave struck in December and then in January 1919. Of all the major cities hit, San Francisco confronted the wave most efficiently, using both masks and vaccines to prevent its spread (Barry, 2005). Local chapters did their best to cooperate with the American Red Cross. According to one report, "Every chapter in Idaho, Oregon and Washington has appointed a committee on influenza" (Kilpatrick, 1919, p. 1). The same was true for coal mining camps in Kentucky, logging camps in Michigan, and in small towns across the United States. In every area, nurses were key to the response, and they responded promptly, without regard to race, class, or color.

1947 Texas City Ship Explosion

In 1947, the Dean of the University of Texas School of Nursing at Galveston wrote about healthcare workers' responses after a ship explosion in Texas City, Texas (Bartholf, 1947), "We were proud of the performance of the whole organization, and particularly of the nurses and doctors—they just clicked and came up to par in a wonderful fashion. I had never seen morale quite so high in this institution" (p. 558). Indeed, nurses and other healthcare personnel often experience a sense of camaraderie after working in a disaster. But this event also shows a more complicated story of competition among healthcare personnel.

In the late 19th and early 20th centuries, disasters mainly resulted from natural events such as hurricanes, disease, tornadoes, earthquakes, and floods. But as industry expanded in the 1900s, industrial accidents increased, with similar devastating results. On April 16 and 17, 1947, what was called the worst industrial catastrophe in U.S. history occurred when ammonium nitrate fertilizer on two merchant ships exploded in the Texas City, Texas docks, killing 405 people, with another 63 unidentified dead (Minutaglio, 2003; Stephens, 1997; Wall, 2008). When the first of the ships, the *Grandcamp*, exploded in the harbor, it caused smoke to rise 2,000 feet in the air and flaming cargo to fly over a one-mile radius. The nearby Monsanto Chemical Plant caught fire from flying steel and burning debris, killing 145 workers. Every fireman who initially responded died, decimating the local fire department. Two planes flying over the docks at the time of the explosion fell from the sky, and windows shattered in Houston, Galveston, and other Texas cities. In addition to the many deaths, 3,000 injuries occurred, one-third of all city dwellings were demolished, and 2,500 people lost their homes (Boyle, 1947; Stephens, 1993; "1200 Feared Dead" 1947).

A major priority after any disaster is the establishment of order out of chaos. With no disaster plan in place, the mayor and police chief had to recruit volunteers, and the disaster response initially was piecemeal. Without a local hospital, Texas City physicians and nurses organized a clearing station where casualties were triaged and the most serious moved to hospitals in surrounding cities and towns. Texas City clinics were full as well, and physicians and nurses worked with no water or electricity. A nurse's aide at one of the local clinics remembered that men from one of the plants came to help, and they worked "like Trojans" (Wheaton, 1948, p. 18).

The resources of other healthcare teams quickly organized and converged on the scene. Alerted by smoke columns across Galveston Bay, orthopedic surgeons, residents, senior medical students, nurses, and nursing students from John Sealy Hospital immediately left for Texas City with plasma, blood, and other supplies. Within an hour after the initial explosion, local American Red Cross chapters began mobilizing. Late in the evening of the first explosion, the Director of Nursing Service from the Red Cross Midwestern Area arrived from St. Louis and started recruiting more than 500 nurses from Texas and nearby states. As in every disaster since Clara Barton's day, many untrained women offered their services, so it became necessary to weed them out by checking credentials (Kernodle, 1949).

In all, 3,000 persons required sudden medical assistance, and after emergency first aid was provided, casualties went to 21 area hospitals. Many were hospitalized at the University of Texas Medical Branch (UTMB) facilities. Survivors began arriving within an hour, and all medical and nursing personnel were placed on 24-hour call. A nurse came in from her vacation and worked in a dispensary set up in the jail. Other nurses, both registered nurses and licensed practical nurses, worked at this dispensary and at the morgue. Soon, several busloads of nurses, under motorcycle escort, came to Texas City and eventually went on to Galveston hospitals (Wheaton, 1948).

John Sealy Hospital handled a total of 498 casualties. Within the first 5 hours, nurses and physicians classified 362 patients in the emergency department, gave them preliminary treatment, and hospitalized them. While physicians performed minor surgery in hallways, volunteer military medical and nursing personnel enabled 10 rooms to be outfitted for surgery. Doctors and nurses operated nonstop over the next 2 days.

Multiple puncture wounds, contusions; cuts from shards of glass; compound fractures; and head, eye, and ear injuries (especially ruptured eardrums) were common. Sixteen patients died from severe head injuries (Blocker & Blocker, 1949; Leake, 1947).

In 1948, the Sisters of Charity of the Incarnate Word told the story of the response of Galveston's St. Mary's Hospital to the Texas City disaster to a writer for *Hospital Progress*, the official journal of the Catholic Hospital Association. St. Mary's benefited from nurses and nurse anesthetists flown in from San Antonio. Sixteen operating rooms were set up, and the sisters opened an unfinished wing to take in 96 patients. During that time 186 patients were detained in the hospital, whereas 8 died (McLeod, 1948). The Red Cross provided 2 billion units of penicillin, 5 million units of tetanus antitoxin, large quantities of whole blood and plasma, streptomycin, sulfa drugs, and gas gangrene antitoxin (Girardeau, 1947).

In 1958 a research associate in the Disaster Research Group of the National Academy of Sciences interviewed several nurses after another disaster and found they were apt to feel insecure when physicians were not around. At the time most nurses were still trained in hospital diploma programs, and they were task-oriented. The data from the Texas City explosion both support and refute this conclusion. Although nurses indeed concentrated on tasks, they also developed a sense of pride when they were able to perform new assessments and expand their nursing roles, both dependent and independent of physicians.

As examples, students from the Schools of Nursing at John Sealy and St. Mary's Hospitals, part of UTMB, worked with teams to care for casualties, both at the scene and in hospitals. Stories from two students reveal they did more than merely assist the physician. One, who constructed her story in the *American Journal of Nursing* (Molsbee, 1947), worked on the pediatric ward at John Sealy Hospital and helped transfer children to other sites to make room for 40 injured adults. Patients came in ambulances, private automobiles, trucks, and milk wagons. Many activities of the nurses who suddenly found themselves in the midst of a disaster were improvised. Although it is not standard practice today, this student learned to fill 20-, 30-, and 50-cc syringes with morphine and give it by changing needles between patients. Nurses did not have regular charts, so they pinned tags on patients' clothes with dose and time they gave the medications (Molsbee, 1947).

A year after the explosion, another student from John Sealy composed a memoir of the events. An operating room supervisor had recruited her to Texas City as the student walked down the steps of the hospital. She was still in her nursing uniform, and, in the first part of the narrative, the form of her language conformed to the image of the compliant student she was taught to be. She said she "didn't have permission from the nursing office" (Givin, 1948, n.p.) to go. The supervisor cried, "It doesn't matter. I give you permission!" This group was one of the first from UTMB to arrive on the scene. Nurses' training in organization and carrying out specific tasks helped them maintain order. The student was able to adapt to the situation and administer first aid to severely burned patients, including giving morphine for pain. In fact, she had an "open order to administer hypodermics of pain relievers as I saw the need. . . . In a situation like this," she wrote, "you are oblivious to anything except doing the job at hand. Somehow, everything you have ever learned in this area comes to the surface and you do the best you can." She worked there for several hours and accompanied a patient back to the hospital in a station wagon, guiding the driver while she held the patient's intravenous infusion. By that time, the hospital grounds were covered with tents, and the Red Cross had arrived (Givin, 1948).

In the above nurse's memoir, her image of a compliant nurse who had to follow orders and adhere to set routines was altered. She wrote, "I later realized there was no way that you could take a holistic view of a patient in a situation like this; it's only the immediate needs that are met. I will never forget that day from the time I felt the vibrations of the explosion coming down those steps of the main building to now when I realize what a confident twenty year old nurse I was." She was amazed at how, when she was at the scene of the disaster, "everything began to fall into place and regardless of rank or race we were a team" (Givin, 1948, n.p.). Thus, as the nursing student reconstructed her story, she moved herself from a peripheral position as a student with little power to a central position, where her words and deeds proclaimed her as equal with the other responders. These included those with higher "rank" such as physicians and people of a different race. Her opportunity to nurse during this disaster led her to repudiate her perceived limitations as a nursing student.

Although the people worked together initially, tensions quickly developed over who would get credit for the rescue work. Regular units of the armed forces arrived on the afternoon of April 16, but they worked independently of the Red Cross. This led the mayor to publicly criticize the Red Cross in the newspaper. He expressed his concern to an official that the Red Cross was "taking credit for everything that is being done in the way of relief" (Givin, 1948, n.p.). For one thing, its workers "went down to the gymnasium morgue and took it over from our people . . . after they had worked there ever since the explosion" (Givin, 1948, n.p.). Furthermore, the Red Cross had called a

press conference that featured physicians it had brought in from the outside. "What about 10 of our local doctors that worked night and day?" the mayor retorted. "What is being said about them to those reporters?" (*Houston Chronicle*, 1947, n.p.). No mention was made of the nurses.

African American and Mexican American residents from El Barrio and The Bottom, the neighborhoods closest to the docks, suffered most from the disaster. Many were left homeless after these areas were utterly destroyed. On April 19 the African American newspaper, the *Informer*, described the disaster, provided photographs, and told stories of dramatic escapes and heroic rescues on the part of African Americans. Black physicians and nurses from Houston cared for African American survivors at John Sealy Hospital, and they also rendered aid at the scene. African American morticians and embalmers came to help, and two ministers from local black churches carried the injured and dying in their cars to hospitals in Galveston (*Informer*, 1947, pp. 1 and 10).

Red Cross nurses worked at the disaster site and in hospitals, and many stayed for 2 months until the regular nursing staff could take over. Red Cross and local public health nurses participated in case-finding activities by making home visits to care for the injured, seeing 2,231 patients in their homes (American National Red Cross, 1947). One of the most difficult tasks was to work with grieving families. City officials set up a temporary morgue in the local high school gymnasium, but they had no system for identifying the dead. Trained nurses accompanied families attempting to locate their missing relatives as they pulled back blankets and viewed the bodies, some so mangled they were never identified (Johnston, 1947).

Even though there were problems with communication and transportation, several groups responded quite well to the disaster, including medical and nursing personnel, because they had the skills and discipline needed for emergencies (Stephens, 1997). Writing after the disaster, Chauncey Leake, Vice-President and Dean of UTMB, noted that the successful responses were a result of the application of military medical principles by a team of skilled specialists in a specialty hospital center. This included first aid by trained rescue personnel; preliminary dressings by general practitioners; rapid diagnosis and sorting by a team of specialty physicians; surgery with careful anesthesia and adequate wound drainage; generous administration of plasma and whole blood; use of penicillin, tetanus, and gas gangrene antitoxins; fluid control; and careful recordkeeping (Leake, 1947). Although this account risks overestimating physicians' importance at the expense of others, nurses no doubt participated in these activities.

Between 1900 and 1947, new research had occurred in blood types, the treatment of gas gangrene, and the use of penicillin and other antibiotics, and Texas City survivors benefited from these discoveries. Emergency medical techniques used in World War II were also put to good use and accounted for a more organized response. At the same time, skill and discipline proved essential to successful disaster relief responses. Particularly for nurses and other healthcare personnel, their jobs required them to deal with emergencies on a day-to-day basis. Although the disaster was new to them, the response process was familiar.

Finally, by 1947 changes were beginning to be seen in nurses' model identities that reflected those of skilled professionals. The writings of nurses who cared for victims in the aftermath of the Texas City disaster revealed self-images of skilled, hard-working, and often exhausted professionals who had opportunities to expand their healthcare roles in new ways. One student nurse chose to remember her experience in the 1947 disaster as a change in how she perceived

herself as a nurse, no longer as a novice but as a competent and decisive professional.

After the Texas City disaster, on May 5, 1947, the Central Committee of the American National Red Cross approved a plan for the enrollment of nurses in the Red Cross Nursing for service to local communities through chapter programs. This plan replaced the type of enrollment in operation from 1905 to 1946, which served primarily as a reserve for the Army and Navy. This would prove beneficial to survivors of disasters in the future.

The Alaska Earthquake of 1964

On March 27, 1964, at 5:36 p.m., the strongest earthquake ever recorded on the North American continent struck Alaska. In Anchorage, the chronicler of Providence Hospital, which became the chief receiving agency of the injured in that city, wrote, "Everyone seemed to sense the need for immediate action and responsibility" (*Chronicles of the Sisters of Providence*, 1964, n.p.).

Known as the Good Friday Earthquake, it had a tremor that lasted approximately 4 minutes, measured 8.6 on the Richter scale, and caused damages estimated at $750 million. It was so powerful that tremors could be felt over a 500,000-square mile area, with shock waves tearing boats from moorings as far away as the Gulf of Mexico. Tsunamis struck all along the western coast of North America from the Arctic to as far south as Crescent City, California. In addition to Anchorage, a number of Alaskan communities such as Seward, Kodiak, and Valdez were affected, as well as several coastal native villages.

The 2-year-old Providence Hospital was the largest private hospital in the state. Owned and operated by the Sisters of Providence, it became the primary medical emergency center for the entire region. The fact that Providence Hospital received minimal damage was extremely important in its response to the disaster. It quickly shifted to emergency power, and its lights drew supplies and personnel from all over the city to its facilities. Two hospitals in the area, the 40-bed Presbyterian and 300-bed U.S. Air Force hospital at Elmendorf, suffered extensive structural damage. Although the Air Force facility evacuated to nearby barracks and the 395-bed U.S. Public Health Service's Alaska Native Hospital, Presbyterian's patients went to Providence Hospital. Because it became obvious that Providence would be the center of medical and nursing attention, there was little need for further coordination of medical care (Haas, 1964).

Hospital staff members mobilized quickly to care for survivors. Sister Barbara Ellen was administrator of Providence, and she and her five sister assistants coordinated the task of keeping the hospital in operation. They had to deal with lack of water and elevator use, no effective sanitation, and no sterilizers. Pharmacy medications had spilled all over the floor, and all phone links were dead (Special Report, 1964). Within a few minutes, an emergency generator restored electricity and heat to vital areas such as the emergency department, surgery areas, nursing stations, and main halls. The U.S. Army provided a generator for the kitchen, and firemen pumped water from a nearby spring into the hospital (*Chronicles of the Sisters of Providence*, 1964).

No nurse left her unit to go to a safer place, and none of the 75 patients in the hospital at the time received injuries from the quake (*Chronicles of the Sisters of Providence*, 1964). Indeed, a survey team of sociologists from the Disaster Research Center, who arrived within 28 hours after the quake, stated, "Few if any persons actually abandoned an ongoing organizational responsibility" (Haas, 1964, p. 26). The physicians responded with their own action plan, and some brought

their families. Key people were pulled to the emergency department, and within 30 minutes the first survivors arrived. Calmness was maintained throughout the hospital, led by Sister Barbara Ellen, who never lost control of the situation (*Chronicles of the Sisters of Providence*, 1964). Indeed, her authority and her maintenance of control in the crisis helped maintain stability throughout the emergency (Fortier, 1964). As the radio broadcasted a need for registered nurses, off-duty Providence personnel came as well as nurses from the evacuated Presbyterian Hospital. Military personnel from Elmendorf Air Force Base and Fort Richardson delivered a 200-bed civil defense hospital to Providence with beds and cots that were set up in the cafeteria, halls, and business office (Langston, 1964; Sister Philias, 1964). Eventually, Providence did not fill to capacity, however, and not all these supplies were needed (Haas, 1964).

The damage to the American Red Cross headquarters in downtown Anchorage delayed its response, but within 24 hours it had mobilized. Sigrid Bullard from Redwood City, California, the Red Cross Nursing Director for the Alaska disaster, put out a call for volunteers, and 45 registered nurses and 27 trained Red Cross nurses aides responded. All the aides and many of the nurses cared for survivors at Providence Hospital throughout the emergency period (Office of Public Information, 1964).

At Providence Hospital, nurses and physicians set up a triage system in the emergency department. Admissions personnel registered 108 people the first night, but only a few were critically injured. In the operating suites flashlights and battery-operated lights were available in addition to the auxiliary power; one doctor delivered a baby by flashlight early Saturday morning when all power briefly failed. Sterilizers were not operational because there was no steam, and nurses washed instruments and sterilized them with Bunsen burners. They had to improvise in other ways, with one using snow as a substitute for hypothermia for a patient undergoing a craniotomy. Others heated water for infant formulas in the doctors' coffee urn, and they used distilled water for drinking purposes (Langston, 1964; Sister Phileas, 1964).

Public health nurses' roles in this disaster included investigating home-based cases, seeking out dislocated families, distributing food and clothing, performing health screenings, and helping survivors find shelter. The morning after the earthquake hit, public health nurses first went to Providence Hospital to see if they were needed. When told that the hospital had sufficient personnel, they went to the state's Civil Defense Headquarters, where they assisted in evacuations (Haas, 1964). Nurses also opened clinics in outlying areas where they provided immunizations. Nurses, including volunteers from Juneau and Fairbanks, aided Anchorage school nurses, as did many retired nurses. One opined, "This was a very exciting experience of community cooperation" (Beltz, 1964). Other school nurses who were able to leave their families responded over the next 2 weeks, caring for more than 300 evacuated Aleuts from Old Harbor and Kaguyak, where a tidal wave had destroyed their villages. Making formula for babies became a full-time job, and eventually Aleut midwives took over the responsibility from the local school nurses (Scott, 1964). Other nursing care required taking vital signs, dispensing medications, and listening to survivors' problems.

Farther away, a public health nurse from the Prince William Sound area was summoned to Anchorage from her post deep in the interior of the state. The village of Chenega was totally destroyed, 23 people died, and all the survivors were forced to move. This nurse and a team of physicians and sanitation engineers visited potential evacuation sites to evaluate available

housing and water supplies for Chenega's residents (Bonehill, 1964).

Red Cross nurses were on the front lines to care for survivors in emergency shelter. Some nurses worked in typhoid immunization clinics and in shelters such as one that housed 166 Aleuts evacuated from Kodiak Island, which had suffered immense structural damage; it was 350 air miles from Anchorage, and it listed 19 dead or missing (Office of Public Information, 1964). This was the area to which Hazel Heywood, then Director of Nursing services for the Red Cross chapter in Milwaukee, Wisconsin, was assigned. Because communications had been knocked out, nurses' only contact with Red Cross headquarters was through the Alaska Communications System, with nurses and others manning the calls as they came through. The disaster teams supplemented the agencies already at the scene. To this end her first job was to relieve the fatigued nurse at a schoolhouse shelter where 600 to 700 people had congregated. Babies needed formulas and clean diapers, and someone was able to bring a washing machine into the schoolhouse. The Red Cross set up its headquarters in a local church in Kodiak and provided nursing coverage for the schoolhouse shelter until April 7. It dispensed groceries and clothes to the needy, helped with housing, and fed evacuees waiting for stateside naval flights. Nurses checked for survivors, a monumental job because there were no transportation facilities, telephones, newspapers, or roads to reach outlying villages on the island (Farley, 1964).

American Red Cross volunteers went to other badly damaged areas. The greatest death toll was in Valdez, where 32 men, women, and children were killed when huge sections of land slid into the sea. A Red Cross representative from San Antonio, Texas, helped care for hospitalized and sheltered survivors there. Fairbanks experienced only a momentary swaying of buildings, and at St. Joseph's Hospital the local Red Cross nursing chairwoman helped screen evacuees from Valdez for communicable diseases and other needs for medical and nursing care (Benson, 1964).

Most of the nurses in Seward, which had been severely damaged, were on duty somewhere, "herding children, gathering families together, setting up first aid stations. . . . The nurses did everything, scrubbed, cooked, set up trays, washed dishes, answered lights, comforted the hundreds who swarmed about the Hospital that first night and all the next day (Blue, 1964, p. 1). A Red Cross nurse from Oregon dealt with disrupted health and sanitation facilities and the dangers of communicable diseases.

Red Cross survey teams made daily trips into the remote, mountainous Alaskan countryside. To obtain information about distant villages, U.S. Public Health Service physicians and Division of Public Health nurses and sanitary engineers also visited sites in Prince William Sound and Kodiak Island. They provided medical and nursing care, preventive measures, health teaching, and further assessments of sanitary conditions. They worked in an advisory role with agencies responsible for the care of refugees, and as they returned to the areas badly damaged or destroyed, they helped in arranging temporary facilities (Office of Public Information, 1964).

Conclusion

Public health nurses' disaster work has a long history. The exemplars presented in this chapter are illustrative of the growing focus on expert practice, and they serve as windows for viewing changes in nursing practices. In the late 19th and early 20th centuries, nurses provided care and comfort measures, as well as fluid and nutrition. In fact, during the yellow fever epidemic and the 1918 influenza pandemic, nursing care

was usually the only treatment for the illness. As the 20th century progressed, nurses began participating in emergency first aid at the scene. They took vital signs, cared for physical and emotional wounds, administered plasma, and gave medications. Nurses, along with others, worked around the clock, often too busy to eat. Although many carried out traditional tasks of easing fears, they also worked with intravenous infusions, surgery, infection control, and pain relief. They possessed the knowledge and discipline needed during emergencies and did the skilled work they were educated to do. In the end, disasters created opportunities for nurses to expand their practice, blurring the disciplinary boundaries between medicine and nursing as they went. Disasters also blurred the boundaries of race and class, as nurses and other responders worked to meet the needs of all people affected by the emergency situation.

After disasters such as 9/11 and Hurricane Katrina, public health nurses looked to lessons learned from the past. Disasters such as these demonstrate the need for qualified nursing, a task that nurses described in this chapter willingly assumed. For example, nurses in these disasters took charge, worked together, worked it out, and participated in case finding. As in the past, public health nurses today take charge of clinics and coordinate activities for vaccinations and the prevention of disease. They establish significant collaborative relationships with the American Red Cross and numerous other state agencies and organizations. They also reduce the impact of the disaster on the community's health and decrease morbidity and mortality from communicable diseases through case finding. Just as in Galveston in 1900 and Anchorage in 1964, today's disasters witness large numbers of individuals in hospitals and shelters. Nurses have to work without electricity and sustain adequate communication at all times. After September 11, 2001, for example, New York hospitals treated many patients with no electricity, gas, phone connections, or computers (Gaskill, 2006). Yet nurses learned, as in the past, that practicing in a disaster was something they could do, and do well. One of the new topic areas in *Healthy People 2020* refers to preparedness (U.S. Department of Health and Human Services, 2010). The objectives under this topic area will offer public health nurses guidance and direction in the event that nurses need to respond again in the future.

References

American National Red Cross. (1947). *A preliminary report on the Texas City explosions.* Texas City file. Rosenberg Library, Galveston, Texas. St. Louis, MO: American National Red Cross, Midwestern Area.

Barry, J. (2005). *The great influenza: The epic story of the deadliest plague in history.* East Rutherford, NJ: Viking Press.

Bartholf, M. (1947). Co-operation. *American Journal of Nursing, 47*(8), 558.

Barton, C. (1900). *To the people of the United States. 1900 Storm online manuscript exhibit, Red Cross Records, MSS # 05-0007.* Retrieved from http://www.gthcenter.org/exhibits/storms/1900/Manuscripts/RecCross_7/index.html

Barton, C. (1904; reprinted 2005). *The Red Cross in peace and war.* Washington, DC: American Historical Press.

Beltz, A. (1964). Greater Anchorage health district. *Alaska Nurse, XIII*(4), 8.

Benson, R. (1964). Fairbanks reports. *Alaska Nurse, XIII*(4), 11.

Bixel, P. B., & Turner, E. H. (2000). *Galveston and the 1900 storm.* Austin, TX: University of Texas Press.

Blagden, J. D. (2000). Letter to family, September 10, 1900. In C. E. Greene & S. H. Kelly (Eds.), *Through a night of horrors: Voices from the 1900 Galveston storm,* (pp. 17–18). College Station, TX: Texas A&M University Press.

Blocker, V., & Blocker, T. G. (1949). The Texas City disaster: A survey of 3,000 casualties. *American Journal of Surgery, LXXVII*(5), 756–771.

Blue, E. (1964). Seward General Hospital. *Alaska Nurse, XIII*(4), 1.

Bonehill, B. A. (1964). Prince William Sound area as seen by a PHN after Alaska's disaster. *Alaska Nurse, XIII*(4), 10.

Boyle, H. (1947). Monsanto explosion offers foretaste of atom bomb. *The Houston Chronicle,* April 18, n.p.

Byerly, C. (2005). *Fever of war: The influenza epidemic in the U.S. Army during World War I.* New York, NY: New York University Press.

Chronicles of the Sisters of Providence. (1964). Seattle, WA: Sisters of Providence Archives.

Crosby, A. (2003). *America's forgotten pandemic: Influenza 1918* (2nd ed.). Boston, MA: Cambridge University Press.

D'Antonio, J., & Whelan, J. (2004). Moments when time stood still: A look at the history of nursing during disasters. *American Journal of Nursing, 104*(11), 66–72.

Dock, L., & Pickett, S. (1922). *History of the American Red Cross.* New York, NY: MacMillan.

Doty, P. M. (1919). A retrospect of the influenza epidemic. *Public Health Nurse, 11*(12), 949–957.

Farley, J. M. (1964). Alaskan earthquake jolts nurse's schedule. *The Milwaukee Journal,* April 26, n.p.

Fayling, L. R. D. (2000). Fear influenza outbreak among sailors may spread. In C. E. Greene & S. H. Kelly (Eds.), *Through a night of horrors: Voices from the 1900 Galveston storm* (p. 91). College Station, TX: Texas A&M University Press.

Fieser, J. (1941). *Report to Mr. Atkinson, January 15, 1941 re: Influenza Epidemic of 1918.* NARA CP Records of the Red Cross, Box 557, 500.2 Influenza.

Fortier, E. J. (1964). *Observations for Sister Philias on Providence Hospital and earthquake.* Seattle, WA: Sisters of Providence Archives.

Gaskill, M. (2006). On their toes. *Nursing Spectrum.* Retrieved from http://include.nurse.com/apps/pbcs.dll/article?AID=2006608280312

Geister, J. (1957). The flu epidemic of 1918. *Nursing Outlook, 5*(10), 582–584.

Girardeau, G. (1947). *Annual report, July 1, 1946 to July 1, 1947. Galveston County Chapter.* St. Louis, MO: American National Red Cross.

Givin, L. P. (1948). *Memoir, Texas City disaster.* University of Texas Medical Branch Library.

Haas, J. E. (1964). Some preliminary observations on the responses of community organizations involved in the emergency period of the Alaskan earthquake. *Disaster Research Center Working Paper #2.* Newark, DE: Disaster Research Center, University of Delaware.

Hilleman, M. R. (2002). Realities and enigmas of human viral influenza: Pathogenesis, epidemiology and control. *Vaccine, 20,* 3068–3087.

Houston Chronicle. (April 21, 1947). Retrieved from http://www.redcross.org/services/nursing/0,1082,0_389_,00.html#develope

Informer. (April 19, 1947). Employee of Texas City café tells of his escape, p. 10.

Informer. (April 19, 1947). Many Negroes killed, scores injured in Texas City blast, p. 1.

Johnson, N., & Mueller, J. (2002). Updating the accounts: Global mortality of the 1918–1920 "Spanish" influenza pandemic. *Bulletin of the History of Medicine, 76,* 105–115.

Johnston, M. E. (1947). Relatives claim dead at morgue. *Houston Post*, April 18, p. 20.

Kernodle, P. B. (1949). *The Red Cross nurse in action, 1882–1948*. New York, NY: Harper and Brothers.

Kilpatrick, E. (1919). *Report of the Northwest ARC Division, 1919*, in National Archives Records Administration, College Park (NARACP), 803.11 epidemics, Box 689, folder 1.

Kreps, G. A. (1990). The Federal Emergency Management System in the United States: Past and present. *International Journal of Mass Emergencies and Disasters, 8*(3), 281.

Langston, D. V. (1964, July 27). Report of a hospital in a disaster area. *Journal of the American Medical Association*, 306–307.

Leake, C. D. (October, 1947). *Copy of military medical principles applied to a civilian disaster*. University of Texas Medical Branch Library.

Markel, H., Lipman, H. B., Navarro, J. A., Sloan, A., Michalsen, J. R., Stern, A. M., & Cetron, M. S. (2007). Nonpharmaceutical interventions implemented by U.S. cities during the 1918–1919 influenza pandemic. *Journal of the American Medical Association, 298*(6), 644–653.

McLeod, T. (1948). When disaster strikes. *Hospital Progress, 408,* 411.

Minutaglio, B. (2003). *City on fire: The explosion that devastated a Texas town and ignited a historic legal battle*. New York, NY: HarperCollins.

Molsbee, A. F. (1947). Students give disaster service in Galveston. *American Journal of Nursing, 47*(6), 414.

Moorehead, C. (1998). *Dunant's dream: War, Switzerland and the history of the Red Cross*. London, UK: HarperCollins.

National Park Service, U.S. Department of Interior. (2006). *Johnstown flood*. Retrieved from http://www.nps.gov/jofl/faqs.htm

Noyes, C. (1918, September 25). *Memo to all division directors*. National Archives Record Administration (NARA). Memo found in CP Box 689 of the Influenza Epidemic records of 1918, Record Group 803.11.

Office of Public Information, Western Area, American Red Cross. (1964). *Nurses answer call quickly for Alaskan disaster duty*. American Red Cross Office, Anchorage, Alaska. n.p.

Rafferty, J. (1974). *Mercy Hospital, 1947–1972: An historical review*. Pittsburgh, PA: Mercy Hospital.

Rubin, C. B. (Ed.). (2007). *Emergency management: The American experience, 1900–2005*. Fairfax, VA: Public Entity Risk Institute.

Scott, E. (1964). School nurses—Anchorage. *Alaska Nurse, XIII*(4), 6.

Sister Philias. (1964). *Three C's for an operating room in disaster*. Seattle, WA: Sisters of Providence Archives, PMCA, Box 32.

Special Report. (1964). Hospitals and the Alaskan earthquake. *Journal of the American Hospital Association, 38,* 23–24A.

Stephens, H. W. (1993). The Texas City disaster: A re-examination. *Industrial and Environmental Crisis Quarterly, 7*(3), 189–190.

Stephens, H. W. (1997). *The Texas City disaster, 1947*. Austin, TX: University of Texas Press.

1200 Feared dead in Texas blasts. (1947, April 17). *New York Times*, n.p.

U.S. Department of Health and Human Services. (2010). *Healthy People 2020*. Retrieved from http://www.healthypeople.gov/2020/default.aspx.

Veenema, T. G. (2007). *Disaster nursing and emergency preparedness for chemical, biological and radiological terrorism and other hazards* (2nd ed.). New York, NY: Springer.

Visiting Nurse Society. (1918). Newspaper clipping from scrapbook. VNS Collection, UPenn CSHN, Barbara Bates Center of the History of Nursing.

Wall, B. M. (2008). Healing after disasters in early 20th-century Texas. *Advances in Nursing Science, 31*(3), 211–224. Excerpts reprinted with permission.

Wheaton, E. L. (1948). *Texas City remembers*. San Antonio, TX: Naylor.

For a full suite of assignments and additional learning activities, use the access code located in the front of your book to visit this exclusive website: http://go.jblearning.com/londrigan. If you do not have an access code, you can obtain one at the site.

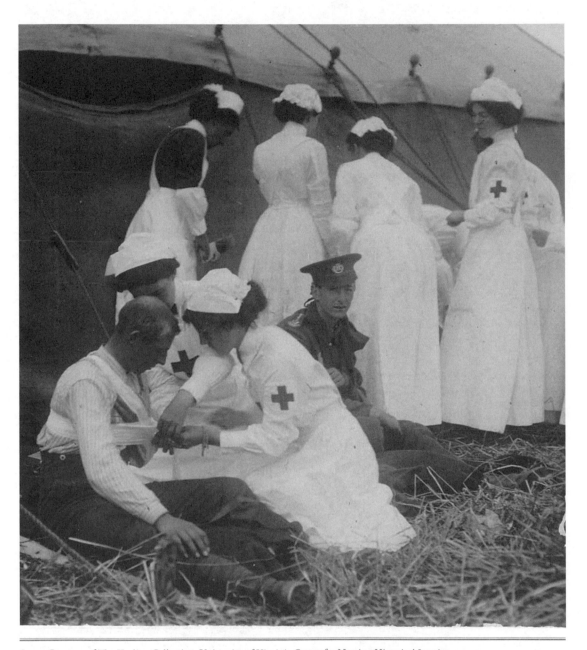

Chapter 16

Emergency Preparedness in the 21st Century: Two Post-9/11 Case Studies

Lucille Ferrara
Keith Veltri
Michela Catalano

The most important aspect of disaster care is pre-disaster planning by the responsible community agencies. This has been demonstrated again and again in such large-scale disasters as tornadoes, hurricanes, transportation accidents, and explosions of inflammable gases, ammunition, plastics, or other highly combustible materials where large numbers of lives are lost and the injured require varying degrees of care (Kinch, 1959, pp. 506–507).

LEARNING OBJECTIVES

By the completion of this chapter, the reader will be able to

- Describe the two methods of point of dispensing (POD) care delivery
- Reflect on the meaning of emergency preparedness in public health
- Discuss the multidisciplinary collaboration needed in emergency preparedness

KEY TERMS

- ❑ push POD model
- ❑ pull POD model

2011 marked the 10-year anniversary of the 9/11 attacks. Our nation, our cities, and our lives were changed forever on that Tuesday morning in September. The events of the day and the atrocities that followed affected us all in different ways. The following chapter is both a reflection as well as a report of the accounts of the aftermath of 9/11 in a New York City (NYC) medical center and the response this medical center had with regard to emergency preparedness not only for the medical center community, but for the community and populations it serves. Two case studies are presented to illustrate the medical center's response to a call to action from the Department of Homeland Security, the Department of Emergency Preparedness for the City of New York, and the NYC Department of Health and Mental Hygiene (DOHMH). Two methods of point of dispensing (POD) care delivery are demonstrated in these cases: the push POD and the pull POD models of rapid immunization and prophylaxis distribution/dispensing. Through these efforts, multidisciplinary collaboration was the common denominator.

Push Point of Dispensing and Pull Point of Dispensing Defined

Two types of POD methods exist: the pull and push POD models. The pull POD model consists of administering mass prophylaxis or vaccines to employees who report to a specific central location. The push POD model utilizes mobile teams to physically bring prophylaxis to the employees, decreasing the amount of time spent away from work. The following case studies illustrate both methods.

The Pull POD: Smallpox Initiative

Background

Bioterrorism was identified as a real threat well before the 9/11 attacks, but increased fear developed following the events of 9/11. Anthrax was the first major bioterrorism event, with cases identified in New York, Washington, D.C., and Florida that were said to have been spread through the mail; this spawned mass hysteria among U.S. citizens. Hospitals began stockpiling Ciprofloxin in order to prepare for a potential anthrax attack/exposure. Emergency Departments were overwhelmed with patients fearing that they were exposed to anthrax and demanding prescriptions for Cipro to protect themselves and their families. The potential exposure of Anthrax through a bioterrorist attack instilled great fear. The real threat and subsequent danger, however, would lie in the potential exposure to smallpox. Smallpox virus, although eradicated worldwide, is still kept alive and viable in the event of an outbreak where vaccine would need to be mass produced. According to the Centers for Disease Control and Prevention (CDC, 2003), "Although smallpox was declared globally eradicated in 1980, there is concern that smallpox virus may exist outside the two WHO-designated repository laboratories" (p.1). This concern about a potential bioterrorist attack prompted the U.S. House of Representatives, House Select Committee on Homeland Security to mandate the smallpox initiative. Unfortunately, the intended response to this initiative was less than what was expected and the initiative failed. Through the efforts of the state and local DOHMH, the plan was to vaccinate 500,000 first responders in 30 days; however, after one year, only 40,000 were actually vaccinated (U.S. House of Representatives,

House Select Committee on Homeland Security, 2004). Three key factors attributed to this failure were identified: insufficient allocation of resources, an inadequate compensation plan for healthcare workers suffering potential side effects from the vaccine, and healthcare workers and the public's perceived lack of urgency with regard to a smallpox threat (U.S. House of Representatives, House Select Committee on Homeland Security, 2004). The following case study describes the smallpox initiative of the NYC DOHMH and the medical center's work in following the directive according to the pull POD model.

The Smallpox Initiative

In October 2002, the NYC DOHMH issued a directive that was part of a federal mandate to vaccinate the 500,000 healthcare workers who would serve as first responders in the event of a bioterrorist attack involving smallpox. Part of this initiative provided education to staff in select hospitals in the NYC area for case identification, surveillance, preparation, and planning in the event of a bioterrorist attack, and to provide training for physicians and nurses to serve as first responders. These first responders would be vaccinated and then trained by the DOHMH staff to be certified as vaccinators as well.

Montefiore Medical Center (MMC) was selected as a site that would provide rapid immunization in the event a smallpox outbreak occurred in the NYC area. Montefiore Medical Center is a not-for-profit academic medical center and the largest healthcare provider in the Bronx, New York, with a total bed count capacity of 1,400. At the time of this initiative, the Montefiore delivery system included three acute-care hospitals: the Jack D. Weiler, Moses, and the Children's Hospital at Montefiore (CHAM). The plan was set up as a tiered method

for rapid immunization. Within the first tier, the initial vaccinations would be provided to the team responsible for overall care and immunization of the healthcare workers who would be providing direct patient care. The second tier would involve the mass immunization of the surrounding community to include all patient populations, both healthy and vulnerable.

The team reported to the NYC DOHMH office in Manhattan to receive special training that included clinic setup, documentation, immunization, and patient education. Once the 2-day training was complete, the staff of the Department of Occupational Health Services (OHS) developed and mobilized the plan. During the first phase of this plan, education to all hospital staff was conducted. During these education/information sessions, smallpox facts, which included detailed information about the vaccine, were provided. At these sessions, staff were given the dates and times that vaccine would be available and administered during the specialty clinic hours. The DOHMH would provide the live smallpox vaccine as well as vaccinators/trainers for the staff during these specialty clinic days. The Occupational Health Staff of MMC would be responsible for all phases of this endeavor. This staff included a physician (also the director), a nurse practitioner, a staff administrator and a secretary; other stakeholders in this effort included nursing administration, infection control, and hospital administration. Educational sessions were held at all three locations. The attendance at these sessions was at best, modest. Additional information was provided through pamphlets and other educational materials provided by the NYC DOHMH. Flyers, emails, and posters were used to communicate the dates, times, and location for the smallpox vaccination clinic. This method of vaccine delivery is an example of a pull POD, where a central location is created to provide mass prophylaxis for an infectious disease exposure (in this case, smallpox). Out of 6,000 direct care providers (nurses, physicians, house staff, and ancillary care) who were targeted and educated, only 10 were vaccinated. Unfortunately, this marginal response became the norm throughout the nation because of the factors described earlier.

The Push POD: The Influenza Vaccine Initiative

Background

After the 9/11 events, the NYC DOHMH recognized the need to develop a uniform procedure in the case of a potential health disaster. During the 2006–2007 fiscal year, the DOHMH requested that all citywide hospitals participate in a POD drill. All participating hospitals were required to have a team of five healthcare professionals, including one pharmacist, one physician, two nurses, and another member of their institution. The drill was to be conducted within a 4-hour interval to simulate a situation of mass prophylaxis using influenza as a surrogate vaccine or pharmaceutical agent needed in the event of a public health emergency. Following the initiative, hospitals were asked to submit their written medication distribution protocol implemented at the institution.

The Influenza Vaccine Initiative

Montefiore Medical Center participated in this initiative and at that time included four acute-care hospitals: the Jack D. Weiler, Moses, CHAM, and its North Division. Developing this initiative represented a formidable challenge, so the MMC utilized the delivery of influenza vaccine during the 2007 season as a surrogate for rapid distribution of potentially needed vaccines

or medications in order to estimate the capacity to respond to biologic emergencies. Also motivating the MMC was the Joint Commission's 2007 (www.jointcommissionreport.org, 2007) issuance of a new standard that required hospitals and long-term care facilities to offer influenza immunizations to all staff members and practitioners. The exercise added to the annual influenza campaign for the medical center staff members. The hospital protocol was reviewed and later approved by the infectious disease division and the emergency preparedness committee. Both OHS and the pharmacy department developed the disaster plan. While many hospitals generally have written emergency preparedness plans in place, most may not have successfully tested the detailed mass prophylactic effort in advance.

Guidelines were established to streamline the organizational processes. During the preplanning stage, it was suggested to select team leaders, establish a planning committee, draft an effective plan of action, establish mobilizing teams, and devise a push POD strategy. The team leaders would then be responsible for managing the entire initiative and liaising between the state and the hospital. The established committee determined the necessities of the exercise and ensured the availability of all essential supplies. The team would be responsible for adequately storing and maintaining influenza vaccine, screening and administering the vaccine, and documenting vaccinated employees. Submission of all documentation, including a list of team leaders, members, and attendance lists of both planning meetings and the POD exercise, were required. Once all required information was obtained, the DOHMH approved state reimbursement for the exercise.

To comply with the request of the DOHMH (www.nyc.gov/health), MMC chose the push POD model for this initiative during one

4-hour period (10 am–2 pm) on October 9, 2007. In order to alert the employees of the institution, emails and posters were created in advance. Throughout the activity, MMC used eight teams, consisting of two vaccinators and one record keeper. Each team used rolling carts to appropriately house all vaccines and supplies needed during the exercise. Vaccines supplied by OHS were originally purchased by the pharmacy department from various manufacturers.

The teams were distributed throughout the inpatient units, outpatient facilities, and emergency departments at the Moses, CHAM, and Weiler divisions. For each team a team leader was designated and provided with a walkie-talkie to enable communication with dedicated command center leaders from the hospital security department. When supplies were low, two runners were designated to report to the pharmacy and/or command center to replenish these necessities. During the drill, employees were continuously informed of the whereabouts of the team by the overhead hospital paging system. Following the 4-hour exercise, all team members reported to the command center for a debriefing.

During the 4-hour test run, the team was able to immunize 942 healthcare workers. Predicting a 24/7 operation in the event of a biological terrorism event, the push POD operation would have the capacity to immunize 12,000 healthcare workers, the approximate population of the hospital, in 48 hours. This exercise was replicated for the 2008 influenza program and the results were identical. This initiative achieved overwhelming success that has been replicated annually.

Thoughts, Reflections, and Lessons Learned

The two case studies presented offer much food for thought. In both scenarios, multidisciplinary collaboration was crucial in the planning and implementation phases. Involving key stakeholders, especially those who serve as decision makers, such as administrators, is another vital component in ensuring program success. The multidisciplinary collaboration, however, is not enough, as was demonstrated in the case of the smallpox initiative. All of the elements were there: collaboration, excellent communication (flyers, posters, emails, information sessions), the plan was followed as prescribed by the directing agency, but the end user (healthcare worker/vaccine recipient) did not participate. As noted earlier, the House Select Committee on Homeland Security offered three compelling factors to explain the lack of participation: inadequate funding, lack of compensation for potential injury, and a lack of perceived threat of exposure. The first two factors are fairly straightforward and self-explanatory but the third factor, lack of perceived threat of a smallpox exposure, is worrisome. The question then is what should be done to better educate healthcare workers and the general public that bioterrorism is real and that it is not a question of if, but when, this will occur. The real lesson learned then is that perhaps more time should be spent on having meaningful discussions, seminars, and campaigns that focus on public awareness of these types of threats.

Or is it more than that? Consider the case of the influenza vaccine initiative: Healthcare workers, as well as the public, have first-hand experience with flu either as a patient, a direct care provider, or in some cases as both. The most compelling lesson learned may be related to the lived experience of the end user (healthcare worker, first responder) in both situations. The public can relate to that which is known and experienced. The United States has not experienced a smallpox epidemic since the 1700s. An influenza epidemic is real, as can be seen in the H1N1 pandemic of 2010. The push POD influenza initiative not only was an overwhelming success but also demonstrated almost the exact outcome each time it was replicated. In addition, is it possible that the model of push POD delivery, taking the vaccine to the people, is another reason for the success of the influenza initiative? A long-standing public health strategy is to bring vaccines to the people, in this case, where they work. Perhaps it was the integration of this public health strategy long used with much success in communities that has the potential for such success in tertiary care settings as well. The significance of this outcome measure warrants further study. Perhaps the findings could offer some recommendations and strategies that may help in ensuring the success of other similar initiatives, such as those dealing with smallpox.

Summary

Two case studies were presented, demonstrating how multidisciplinary collaboration, effective communication, education, and repetition are vital to the successful implementation of any initiative. Emergency preparedness is a phrase that is used and quoted frequently but one that should not be thought of as simple. Many levels and layers of complexity create and define what constitutes being truly prepared. Depending on the source, our nation is neither completely prepared nor completely unprepared for a bioterrorist attack. Many factors such as funding, compensation for injury, and perceived usefulness constitute major roles in ensuring the success of initiatives involving vaccine administration and chemical prophylaxis. One area worth exploring and targeting is public awareness of the "realness" of bioterrorism and its inevitability. Another is being aware of how the method of delivery of care is being developed. Bringing care to the people where they work may be a key public health strategy to be implemented in tertiary care. Being prepared, according to Merriam-Webster, means: "to make ready beforehand for some purpose, use or activity; to work out the details of; plan in advance; to get ready" (2011, n.p.). That said, are we prepared?

References

Centers for Disease Control and Prevention (CDC). (2003). Executive Summary. *Smallpox Response Plan and Guidelines.* Retrieved from www.bt.cdc.gov/agent/smallpox/response-plan/files/exec-sections-i-vi.pdf

Guidelines for Core Deliverable H-Push Pod, The City of New York. http://www.nyc.gov/health

Joint Commission. (2007). *Improving America's Hospitals, The Joint Commission's Annual Report on Quality and Safety,* Retrieved from www.jointcommission report.org

Kinch, A. (1959). Bellevue responds when disaster strikes in New York City. *American Journal of Nursing, 59*(4), 504–509.

Merriam-Webster Online Dictionary. (2011). Retrieved from http://www.merriam-webster.com

U.S. House of Representatives, House Select Committee on Homeland Security. (2004). *A biodefense failure: The national smallpox vaccination program one year later.* Washington, DC: Author.

For a full suite of assignments and additional learning activities, use the access code located in the front of your book to visit this exclusive website: http://go.jblearning.com/londrigan. If you do not have an access code, you can obtain one at the site.

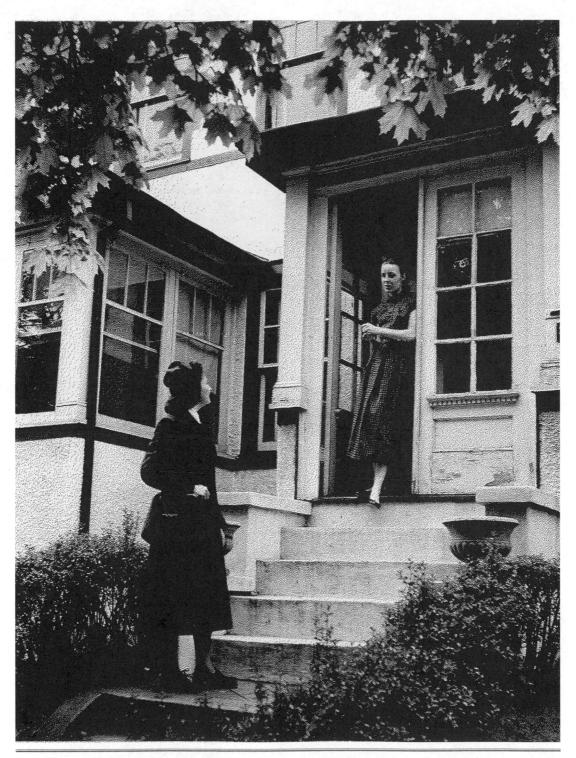

Source: Courtesy of the Visiting Nurse Service of New York.

Chapter 17

Nursing Education and Public Health Nursing

Cathleen M. Shultz
Karen Kelley

By 1950, more than 17 years would have been added to the average span of American life.... It could not have been accomplished without skilled nursing for the sick; the participation of nurses in immunization and case-finding programs; persuasive teaching of health principles by nurses in homes, schools, hospitals, industries, clinics, and health centers; and the public information for groups of community leaders (Roberts, 1954, p. 4).

LEARNING OBJECTIVES

At the completion of this chapter, the reader will be able to

- Identify three challenges related to public health and nursing education.
- List two of the public health clinical experiences described in this chapter.
- Describe the intervention wheel strategies applied in at least one of the public health clinical experiences identified above.
- Explore additional creative public health clinical experiences.

KEY TERMS

- ❏ Essentials of Baccalaureate Nursing Education for Entry Level Community/ Public Health Nurses
- ❏ Institute of Medicine reports for nursing education
- ❏ Population-focused care
- ❏ Service learning
- ❏ Social justice
- ❏ Teaching–learning strategies

Nursing is in an ideal position to respond to numerous challenges facing the healthcare system today. The list of challenges related to the health needs of our nation and our global neighbors is nearly endless: skyrocketing costs of health care and the resultant need for a renewed emphasis on prevention and health promotion measures, healthcare inequalities and disparities, the epidemic of childhood obesity, immigration, the increasing complexity of care for those with chronic illness, anticipated pandemics, emerging and reemerging infectious diseases, threats of bioterrorism, the burden of disease, the enormous expansion of technology, the human immunodeficiency virus (HIV)/acquired immune deficiency syndrome (AIDS) epidemic, unemployment, homelessness, violence, increasing globalization, and increasing evidence of the major impact that the economic and social environments have on health, to name some of these challenges. As the nation responds to the healthcare system crises, public health has regained attention as a viable response to meet many of these challenges. Nurses are a large workforce with a lengthy history of practicing in public health settings. Many nurses practice in positions that place them in people's homes, schools, workplaces, houses of worship, public clinics, and other settings where public health expertise is needed.

Although barriers exist to specializing in public health nursing, it is imperative that nursing education programs prepare graduates who are skilled in use of public health practices, able to work as a member of multidisciplinary public health teams, are knowledgeable of the determinants of health affecting populations, and know how to integrate this knowledge into interventions that positively impact the health of individuals, families, and communities. This chapter explores the educational mandates for nursing students as related to public health, educational challenges, and practical learning exemplars that integrate these into learning experiences that can develop public health skills, knowledge, and aptitudes in nursing students—in other words, "applying and doing" in nursing education. Graduates must be prepared as professionals ready to meet rapidly changing healthcare system demands.

Challenges to Nurse Educators

Nursing and nursing education have come full circle. History seems to repeat itself, but the context changes. From the early days of the colonies to the present, the United States has struggled with its nursing numbers, the preparation of its nursing workforce, and containment and conquering of its infectious diseases and other major causes of maiming and death. Our state and federal governments coasted through the last five decades and reduced resources that were needed to build a strong public health workforce and infrastructure, which are now costly to reconstruct and repair. There is a pressing need to graduate nurses capable of understanding and meaningfully contributing to the public's health. As mentioned elsewhere in this text, leaders such as Florence Nightingale, Lillian Wald, and Clara Barton pressed to create, implement, and sustain public health initiatives that changed health and disease practices for decades after their deaths. They modeled perseverance and courage and met the challenges of their times. They were among the first nurse systems thinkers.

Historically, public health nurses were valued by society and functioned autonomously. They practiced in settings and with populations that were of minimal interest to other healthcare disciplines. Traditionally, public health nursing care encompassed the unempowered and the invisible—women, children, the poor, immigrants, and other disenfranchised groups. Gradually, practice shifted from personal healthcare services, such as home care, to public health issues and activities. It is beyond the scope of this chapter to comprehensively explore major discoveries and movements that altered public health needs and practices. Dramatically, the cataclysmic events that redirected the nation's public health policies, urgencies, and attention were the terrorist attacks on the World Trade Center and the Pentagon and the brave passengers of a hijacked airliner that crashed near Shanksville, Pennsylvania, on September 11, 2001. Thousands were killed and even more were injured or sustained chronic conditions because of their part in that day's activities. Shortly thereafter, the anthrax exposures of thousands in New York, Florida, and Washington, DC, forced a reexamination of the weakened public health infrastructure and ultimately the preparation of nurses for a timely response to population needs.

The Institute of Medicine (IOM, 2003) developed seven public health priorities, which are summarized in **Box 17-1**. Nursing education programs are addressing these priority needs as well as other initiatives such as disaster preparedness. Public health issues are competing with bioterrorism activities for resources. The worldwide economic depression remains

Following a tornado, these lone steps mark a reminder of the homes that were present hours before. Inhabitants are at a local shelter receiving health care and aid from nursing students and relief organizations.

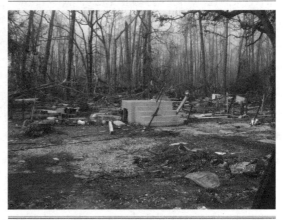

Source: Courtesy of Cathleen Shultz.

unresolved, and its full effects are yet to be seen. Regardless of the pressures felt by nurse educators and nursing students, preparation for effective public health needs is central to developing and sustaining a prepared nursing workforce and a healthy population.

Responding to the Public Health Needs

Teaching IOM: Implications of the Institute of Medicine Reports for Nursing Education, based on the series of **IOM reports for nursing education** aimed at improving the safety and overall quality of health care in the United States, addresses areas of interest to nurse educators in preparing students in public health (Finkelman & Kenner, 2007). The IOM (2003) report views education of health professionals as a "bridge to quality care" (p. 9) and states that education must change to meet the needs of current and future healthcare systems.

Box 17-1 Institute of Medicine's Seven Public Health Priorities

1. Understand and emphasize broad determinants of health
2. Create a policy focus on population health
3. Strengthen the public health infrastructure
4. Build partnerships
5. Develop systems of accountability
6. Emphasize evidence-based practice
7. Enhance communication

Source: IOM, 2003.

The authors provide understanding that adding content is nearly impossible in already overfilled curriculums but offer that threads such as cultural competence and informatics (Shultz, 2009b) can be woven into other public health learning activities, allowing the student to gain the knowledge and experience its application. Suggestions also involve students from different health-related professions located in the academic institution to have joint educational opportunities.

In addition to legislative expectations such as a state's nurse practice acts, nursing program approval standards and health laws, and other requirements such as clinical agency expectations, numerous organizations, such as accrediting bodies, affect nursing education in the United States. National initiatives that push for increased competence in gerontology, women's health, safety, healthy work environments, and end-of-life

practices add to the challenges facing nursing students and educators. Currently, programs' lengths and types are defined by law and graduates enter practice after passing the National Council Licensure Examination, which tests practice expectations, within 6 months of graduation. Faculty must create learning activities that quickly involve students in increasingly complex case situations to graduate competent, dedicated, lifelong learners.

Students at all educational levels need exposure to relevant definitions of nursing, public health, and public health nursing and an understanding of public health nursing as a specialty (Table 17-1). Beyond basic understandings, faculty program decisions involve collectively selecting methods to incorporate learning public health concepts and nursing roles (Table 17-2). Faculty may choose a public health total curriculum, a multicourse focus, or a single-course

Table 17-1 Relevant Nursing Public Health Definitions

Term	Definition
Nursing	The protection, promotion, and optimization of health and abilities, prevention of illness and injury, alleviation of suffering through the diagnosis and treatment of human response, and advocacy in the care of individuals, families, communities, and populations (American Nurses Association, 2003, p. 6; 2004, p. 7)
Public health	Science and art of preventing disease, prolonging life, and promoting health and efficiency through organized community effort (Winslow, 1920, p. 30)
Public health practice	What we as a society do collectively to ensure the conditions in which people can be healthy (IOM, 1988, p. 1; 2003, p. 28)
Public health nursing	A practice that is affected by ". . . biological, cultural, environmental, economic, social, and political factors. As part of the healthcare system public health nursing practice is responsive to these factors through working with the community to promote health and prevent disease, injury, and disability" (American Public Health Association, 2011, para. 2) A specialty practice of nursing defined by scope of practice and not by practice setting (Council on Linkages Between Academia and Public Health Practice, 2001; Quad Council of Public Health Nursing Organizations, 1999)
Public health nursing specialty	Contains 8 core foundation principles of public health nursing identified and discussed in the *Public Health Nursing: Scope and Standards of Practice* (American Nurses Association, 2007; Association of Community Health Nursing Educators, 2003)

Table 17-2 SELECT EXAMPLES OF PUBLIC HEALTH CONCEPTS AND PUBLIC
HEALTH NURSING ROLES

Public Health Concepts	Public Health Nursing Roles and Duties
Population-focused care	Advocate
Disaster planning and response	Collect, monitor, and analyze data
Public health surveillance	Case manager
Outbreak investigation	Health policy and legislation involvement
Community and population assessment	Referral resource
Use of evidence-based interventions	Literacy assessor
Infectious disease prevention, recognition, and care	Educator
Vulnerable populations	Identify community needs
Partnerships	Create and implement educational activities
Health agency roles (federal, state, local)	Direct primary caregiver
Epidemiology—the scientific core	Organize public health services
Service learning	
Social justice	
Violence	
Cultural competency	

focus. Complex learning, such as public health nursing, most often takes time. An early curriculum introduction to the concepts and roles fosters deeper understanding before graduation. The greater the lack of experienced public health nursing clinicians, the more faculty will need to creatively develop relationship-based clinical experiences.

Integrating Learner Knowledge, Skills, and Aptitudes to Develop Public Health–Focused Nursing Care

Because of the limited time for educational experiences (both didactic and clinical), there is a need to create learning experiences that meet multiple outcome objectives. Carter, Kaiser, O'Hare, and Callister (2006) urged **teaching–learning strategies** based on public health nursing practice (Quad Council of Public Health Nursing Organizations, 1999, public health nursing competencies (Quad Council, 2004), and **Essentials of Baccalaureate Nursing Education for Entry Level Community/ Public Health Nurses** (Association of Community Health Nursing Educators, 2000). Program, course, and class decisions affecting learning rest with faculty. Exemplar teaching and learning examples are provided in the narrative that follows. They are modifiable depending on learner expectations and placement of the learning strategies in the nursing program.

Where possible, faculty align clinical assignments directly to theory application. For situations where finding appropriate clinical experiences is difficult, either clinical experiences or simulations are created. Theory and application are at the individual, family, and community levels. Many class activities are discussed at the national and global levels, with some students participating in international experiences. Application of national and global issues to the local situation is made. Nurse educators, from novice to expert, build real-world learning activities that use cognitive, affective, and psychomotor skills. Evidence-based teaching, learning, and evaluation methods are increasing in numbers and scope as the science of nursing education is pursued (Shultz, 2009a). Many of these are applicable to teaching public health nursing that faculty are urged to use and further research.

In the beginning of the public health-focused nursing course, students are introduced to the learning outcomes. For most students, viewing the community as the client is difficult to grasp, as is the idea of **population-focused care**. As the semester's content outline, clinical rotations, and learning assignments are reviewed, the students begin the journey of combining concepts that seem to be unrelated, such as healthcare financing and epidemiology, into what they will come to know as public health nursing. As each content area is covered, the learning links between them are explained and experienced. By the end of the semester, bridges between those links are stronger and the students view the interrelated concepts of public health more clearly.

An example of an assignment that encourages these connections involves the students locating and presenting a current event article in class. They prepare the public health news item for display on the classroom's bulletin board after the in-class verbal presentation. Connections to the various concepts in public health are made during the classroom discussion. The assignment increases student awareness of media interpretations of health-related news items and their relevance to nurses. An example is the media events announcing the severe acute respiratory syndrome, caused by a virus that led to illness and death for many in 2003. From China, the disease spread rapidly to other countries by airline passengers traveling internationally. In this situation, the media coverage lasted several months and was timely for class discussions. News items that involve health promotion and prevention studies are especially useful for class discussions because of the nature of these studies and the amount of rapidly conflicting information that often appears simultaneously.

Early in the semester, healthcare financing, healthcare systems, health policy, and political issues are taught. Emphasis is on their interconnectedness and the dramatic influences they bear on health status and needs. Extensive discussion regarding effects on vulnerable populations and concern for social justice dominate learning. At this section's conclusion, students produce an in-class debate on the pros and cons of universal health care. It is typically a lively debate. Preparation requires knowledge of public health concepts and assigned readings. In a reflective summative evaluation of the activity, students report a broader view of the issue and additional insight into how populations and the healthcare system are affected.

Public Health Clinical Experiences

Clinical experiences involve nursing in schools, local health departments, rural health clinics, home health settings, screenings (hearing, vision, scoliosis, body mass index, laboratory, and wellness focused), area agencies on aging, and disaster management simulation (Bambini, Washburn, & Perkins, 2009). Students use clinical experience guidelines for each separate experience (see example in **Figure** 17-1). Each requires a student self-assessment (establishes goals and monitors progress toward them), which is a technique that enhances self-directedness (Nicol & Macfarlane-Dick, 2006). Fitzpatrick (2006) determined that self-assessment positively influences students' development, particularly their sense of autonomy and thinking skills (Maclellan & Soden, 2006). When shared, faculty members gain insight into students' thinking (Davies, 2002), and it becomes a mechanism for personalized feedback (Cato, Lasater, & Peeples, 2009).

The goal of each experience is to develop clinical judgment (Tanner, 2006), which facilitates students thinking like a public health nurse. The reflective self-assessment activity incorporates the four phases of Tanner's clinical judgment model (noticing, interpreting, responding, and reflecting) with students describing their responses to clinical situations using behavioral descriptors. The learning strategy fosters clinical judgment (Craft, 2005; Lasater, 2007a, b; Lasater & Nielsen, 2009; Nielsen, Stragnell, & Jester, 2007).

Creating Clinical Experiences: Wellness Screening

With the increasing emphasis in the United States on controlling healthcare costs, a growing interest in prevention is occurring in all sectors of health care. Both governmental and private stakeholders are urgently implementing ways to control costs. Public health professionals have long advocated prevention as a way to meet that goal. Students in the community health nursing

course learn a variety of skills and concepts that consider both risk factors and interventions at the primary, secondary, and tertiary levels of prevention.

Each semester the public health nursing students conduct a wellness screening for faculty, staff, and students at the university. The screening involves two interactions between students and participants. The first interaction involves actual screening assessments. Participants choose from a selection of laboratory tests including lipid panels, high sensitivity C-reactive protein, complete blood counts, glucose, hemoglobin A1c, complete metabolic panels, prostate-specific antigens, testosterone levels, arthritis profiles, vitamin D levels, thyroid screens, and HIV. Body fat analysis and health risk appraisals are also offered. In clinical conferences the students learn which screenings, such as lipid panels, are recommended for the general population and which are targeted screenings based on risk factors. This provides an excellent application of screening theory. The students then learn to analyze results and provide written counseling to each participant. With guidance they recommend additional screenings such as mammography or colonoscopy based on the age and sex of the participant. Students ensure that all screenings are returned from the laboratory and organize and package the results. From this experience students learn many skills and abilities needed to manage a screening program; these skills include clinic setup, managing traffic flow, involvement with forms that order and report results, and dismantling the clinic. The following week, students are available for participants to receive results, be counseled regarding recommended lifestyle changes, and refer to local health providers as needed.

The nursing program partnered with a local wellness company affiliated with a certified

Figure 17-1 Sample clinical experience journal template.

Clinical Experience Journal

Clinical Experience in: Local Health Department

Date:_____ **Setting**: <insert name of agency> **Location**: <insert town or city> .

This clinical experience is guided by your clinical teacher and supervised by agency personnel. The clinical teacher will visit the site during the experience and is available during the experience by phone or text at <insert number> or <insert email address>.

You are expected to complete preparatory materials prior to the experience, participate in nursing care at the agency, and meet this experience's learning objectives. Following the experience, complete a reflective self-assessment evaluation of your experiences. Evaluation is comprehensive and is also completed by agency personnel and the clinical teacher.

Purposes of the Experience:
- To participate in public health nursing at a local health department
- To determine services offered at a local and state health department

Preparation:
Review the State Department of Health (SDH) website. What programs are offered by the SDH? What is the structure of the organization? How is the SDH funded?

Objectives:
1. Describe the major health promotion and disease preventing programs delivered at the HD (family planning, WIC - Women, Infants and Children, Immunization, Communicable Disease, TB, STD, Breast Care). List the requirements for participation in each program, how is it funded, the cost to the participant, what specifically is provided, and describe what occurs during a visit for each of these major programs. What is the protocol if someone is/has a positive TB test? Is HIV positive? Tests positive for syphilis? What immunizations are required? Offered?
2. Describe the cultural diversity of the health unit's target population. How is this diversity being addressed? (Review population statistics for the county.)
3. Use the nursing process to assess, plan, implement and evaluate public health care given to members of the community during your experience. Identify public health nursing roles observed and examples of each.
4. Discuss what referrals are most often needed by patients. How are they made?
5. Describe the process used for reportable diseases. How is the information gathered and reported?
6. What skills did you perform? Describe how you maintain safe nursing practice? Specifically, be prepared to do venipunctures, injections, urine pregnancy tests, fingersticks, assist with pelvic exams, etc.
7. Describe the computer charting and database for record keeping, including vaccination records. Accurately document any findings. Discuss how charting is related to reimbursement for the health unit.
8. Demonstrate professional and ethical standards. Discuss specific issues encountered and their method of resolution.
9. Incorporate teaching/learning principles to provide education to patients and family members. Give examples of education offered at the health department. Also discuss education programs implemented at the community level from the local HD and from the state health department. Select a written health education tool and determine its reading level.
10. Give examples of primary, secondary, and tertiary prevention measures offered at the HD.

Self-assessment evaluation of clinical experience: <Insert Clinical Judgment Rubric>

Arrival Time: _____   Departure Time: _____

---

laboratory to provide the wellness clinic on campus. Approximately 200 people participate each semester. The nursing program works with the campus human resources department, and the cost to those on the university's insurance plan may be reimbursed through an employee wellness benefit. Students experience an example of healthcare financing previously discussed in class and the cost-saving benefits that would appeal to a company that chooses to implement wellness programs. The students learn basic phlebotomy skills and draw blood samples. The experience emphasizes prevention and health promotion and how lifestyle affects biophysical indicators of health.

Nursing student participant in a campus wellness screening clinic.

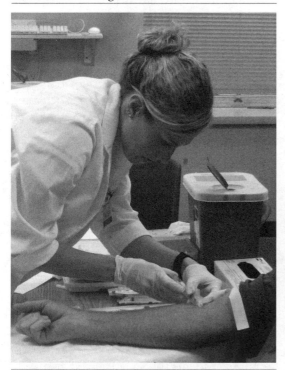

Source: Courtesy of Cathleen Shultz.

Before the wellness screenings, students prepare an educational poster that addresses Healthy People Objectives that are applicable to the target audience for the screening. The students must then consider the audience attending the wellness screening, obtain educational material to supplement the poster, and develop a distributable fact sheet to expand the poster's information. They search the Internet to find reliable sources to order educational materials. They must consider relevance to their poster topic, the cost, time for delivery, and any copyright issues with use. When screening participants wait for appointments, consume donated breakfast foods and drink, and exit the screenings, they visit the displayed posters. Campus wellness screenings were started by the nursing faculty over two decades ago, and there exists a loyal, repeat clientele who depend on these cost-saving services.

Wellness screening clinic poster created by students. The 3D colon model is constructed from fabric with marbles mimicking locations of tumors.

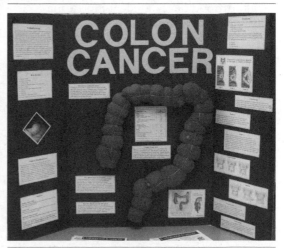

Source: Courtesy of Cathleen Shultz.

Simulation Experiences

DISASTER DRILL

Veenema (2006) reinforces that, as the largest sector of the healthcare workforce in the United States, nurses must be prepared in all aspects of disaster management. Although this article explores formal certificate and degree programs to train nurses in various aspects of disaster management, it also notes the overall importance of preparing nurses to effectively communicate with the wide variety of disciplines represented in disaster management teams. The skills to collaborate, assess, plan, problem solve, and make decisions are noted as essential for nurses being fully prepared to respond to disasters. Landry and Stockton (2008) describe adding disaster management content to undergraduate nursing education and emphasize the importance of including both theory content and hands-on simulated practice.

Disaster Drill/FEMA Course Online   The nursing program had initiated simulated

A damaged church building remains in a neighborhood devastated by Hurricane Katrina in Louisiana.

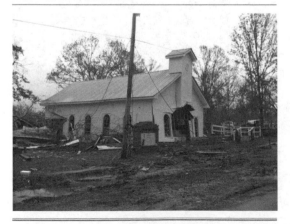

Source: Courtesy of Cathleen Shultz.

disaster drills for student learning in the community health nursing course and another senior clinical course in the past. Over time, and especially after 2001, the drill has morphed into a university–community partnership experience with win–win results. Hundreds of students, community agencies, and personnel now participate and the event is described in the following narrative.

Each spring semester the university conducts a disaster drill where nursing students and other community agencies respond to simulated events such as tornadoes and fires affecting a dorm or other campus buildings. Initiated by the College of Nursing as part of the public health nursing course, the drill has merged into a university- and community-wide event. The merger began as a conversation between nursing and theater faculty. Both disciplines realized the learning value potential of the experience for students. The first interdisciplinary drill was planned in the fall of 2001, and, because of the timing related to the events of September 11, interest and participation grew rapidly. Community agencies now participating include the local police, fire, emergency medical services, and hospital. Fire trucks, police cars, and ambulances and the uniformed responders add to the authenticity of the experience. These community agencies use the drill as training for their personnel, which provides increased community preparedness for actual events as well. The Public Safety Office coordinates university participation, and nursing faculty coordinate the participation of health-related academic areas. The local hospital receives "victims" and uses these victims to have a mass casualty drill for the emergency department. Senior nursing students in the public health nursing course plan the injuries and evaluate the response. Senior nursing students in an advanced medical–surgical nursing course respond to triage and treat victims. They bandage wounds, simulate starting intravenous fluids, and perform other emergency care at the scene. They provide information as to the number of victims and conditions to the medical officer in charge of the scene and observe the communication within the Incident Command System.

The theater students add an essential element of realism to the drill by accurately portraying victims and applying stage makeup to create very realistic injuries. The public health nursing students also learn the details of how the injury will appear and what signs and symptoms would be expected so they can portray the injuries appropriately and advise the theater students. The physician assistant and pharmacy students on campus also serve as victims and responders. Working with interdisciplinary teams is practiced under simulated but intense situations. Journalism and public relations students participate and the health-related students practice relating to the media. A first aid course is completed during a clinical day before the drill. Students view firsthand the Incident Command System operationalized on a local level, which they cover in class before the drill. They also complete the Introduction to the Incident Command System online Federal Emergency Management Agency (FEMA) course certification (http://www.fema.gov/emergency/nims/IncidentCommandSystem.shtm) as part of the preparatory work for the clinical experience.

The disaster drill is a simulated experience that provides opportunity to meet a variety of objectives. The most obvious is the clinical application of disaster management theory. Critical thinking is necessary to appropriately triage and treat victims. The students, through clinical conference discussion, also are aware of the positive influences that the drills have on preparedness for the university and the community. One of the first results was the creation

of an Emergency Management Committee for the university. A nursing faculty is on this committee that has members, both academic and administrative, from many areas of the university. During one drill, which simulated a dorm fire, the fire department had difficulty with master key access to all rooms during the search and rescue phase of the drill. This resulted in their recommendation to install Knox boxes, which allow the fire department access to entire buildings during an emergency. After these boxes were installed on campus buildings, the fire department then discussed the key difficulty with other community businesses and industries; many had Knox boxes installed as well. Each time the drill is conducted on campus, ways to increase safety are found and most are implemented. The drill enables the community to meet FEMA standards and the university to obtain excellent disaster management standards. Debriefing follows the drill to evaluate the response. University-involved academic areas and departments, as well as community agencies, participate to create an excellent way to maximize the learning experience.

Immunization Clinic

Students participate in the local health department's annual influenza immunization clinic. This clinic is also used by the department of health as a mass vaccination drill to prepare for a bioterrorism event. The dual purpose event provides an effective immunization learning opportunity. Many community members receive flu vaccine free of charge and the health department prepares for a disaster. Students work directly with the nurses at the local health department for this event. The students complete screening forms, educate patients, and administer the immunizations. They learn both concepts and skills related to mass vaccination and immunization status of populations.

Interdisciplinary students triage those injured in a simulated community disaster drill that meets community emergency management requirements.

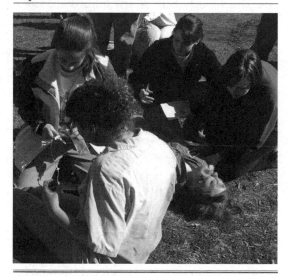

Source: Courtesy of Cathleen Shultz.

Service Learning

Lawler (2008) explored the development of professional nursing values through service-learning experiences. She noted the importance of reflection to the process of **service learning** and that guided reflection and discussion, facilitated by faculty, are crucial to students developing a deeper and broader understanding of the complex social issues commonly found in those utilizing services such as those found in public health nursing. Her findings supported the development of professional values, including **social justice** (Lawler, 2008). Describing a clinical experience that placed nursing students in a setting where they would be in direct and personal contact with those who are poor, DeLashmutt and Rankin (2005) noted that novice students' understanding "about poverty's impact on physical, mental and

spiritual well-being is usually inadequate and undeveloped" (p. 143). At the conclusion of the experience, nursing students demonstrated a much better understanding of the complex nature of poverty and the effective interventions to assist those who are poor.

Students must develop an understanding of poverty to effectively work with the poor who frequently engage public health services. In *Bridges Out of Poverty*, Payne, DeVol, and Smith (2001) outlined typical resources, such as financial, but focused on additional resources, such as emotional, mental, spiritual, coping strategies, knowledge of hidden rules of the social classes, and support systems, that those experiencing poverty frequently lack. The book provides practical ways professionals can assist individuals in acquiring missing resources so that students can effectively engage those in poverty in their health care and assist those in poverty to interact with and hopefully transition into a middle class work environment.

Faith-Based Clinic

A decade of planning that involved nursing faculty resulted in the opening of a free-standing clinic, staffed by various healthcare and other volunteers, within a mile of the university. Clinical experiences at the faith-based clinic for uninsured, low-income individuals provide opportunities for students to meet impoverished individuals who are the faces of the statistics and issues discussed in class. Many clients are homeless, experiencing intimate partner violence, or addicted to substances. Immigrant populations also attend this clinic, allowing an opportunity to develop skills in cultural competence. As the semester progresses, examples of poverty and related issues are from the students' clinical experiences. Connections are made between the determinants of health and poor health status. Students compare the health status of this

Faith-based clinic that provides interdisciplinary services to low-income, uninsured individuals.

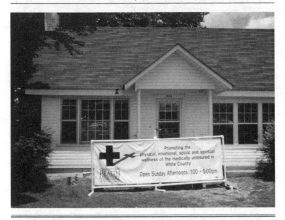

Source: Courtesy of Cathleen Shultz.

population with the wellness screening clinic participants. The differences are dramatic, making for meaningful learning experiences.

School Health Screenings

The students spend one or more clinical days assisting school nurses in the community area with the state-required screenings of hearing, vision, scoliosis, and body mass index. The students quickly realize the value of this service to the school nurses, the students at the school, and the community-at-large. They appreciate the difficulty of school nurses providing multiple required screenings in underfunded settings without assistance. The experience allows for meeting multiple objectives. An interesting related clinical conference focuses on the discrepancy between laws that are passed to mandate screenings and the frequent nonallocation of funding for adequate personnel to conduct the screenings. Outcomes data on the effectiveness of each type of screening program are researched and discussed during conference so that the student can evaluate whether the

screening is necessary based on those findings. The political process to make any needed future change is explored to further model the public health nursing role of advocacy. In this rural setting, over 30 years of nursing students' active involvement in school health have dramatically increased school children's overall health while meeting nursing student learning needs.

Paradigm Shift From Local to Global Worldview

Nurses practicing in future settings will be required to change their thinking paradigm from a local to a global worldview. Recognizing this need, faculty members have identified concepts and learning experiences to prepare graduates for the changing world. The umbrella concepts are social justice, healthcare missions, culture of poverty, global learning, and systems thinking.

Social Justice

A study on developing competencies in social justice, equity, and the social determinants of health explored how nursing education programs developed knowledge and skills in these three areas (Cohen & Gregory, 2009a, 2009b). Findings supported that content should be included in theory; further, these concepts also need to be embedded throughout the curriculum and exposed to areas in clinical experience where these factors can be explored. These are included in most clinical experiences in the community health nursing course. Elective courses are offered that strengthen this content.

Boutain (2008) describes the education of nursing students in social justice as "an urgent, yet complex undertaking" (p. 2). She describes student learning experiences about social justice in three stages: "1) social justice knowledge development, 2) social justice knowledge integration and issue identification, and 3) social justice action" (p. 3). Stages are described as built into the curriculum, and by the end of the senior community health nursing course, students were expected to take action on a social justice concern. A method of evaluation is described. "Without the action component, social justice teaching cannot be viewed as trans-formative" (Boutain, 2008, p. 1). In developing a model of faculty scholarship, Boyer (1990) suggested that academia explore ways to respond to social needs. He stated that the reality of the many social crises cause academicians to ask if all the resources of higher education could be of greater service to the nation and to the world.

The goal of educating nursing students about issues of social justice is that the knowledge they gain and the experiences they have will be transformative, becoming part of their lifelong practice. Like past leaders, nurses who actively work to promote social justice are needed to address the many social ills of today (Boutain, 2005). With nurses on the front lines in pub-lic health agencies in communities across the nation and the world, they are ideally placed for service. Having skill sets not just to care about the issues, but to address them effectively, is critical. Skills in community assessment and building community partnerships provide the groundwork for intervention, whereas skills in advocacy and engaging in the political process can be used to bring change to systems. Skills to work with those who are vulnerable enable nurses to develop interventions with individu-als, families, and communities most at risk.

Healthcare Missions

Since the mid-1970s, when the nursing program began, students and faculty have participated in domestic and international health mission expe-riences. The program now co-offers an interdis-ciplinary health missions minor and numerous

Newborn care in a Ghana hospital.

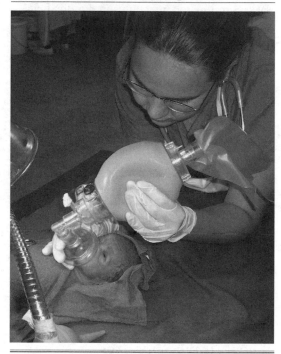

Source: Courtesy of Cathleen Shultz.

courses that can be taken by majors from other disciplines. Some of the courses also meet global literacy degree requirements. One of these elective courses is "Healthcare Missions," which many students choose to take. This course is taught by nursing faculty experienced in provid-ing health care in the developing world and is co-taught by a missions faculty member who has experience in development work in these coun-tries. The class includes content on global health issues such as tuberculosis, AIDS, and malaria, emphasizing their devastating impact on devel-oping countries. Learning activities such as how to make the World Health Organization's oral rehydration solution, treat parasites, and use of culturally appropriate skits to provide health teaching that might not be taught in traditional nursing courses in the United States are explored. As part of the course, students complete a weekend immersion experience a few miles from campus at the university's global village, where they practice bartering skills; cook with very limited ingredients and facilities; live in authentic housing such as an African hut, a Mexican barrio, or an Appalachian shack; and learn development strategies while working through cultural barriers.

Culture of Poverty

This elective course provides in-depth insight into understanding poverty and the worldview of those who are poor and the skills needed to effectively engage with those who are poor. Emphasis is on the culture of generational poverty, but situational poverty is also explored. Poverty, from U.S. and global perspectives, is analyzed for impact. Practical methods to understand and develop interventions to work with those who are poor are explored in depth with strategies such as the use of microdevelopment loans. An excerpt from the introduction of one course textbook states the urgency of community problems and why education in sustainable, effective solutions is necessary:

> *The economic insecurity of low-wage and the middle class threatens the viability of our communities. When members of the middle class flee the cities, taking the tax base and spending power with them . . . when Main Street empties of viable businesses and refills with pawn shops, used clothing stores, social service storefronts, and payday lenders . . . when people can't afford to stay in the community to raise their children because of the lack of well-paying jobs. . . .and when the free and reduced-price lunch rate at the schools hits 50%, our communities are becoming unsustainable. (Payne, DeVol, & Smith, 2001, p. 5)*

Emphasis is on the connection between poverty and health status.

Global Learning

The College of Nursing offers three annual international experiences in which students can participate. One is a spring break trip to Haiti where the students participate in community primary care clinics; the College of Nursing partners with a larger group from several area churches for this experience. Nursing faculty accompany the students, as do a variety of other professionals. During the spring semester the students also have an opportunity to go with a faith-based group on a medical mission trip to Guatemala. The group has an established hospital and clinics and coordinates multiple healthcare mission trips during the year. The recent focus of the students' experiences were gynecological surgery and plastic surgery for children with cleft lip and palates. The students work with nurses and provide around-the-clock postoperative care

Assessing a sick child's ears in a Tanzania clinic.

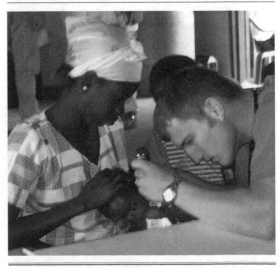

Source: Courtesy of Cathleen Shultz.

for those undergoing surgeries. One memorable story and photograph captured students and patients who were recovering from gynecological surgeries forming a "conga line," led by the volunteer nurses and nursing students, to provide postoperative ambulation.

In the summer, the College of Nursing selects a site in Africa where students go with a faculty member with advanced practice credentials who has long-term experience working as a nurse in Africa. In this immersion experience, the students work in clinics and a mission hospital while gaining experience in pediatrics and labor and delivery. They also obtain firsthand experience with global health issues such as poverty, HIV/AIDS, tuberculosis, malaria, and parasites. Students see death in those who are young and wrestle as never before with why the inequalities exist. Some of these sites have been managed for one to two decades, and long-term health improvements have been realized. Students receive ongoing preparation for months before entering another culture and are debriefed to assist with acculturation upon return.

These trips are all voluntary, but many students do choose to go and bring back those experiences they then share with other students, thus enriching the classes on global health issues. The programs aid all students in experiencing the ties to our global neighbors. Over 80% of the nursing majors voluntarily participate in healthcare missions and global learning, both of which develop their public health nursing knowledge, abilities, and aptitudes.

Systems Thinking

As the semester progresses, linking the information together and guiding the student to make the connections is an educational objective. By the end of the course, the student is expected to make the connections between the determinants of health and health status. The clinical project that ties all these concepts together is the community assessment. The students, through collaborative learning strategies, work on this all semester in groups of four or five. They divide the assessment data to be gathered and then, during the semester, have meetings with faculty who guide them in connecting theory to their findings, evaluating the strengths and weaknesses of the community, and establishing priority health-related problems. Goal setting at the population level is a complex process usually requiring faculty guidance. During this process students become able to develop interventions and population-focused plans of care.

Debriefing

Debriefing after public health nursing experiences occurs during clinical conferences. Debriefing, and evidence-based teaching and learning strategy, has historically been used in nursing education as a method to focus on learning outcomes and intended objectives of experiences (Jeffries & Rogers, 2007). The practice of debriefing varies by teacher. When debriefing involves reflection, students analyze accomplishments and events and think about enhancing and creating more skillful nursing practice. The process involves active engagement and maturing as a learner who evaluates self and others.

Dreifuerst (2009) identifies the attitudes of debriefing as reflection, emotion, reception, and integration and assimilation. Reflection involves reexamining the experience. Exploring and releasing emotions related to learning enhance experiences, but they can also inhibit learning if distraction from active engagement takes place. Teachers facilitate emotional expressions to promote reflective learning. Reception, as openness to feedback, addresses knowledge, skills, and aptitudes. This is a meaningful time to coach students to be open to receive feedback. Using formative feedback for critique and correction makes affective learning more visible (Kuiper, Heinrich, Matthias, Graham, & Bell-Kotwell, 2008). Integration of the experience may be the most difficult because it urges the learner to frame (i.e., attribute meaning to a set of facts [Pesut, 2004]) learning, usually for clinical settings, into the nursing process of the public health nurse. This sets the stage for accommodation and assimilation, the transfer of learning and experiences from one situation to the next. Anticipation, asking "what if" as a process of accommodation, represents higher order clinical judgment and reasoning based on meta-cognition (Benner, Stannard, & Hooper, 1996; Pesut, 2004; Tanner, 2006). "What if" questions that change the details and nursing process frame encourage students to think beyond the boundary of the experience and anticipate the next question. All defining attributes work in tandem during debriefing and optimize the clinical experiences. Omitting, minimizing, or discounting debriefing attributes may be harmful to student learning and future development within a program.

Nurse Educators: Embracing Public Health in Teaching, Learning, and Evaluation

Much of the clinical faculty responsibility lies in creating learning situations that facilitate public health learning outcomes. Clinical experiences can be developed in an educational culture that encourages partnerships with resources and support. Creating positive relationships with agency staff is an essential faculty skill. Because of the nature of clinical experiences related to public health, many of the experiences are mentored. For students to have positive experiences and therefore develop an interest in public health, they must have meaningful, engaging learning experiences. The importance of positive learning environments cannot be overstated. Because of the rural locations or nature of the public health experiences, students may be without peers or faculty present in the agency. If students do not feel welcomed by staff who convey that they want them there, and are willing to help them learn, they will have a less than optimal learning experience. Positive relationships with clinical agency staff assist nurse educators in planning learning and receiving student performance evaluations.

Created and simulated learning experiences require a great deal of time and coordination between academic and administrative departments at the university and community agencies. Faculty who teach these types of clinical experiences must be flexible, have excellent organizational abilities, and be able to make adjustments quickly. When such a large number and variety of people and agencies are involved with learning, rescheduling or changing plans is almost a certainty. So that students are not overwhelmed, the faculty ensures that all plans and changes are clearly communicated to students and that expectations are clear. Being actively engaged in university committees that are involved in the wellness program and emergency management are crucial to planning the wellness screenings and the disaster drill. Much work done by these committees has positively impacted the university and created excellent learning opportunities for the students that continue to improve.

Faculty who are fully engaged in the faculty role continue to develop while teaching. In addition to competence attainment for specialty practice, faculty members can use evidence-based teaching, learning, and evaluation practices. Although the latter task may seem daunting, attempting and refining select teaching practices through the annual review process builds one's expertise. The authors of this chapter have summarized essential teaching resources to strengthen development of learning and evaluating public health nursing content and experiences. Clearly these are fostered in a civil, healthy work environment.

Conclusion

Critical to developing a future public health nursing workforce is the response of nursing education programs to public health needs. While acknowledging barriers to preparing fully specialized public health nurses, nursing faculty are encouraged to address the basic elements in all nursing programs. Through a review of major national documents used as a public health approach framework, evidence-based teaching

and learning strategies are shared. Most have been developed over decades with seasoned faculty and willing students.

An overview of faculty and curriculum activities includes decisions to be made at the program, course, and learning experiences levels. Specific learning strategies, such as the clinical self-assessment journal, simulation, and clinical experiences that foster clinical reasoning and judgment while incorporating public health concepts and nursing roles, are discussed. Student knowledge, skills, and aptitudes development as public health nurses are encouraged in each learning experience.

A major goal of teaching public health nursing is shifting the learner's thinking paradigm from a local to a global worldview.

Equally important is relating that global world-view back to the local level; in other words, the world is now local. Strategies are discussed using these concepts: healthcare missions, culture of poverty, global learning, systems thinking, and debriefing. By incorporating a variety of community agencies and experiences, students see the network of agencies, organizations, professionals, and others in the communities that comprise the local public health system.

In Boyer's (1990) work on models of scholarship, he describes the scholarship of integration that illuminates the faculty role in teaching public health nursing, "making connections across the disciplines, placing the specialties in larger context, illuminating data in a revealing way...what we mean is serious, disciplined

work that seeks to interpret, draw together, and bring new insight to bear on original research" (pp. 18–19).

The connectedness of things is what the educator contemplates to the limit of his capacity. No human capacity is great enough to permit a vision of the world as simple, but if the educator does not aim at the vision no one else will, and the consequences are dire when no one does. (Mark Van Doren, in Boyer, 1990, p. 19)

Public health and nursing are both complex disciplines. Integration of the knowledge of both is necessary for the nurse educator teaching public health nursing. Nurses need the skills to look at entire systems and see how they affect populations and individuals.

References

American Nurses Association. (2003). *Nursing's social policy statement* (2nd ed.). Silver Spring, MD: Author.

American Nurses Association. (2007). *Public health nursing: Scope and standards of practice*. Silver Spring, MD: Author.

Association of Community Health Nursing Educators. (2000). *Essentials of baccalaureate nursing education for entry level community/public health nurses*. Pensacola, FL: Author.

Association of Community Health Nursing Educators. (2003). *Essentials of master's level nursing education for advanced community/public health nursing practice*. Lathrop, NY: Author.

Bambini, D., Washburn, J., & Perkins, R. (2009). Outcomes of clinical simulation for novice nursing students: Communication, confidence, clinical judgment. *Nursing Education Perspectives, 30*(2), 79–82.

Benner, P., Stannard, D., & Hooper, P. L. (1996). A "thinking-in-action" approach to teaching clinical judgment: A classroom innovation for acute care advanced practice nurses. *Advanced Practice Nursing Quarterly, 1*(4), 70–77.

Boutain, D. M. (2005). Social justice as a framework for professional nursing. *Journal of Nursing Education, 44*(9), 405–408.

Boutain, D. M. (2008). Social justice as a framework for undergraduate community health clinical experiences in the United States. *International Journal of Nursing Education Scholarship, 5*(1), 1–12.

Boyer, E. L. (1990). Scholarship reconsidered: Priorities of the professoriate. San Francisco, CA: Jossey-Bass.

Carter, K. F., Kaiser, K. L., O'Hare, P. A., & Callister, L. C. (2006). Use of PHN competencies and ACHNE essentials to develop teaching–learning strategies for generalist C/PHN curricula. *Public Health Nursing, 23*(2), 146–160.

Cato, M. L., Lasater, K., & Peeples, I. (2009). Nursing students' self-assessment of their simulation experiences. *Nursing Education Perspectives, 30*(2), 105–108.

Cohen, B. E., & Gregory, D. (2009a). Community health clinical education in Canada. Part 1. "State of the art." *International Journal of Nursing Education Scholarship, 6*(1), 1–17.

Cohen, B. E., & Gregory, D. (2009b). Community health clinical education in Canada. Part 2. Developing competencies to address social justice, equity, and the social determinants of health. *International Journal of Nursing Education Scholarship, 6*(1), 1–15.

Council on Linkages Between Academia and Public Health Practice. (2001). *Core competencies for public health professionals*. Washington, DC: Public Health Foundation.

Craft, M. (2005). Reflective writing and nursing education. *Journal of Nursing Education, 44*(2), 53–57.

Davies, P. (2002). Using student reflective self-assessment for awarding degree classifications. *Innovations in Education and Teaching International, 39*(4), 307–319.

DeLashmutt, M. B., & Rankin, E. A. (2005). A different kind of clinical experience: Poverty up close and personal. *Nurse Educator, 30*(4), 143–149.

Dreifuerst, K. T. (2009). The essentials of debriefing in simulation learning: A concept analysis. *Nursing Education Perspectives, 30*(2), 109–114.

Finkelman, A., & Kenner, C. (2007). *Teaching IOM: Implications of the Institute of Medicine reports for nursing education*. Silver Spring, MD: American Nurses Association.

Fitzpatrick, J. (2006). An evaluative case study of the dilemmas experienced in designing a self-assessment strategy for community nursing students. *Assessment & Evaluation in Higher Education, 31*(1), 37–53.

Institute of Medicine (IOM). (1988). *The future of public health*. Washington, DC: National Academies Press.

Institute of Medicine (IOM). (2003). *The future of public health in the 21st century*. Washington, DC: National Academies Press.

Jeffries, P. R., & Rogers, K. J. (2007). Theoretical framework for simulation design. In P. R. Jeffries (Ed.), *Simulation in nursing: From conceptualization to evaluation* (pp. 21–33). New York, NY: National League for Nursing.

Kuiper, R., Heinrich, C., Matthias, A., Graham, M. J., & Bell-Kotwell, L. (2008). Debriefing with the OPT model of clinical reasoning during high fidelity patient simulation. *International Journal of Nursing Education Scholarship, 5*(1), Article 17.

Landry, L. G., & Stockton, A. (2008). Evaluation of a collaborative project in disaster preparedness. *Nurse Educator, 33*(6), 254–258.

Lasater, K. (2007a). Clinical judgment development: Using simulation to create an assessment rubric. *Journal of Nursing Education, 46*(11), 496–503.

Lasater, K. (2007b). High-fidelity simulation and the development of clinical judgment: Students' experiences. *Journal of Nursing Education, 46*(6), 269–276.

Lasater, K., & Nielsen, A. (2009). Reflective journaling for clinical judgment development. *Journal of Nursing Education, 48*(1), 40–44.

Lawler, K. B. (2008). *Service-learning and the development of professional nursing values in adult undergraduate students*. Retrieved from http://proquest.umi.com/pqdweb?index=null&did=1609700001&SrchMode=5&Fmt=2&re

Maclellan, E., & Soden, R. (2006). Facilitating self-regulation in higher education through self-report. *Learning Environments Research, 9*, 95–110.

Nicol, D. J., & Macfarlane-Dick, D. (2006). Formative assessment and self-regulated learning: A model and seven principles of good feedback practice. *Studies in Higher Education, 31*(2), 199–218.

Nielsen, A., Stragnell, S., & Jester, P. (2007). Guide for reflection using the clinical judgment model. *Journal of Nursing Education, 46*(11), 513–516.

Payne, R. K., DeVol, P. E., & Smith, T. D. (2001). *Bridges out of poverty: Strategies for professionals and communities*. Highlands, TX: AHA Process.

Pesut, D. J. (2004). Reflective clinical reasoning. In L. Hayes, H. Butcher, & T. Boese (Eds.), *Nursing in contemporary society* (pp. 146–162). Upper Saddle River, NJ: Pearson-Prentice Hall.

Roberts, M. M. (1954). *American nursing: History and interpretation*. New York, NY: Macmillan.

Quad Council of Public Health Nursing Organizations. (1999). *Scope and standards of public health nursing practice*. Washington, DC: American Nurses Association.

Quad Council of Public Health Nursing Organizations. (2004). Public health nursing competencies. *Public Health Nursing, 21*(5), 443–452.

Shultz, C. M. (Ed.). (2009a). *Building a science of nursing education: Foundation for evidence based teaching-learning*. New York, NY: National League for Nursing.

Shultz, C. M. (2009b, April/May). Preparing to work in an informatics-based world. *Imprint*, 36–39.

Tanner, C. A. (2006). Thinking like a nurse: A research-based model of clinical judgment. *Journal of Nursing Education, 45*(6), 204–211.

Veenema, T. G. (2006). Expanding educational opportunities in disaster response and emergency preparedness for nurses. *Nursing Education Perspectives, 27*(2), 93–99.

Winslow, C. E. A. (1920). The untilled fields of public health. *Science, New Series, 51*(1306), 22–33.

For a full suite of assignments and additional learning activities, use the access code located in the front of your book to visit this exclusive website: http://go.jblearning.com/londrigan. If you do not have an access code, you can obtain one at the site.

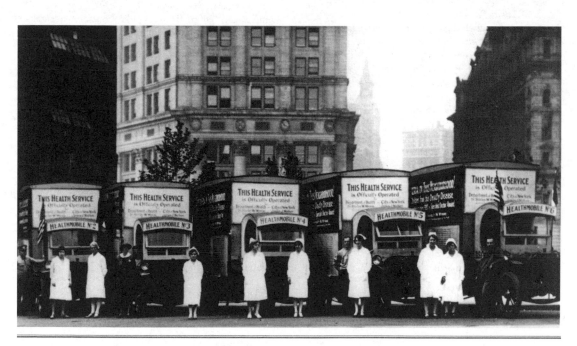

Source: Courtesy of the Visiting Nurse Service of New York.

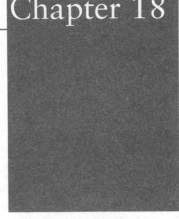

Chapter 18

Conversation About Primary Health Care

Marie Truglio-Londrigan
Joanne Singleton
Sandra B. Lewenson
Liliana Lopez

It is true that in the future as in the past, the course nursing takes will be determined to a great extent by social forces and conditions which no one can entirely for see or control. But the nursing group, by thoughtful planning and well-directed effort, can do much to influence its own destiny and it is not too much to say that it may also influence the destiny of the human race (Dock & Stewart, 1938, p. 354).

LEARNING OBJECTIVES

By the completion of this chapter, the reader will be able to

- Discuss the difference between primary health care and primary care
- Describe how the Declaration of Alma-Ata influenced primary health care

- Debate the challenges to the delivery of primary health care

KEY TERMS

- ❏ Cultural authority
- ❏ Declaration of Alma-Ata
- ❏ Primary care

- ❏ Primary health care
- ❏ Social legitimacy

When the authors of this text began to contemplate what type of content would be presented within its pages, it was clear that the focus would be on the public and how healthcare practitioners may work together with the public in the achievement of one primary goal: health for all Americans. The areas to be discussed would be the science of public health as well as the types of interventions that are necessary for the attainment of our goal. The implementation of these interventions in a collaborative way with the public, however, is not enough. What we need, as a nation, is to shift our worldview so that we first acknowledge that there are ways of practicing other than our present day medical care model, which is *not* synonymous with health care, and then to have the courage to navigate these uncharted waters.

When President Barack Obama signed the Patient Protection and Affordable Care Act (PPACA) in 2010, the possibilities of what may be for our healthcare system shifted. For some, the imbalance is unsettling; for others, there is excitement. There is acknowledgment among all that this PPACA "does not focus solely on physician-provided medical care to individual patients. Instead, the statute is suffused with provisions that promise to elevate the status of, and national commitment to, disease prevention wellness promotion, and population based interventions" (Deville & Novick, 2011, p. 102).

The authors of this text and of this chapter embrace this shift. It is our belief that the path we must walk is a path known as **primary health care**. This idea of primary health care has already been discussed elsewhere in this text, so the purpose of this chapter is to reconsider primary health care in light of this previous discussion. We invite the reader to consider all aspects of public health and primary health care in relationship with nursing's role in making this shift.

The Declaration of Alma-Ata

In 1978, the saying "Health for All" was coined by the World Health Organization (WHO) and the idea of primary health care was derived as the means of achieving this goal. So strong was this belief that at the International Conference on Primary Health Care (1978) the **Declaration of Alma-Ata** expressed a call to action by all governments and world communities to promote and to protect all people. This Declaration contains 10 principal points, the 6th and 7th of which speak specifically to the idea of primary health care. The entire Declaration may be viewed in **Box 18-1**.

A careful review of this document informs the reader of the worldview of those who had a vision and put that vision into words so that others may place these words into actions. First and foremost, health is seen as a basic human right that requires the action of many, but it also recognizes that there are inequities that are unacceptable and a concern to all. The declaration acknowledges that health for all is essential to economic and social development and enhances quality of life. Furthermore, the declaration is clear that "the people" need to be active participants in the attainment of this health both individually and collectively. Additionally, not only are people key to the attainment of health, but governments are responsible for the health of their own people and that these governments must formulate policies that will facilitate and sustain primary health care. Finally, primary health care is seen as the key to attaining the health of the people.

Primary Health Care

As mentioned in the previous paragraph, the sixth and the seventh principal points speak

Box 18-1 Declaration of Alma-Ata

Declaration of Alma-Ata International Conference on Primary Health Care, Alma-Ata, USSR, September 6–12, 1978

The International Conference on Primary Health Care, meeting in Alma-Ata this twelfth day of September in the year Nineteen hundred and seventy-eight, expressing the need for urgent action by all governments, all health and development workers, and the world community to protect and promote the health of all the people of the world, hereby makes the following

Declaration:

I

The Conference strongly reaffirms that health, which is a state of complete physical, mental and social wellbeing, and not merely the absence of disease or infirmity, is a fundamental human right and that the attainment of the highest possible level of health is a most important world-wide social goal whose realization requires the action of many other social and economic sectors in addition to the health sector.

II

The existing gross inequality in the health status of the people particularly between developed and developing countries as well as within countries is politically, socially and economically unacceptable and is, therefore, of common concern to all countries.

III

Economic and social development, based on a New International Economic Order, is of basic importance to the fullest attainment of health for all and to the reduction of the gap between the health status of the developing and developed countries. The promotion and protection of the health of the people is essential to sustained economic and social development and contributes to a better quality of life and to world peace.

IV

The people have the right and duty to participate individually and collectively in the planning and implementation of their health care.

V

Governments have a responsibility for the health of their people which can be fulfilled only by the provision of adequate health and social measures. A main social target of governments, international organizations and the whole world community in the coming decades should be the attainment by all peoples of the world by the year 2000 of a level of health that will permit them to lead a socially and economically productive life. Primary health care is the key to attaining this target as part of development in the spirit of social justice.

VI

Primary health care is essential health care based on practical, scientifically sound and socially acceptable methods and technology made universally accessible to individuals and families in the community through their full participation and at a cost that the community and country can afford to maintain at every stage of their development in the spirit of self-reliance and self-determination. It forms an integral part both of the country's health system, of which it is the central function and main focus, and of the overall social and economic development of the community. It is the first level of contact of individuals, the family and community with the national health system bringing health care as close as possible to where people live and work, and constitutes the first element of a continuing health care process.

VII

Primary health care:
1. reflects and evolves from the economic conditions and sociocultural and political characteristics of the country and its communities and is based on the application of the relevant results of social, biomedical and health services research and public health experience;

(continues)

Box 18-1 *(continued)*

2. addresses the main health problems in the community, providing promotive, preventive, curative and rehabilitative services accordingly;
3. includes at least: education concerning prevailing health problems and the methods of preventing and controlling them; promotion of food supply and proper nutrition; an adequate supply of safe water and basic sanitation; maternal and child health care, including family planning; immunization against the major infectious diseases; prevention and control of locally endemic diseases; appropriate treatment of common diseases and injuries; and provision of essential drugs;
4. involves, in addition to the health sector, all related sectors and aspects of national and community development, in particular agriculture, animal husbandry, food, industry, education, housing, public works, communications and other sectors; and demands the coordinated efforts of all those sectors;
5. requires and promotes maximum community and individual self-reliance and participation in the planning, organization, operation and control of primary health care, making fullest use of local, national and other available resources; and to this end develops through appropriate education the ability of communities to participate;
6. should be sustained by integrated, functional and mutually supportive referral systems, leading to the progressive improvement of comprehensive health care for all, and giving priority to those most in need;
7. relies, at local and referral levels, on health workers, including physicians, nurses, midwives, auxiliaries and community workers as applicable, as well as traditional practitioners as needed, suitably trained socially and technically to work as a health team and to respond to the expressed health needs of the community.

VIII

All governments should formulate national policies, strategies and plans of action to launch and sustain primary health care as part of a comprehensive national health system and in coordination with other sectors. To this end, it will be necessary to exercise political will, to mobilize the country's resources and to use available external resources rationally.

IX

All countries should cooperate in a spirit of partnership and service to ensure primary health care for all people since the attainment of health by people in any one country directly concerns and benefits every other country. In this context the joint WHO/UNICEF report on primary health care constitutes a solid basis for the further development and operation of primary health care throughout the world.

X

An acceptable level of health for all the people of the world by the year 2000 can be attained through a fuller and better use of the world's resources, a considerable part of which is now spent on armaments and military conflicts. A genuine policy of independence, peace, détente and disarmament could and should release additional resources that could well be devoted to peaceful aims and in particular to the acceleration of social and economic development of which primary health care, as an essential part, should be allotted its proper share.

The International Conference on Primary Health Care calls for urgent and effective national and international action to develop and implement primary health care throughout the world and particularly in developing countries in a spirit of technical cooperation and in keeping with a New International Economic Order. It urges governments, WHO and UNICEF, and other international organizations, as well as multilateral and bilateral agencies, nongovernmental organizations,

Box 18-1 (*continued*)

funding agencies, all health workers and the whole world community to support national and international commitment to primary health care and to channel increased technical and financial support to it, particularly in developing countries.

The Conference calls on all the aforementioned to collaborate in introducing, developing and maintaining primary health care in accordance with the spirit and content of this Declaration.

Source: World Health Organization [WHO]. (1978). *Declaration of Alma-Ata.* Retrieved from www.euro.who.int/__data/assets/pdf_file/0009/113877/E93944.pdf

---

specifically about primary health care. The Alma-Ata Declaration of 1978 formally defined primary health care as:

essential health care based on practical, scientifically sound, and socially acceptable methods and technology made universally accessible to individuals and families in the community through their full participation and at a cost that the community and country can afford to maintain at every stage of their development in the spirit of self-reliance and self-determination. It forms an integral part both of the country's health system, of which it is the central function and main focus, and of the overall social and economic development of the community. It is the first level of contact of individuals, the family, and community with the national health system bringing health care as close as possible to where people live and work, and constitutes the first element of a continuing health care process. (WHO, 1978, para. 6)

The Declaration is very specific when it comes to primary health care and highlights several additional areas of interest. These include the notion that primary health care:

- Reflects the culture of the nation and its people; therefore, the development of

health initiatives takes place with the people and where the people are. In this way, these health initiatives will be culturally sensitive and appropriate, thus making them congruent with the people and their ideas, values, and beliefs.

- Addresses all areas of health including health promotion, disease prevention, and curative care, including the availability and accessibility of needed medications and immunizations as well as rehabilitation. In this way, primary health care is seen as a philosophy and a way to practice that is inclusive of all contexts, not just the community.

- Includes education toward the attainment of health as well as essentials for public health, such as clean water, sanitation, and nutrition. Education must reflect cultural ideas, values, and beliefs as well as focus on educational strategies that are congruent with the population and their needs.

- Involves more than healthcare practitioners and is inclusive of multiple sectors of the community and thus multiple partners.

- Requires maximum participation and partnering with individuals, families, communities, and populations. This partnering may be a challenge, but it reflects a true working relationship where all individuals are considered essential and all voices are heard—where all people assume responsibility in shared decision making in the development of health initiatives and the movement toward stated goals.

Take a few minutes and, as a group, critically examine the Declaration provided for you in Box 18-1, specifically points six and seven. Think about the type of care you have seen rendered in your past clinical experiences. Identify one specific care initiative and answer the following questions:

- In what ways is that care initiative reflective of the Declaration and primary health care?
- In what ways is that care initiative ineffective?
- Can you take one of your clinical experiences and shape and shift it so that it is reflective of the worldview and practices of primary health care?

What Has Been Our Progress?

It has been over 30 years since the introduction of the Declaration of Alma-Ata, and many have questioned how far we have come as a nation and globally. While it is true there have been changes and improvements with water access, sanitation, and antenatal care, there have been other areas where progress has not been as aggressive. For example, health and the attainment of health have been unequal across countries, and the identification of inequalities within countries is noted (WHO, 2008). If one considers the United States as an example, would you say that health and access to health is equitable across all populations? Several trends represent barriers to the attainment of health for all; these are noted in Box 18-2.

There are initiatives, within certain countries, that have attempted to meet the challenge of ensuring their people have health care. **Table 18-1** provides several exemplars of such endeavors. Take a few minutes to read these exemplars. Do you see elements that are reflective of the Declaration and of primary health care? A space has been provided for you in the table to draw out these elements for discussion.

We can see from the exemplars that the worldview and philosophy of primary health care considers health care to be more than the medical treatment of disease: it takes into consideration prevention and is responsive to the unique needs of the community and the vulnerable members of that community. Primary health care is broader and also focuses on fair and equal access to housing, education, and employment for each citizen (Heggenhougen, 1984).

Box 18-2 Challenges Toward the Achievement of Health

Aging Population
Worldwide Transmission of Communicable
  Diseases
Burden of Chronic and Noncommunicable
  Disorders
Climate Changes
Food Security
Social Tensions
Economic and Political Crises That Challenge
  Access and Delivery of Services
Failure of Health Sectors to Anticipate and
  Respond to Health Challenges
Under-resources in Countries

Source: Adapted from World Health Organization. (2008). *The world health report 2008: Primary health care now more than ever.* Geneva, Switzerland: Author.

Table 18-1 EXEMPLARS OF PRIMARY HEALTH CARE

Exemplar	Elements Reflective of the Declaration and Primary Health Care

New York City
Mobile Health Van

The purpose of the mobile health van program is to reach out to the underserved and uninsured population living in shelters and poor areas of New York City. It is imperative to go to the specific sites or buildings where people live to provide services to people who may not have access to medical care, who choose not to get care in a traditional health setting because the services or the context of the services are not acceptable, or who may lack the monetary funds to afford transportation to access these needed services. Once registered in the mobile van, patients can go back to their buildings to wait to be seen. Not having to wait in a clinic setting or in the van is very convenient for the patients because they can just wait in their apartment to be called. The mobile van provides all the primary care services found in any clinic setting. It is staffed by a driver, nurse (LPN), and family nurse practitioner who is bilingual (English and Spanish) and who has made herself available anytime with the use of a cell phone.
These services include regular physicals, school or employment physicals, immunizations, internal medicine, women's health, pediatrics, treatment for adolescents, etc. Any referrals are done accordingly.
Patients are coming back keeping their appointments, and bringing their entire families (Lopez, Personal Communication, June 2011).

Thailand

Primary Health Care in Thailand has been deemed a success. Part of the reason for this success has been attributed to the role of community volunteer. These volunteers included Buddhist Monks at the temples of Thailand, many of which are located in rural areas. In the 1990s, there was a change in how the people of Thailand lived their lives. The monks had to reflect on how they were providing help to their people. Based on these reflections, the monks continue to provide services to the population with added emphasis on health promotion and disease prevention. Communities are encouraged to participate in these services as other community members are active in the volunteer work (WHO, 2011).

(continues)

Table 18-1 (continued)

Exemplar	Elements Reflective of the Declaration and Primary Health Care
The Cuban National Health System	

The development of the Cuban health system began after their revolution, starting in the rural areas making progress toward the urban areas; since then, there has been a continual evolution of the national system toward primary health care. The Cuban National Health System is organized into three levels. The first level is seen as the point of entry where primary care is offered by a physician and nurse. The team sees their patients at the clinic at one point in the day and makes home visits at other times. These primary care clinics are known as neighborhood clinics, which are located throughout Cuba. Many doctors and nurses live in the environment in which they practice. The nurse and the doctor, together along with other members of the team, see to environmental, psychological, and social issues. These other professionals may include social workers, sanitation workers, and others who can attend to issues outside of physical health. The second level of care involves making acute and long-term care available. The third level of care is the more specialized care (Feinsilver, 1993; Whiteford & Branch, 2008). Part of this community system involves the local health brigade members who must attend classes to learn how to work with the people in the neighborhood and serve to "facilitate community participation in health promotion campaigns" (Whiteford & Branch, 2008, p. 44).

This worldview was further expanded upon by Rifkin and Walt (1986), who noted that primary health care consists of not only medical services, but also cultural, economic, and environmental factors that facilitate or prevent the onset of illness. Furthermore, these authors identified several important distinctions that need to be considered when speaking about primary health care: (a) health for all and the attainment of such will take place when there is equitable distribution of social rights and privileges, (b) the importance of access to basic goods such as food, shelter, education, and employment, and (c) the need to understand the importance of community involvement and a multi-sectorial approach to health issues. Primary health care is community-based and aims to promote self-efficacy; therefore, we may see that primary health care is not merely improvements in the provision of health services; it is also "understanding and improving the range of social, political, and economic factors which ultimately influence the improvement of health status" (Rifkin & Walt, 1986, p. 561). This view was later supported by Heggenhougen (1993) who spoke to the need to shift away from the unidimensional medical understanding of health and illness to one that understood the importance of the biological, environmental, and sociocultural factors and how these may either disturb or enhance health. More recently, the WHO (2008) developed a comprehensive report discussing the need for reform in several areas if we are to shift away from this unidimensional way of practicing. These areas included service delivery reform, public policy reform, leadership reform, and universal coverage reform.

Why the Struggle?

While it is clear that there has been progress and it appears that primary health care continues to be relevant, there are still challenges ahead. In the U.S. healthcare system, primary health care does not seem to be the driving force. We still hold on to a system that focuses on specialized curative care with an approach to disease control that sponsors short-term results and fragmentation of service delivery (WHO, 2008). Part of the reason for this struggle is that despite the 30-year history of primary health care, the term still creates confusion for some. Gordon and Plamping (1996) discussed the lack of a shared understanding of primary health care and indicated that one of the reasons for this is that hospital care is much more visible and demonstrative and that primary health care is much more complex. For example, consider some of the points that are made in the definition of primary health care. When a definition speaks to the importance of culture in primary healthcare initiatives, what does this mean? Are we really culturally and socially astute? Do we really conduct cultural assessments of the communities and people we are working with? Do we really understand the

communities' culture or the people's culture? Are we really sensitive to their needs? When we develop health initiatives, are they really culturally congruent? When we develop community initiatives where community participation is key, whose community are we referring? Is it the community as defined by the people or is it a community defined by the administrators of a hospital or some other external group (Wayland & Crowder, 2002)? When we speak about community participation, what do we mean by this? Do we really understand the importance of this type of participation? Do we understand how to initiate partnerships and coalitions and sustain those partnerships? What about communication and shared decision making in these partnerships? Do we understand the skills that are inherent within these words? Are we ready to live in a world where we share and facilitate the empowerment of the people? The purpose of these questions is to illustrate the complexity of the primary healthcare worldview and to also demonstrate that the values inherent within this worldview may be values not everyone may be comfortable acknowledging and accepting.

Values are important to consider. They are concepts and ideas that we hold dear, and they "serve as standards for how we understand ourselves and the world around us, and we often use them as a basis for our decisions and actions" (Heard, 1990, p. 1). In American culture, certain values are more dominant than others. Beauchamp (1985) noted that in the United States, the dominant language of politics is that of individualism, while the community is considered secondary. Individualism is rooted deeply in our historical consciousness. Individualism focuses on "the human condition as it exists apart from others and serves to promote ideas of personal freedom, self-improvement, privacy, achievement, independence, detachments, and self-interest" (Heard, 1990, p. 3). The second value, known as community, sets forth a view of people "within the context of human relationships. It concentrates on qualities that people have through their associations with others such as intimacy, benevolence, fellowship, belonging, dependence, social involvement, and the public good" (Heard, 1990, p. 3). To further explain this, contemplate the term of equity—so essential for primary health care—identified earlier in this text. If we speak of equity of services and enhancing access, we must also ensure social and economic justice for all. Now reflect on "health for all" with equity of services along with the attainment of social and economic justice. From what values do these emanate? When one considers this question, some will select the value of community, especially because that particular value speaks to the public good. Now, consider the Declaration of Alma-Ata and specifically point number five, which speaks to the responsibility of the government in ensuring the health of its people. Given the emphasis on the value of individualism within the American culture and the American government, this informs us as to why some people who have a stronger leaning toward the values of individualism may have difficulty welcoming the idea of primary health care.

Analyzing the two values of individualism and community, we can see the tension that exists between them because they both are present in our American culture. This does not mean that a transformation in our social consciousness is impossible, but it does mean that it will take a willingness to listen and an openness to the idea of primary health care for there to be a shift in worldviews or a cultural transformation in our ideas. Remember that with this shifting of worldview, there is an opportunity for acceptance of primary health care, which will lead to a sharing of power and a much-needed restructuring and redistribu-

tion of care and services. Heggenhougen (1984) noted primary health care will "ultimately lead to a reduction in the greater benefit for the few to the greater benefit for the many" (p. 217). How do you suppose this is received by the few? According to Cueto (2004), there is increasing resistance among some professionals because "they fear losing privileges, prestige, and power" (p. 1872). Our present healthcare system is steeped in our own American culture, with certain values being stronger than others. Taking this into account, any alteration in our worldview will require a shift toward seeing that health for all citizens is a fundamental right that can take place only with the restructuring of our healthcare system.

A final point to be made about the struggle for primary health care refers to the confusion that exists between it and the term **primary care**. They are not one and the same, although the similarities in their names may cause individuals to believe that they are. "Primary care is often used interchangeably with primary medical care as its focus is on clinical services provided predominantly by [general practitioners], as well as by practice nurses, primary/community health care nurses, early childhood nurses and community pharmacists" (The University of New South Wales, 2010, para. 3). According to a report of the National Primary Health Care Conference of 2004, primary care:

> *deals mainly with the prevention and treatment of sickness.... Primary care may involve immunization, preventative advice (stop smoking, get some exercise), diagnosis and treatment of illness, but it stops short of a comprehensive, intersectional approach to producing or enhancing health. Perhaps most importantly, primary care is focused on individuals and families, but not the community as the unit of intervention. (Edwards et al., 2004, p. 4)*

Primary care serves the necessary purpose of treating the patient based on a model that "involves a single service or intermittent management of a person's specific illness or disease condition in a service that is typically contained to a time-limited appointment, with or without follow-up and monitoring or an expectation of provider–client interaction beyond that visit" (Keleher, 2001, p. 59). Hence, in the United States, primary care "remains a medical model" (Murray, 2011, p. 3). This primary care has served us well, and because of this accomplishment of our medical care system, physicians have achieved **cultural authority** that has also lead to the establishment of **social legitimacy** (De Ville & Novick, 2011, p. 106), making it difficult to shift worldviews that may be more in line with primary health care.

Contemplating these two ideas—primary care and primary health care—the authors of this chapter wonder if the shifting of this worldview encompasses a shift to broaden our vision rather than to look in a new direction. Primary care is a way of practicing between the practitioner and the individual or family. As practitioners conduct their practice, there is a need for them to broaden their view and see beyond the individual or family sitting in front of them. This broadening of their worldview presents them with a vision of a population of people who can participate in making decisions that pertain to their care and the potential for an intersectoral collaborative practice that together works toward primary healthcare initiatives. This shift also includes a conscious awareness of the need to balance the values of individualism and community in such as way that fits the cultural identity of this nation. **Figure** 18-1 offers a visual depiction of this model.

The Teaching of a Philosophy

The section above provides a brief overview as to some of the reasons why there has been difficulty with our culture's ability to embrace the philosophy of primary health care. This is a text that focuses on population-based care and public health nursing for educational purposes. The authors of this chapter see in the field of education a way and means to introduce to the reader this worldview for consumption and for emulation. Has nursing generally and have nurses individually conducted their practice according to the principles of primary health care? How does one teach this philosophy? According to Cueto (2004), one of the struggles of medicine in the acceptance and application of primary health care is in the fact that "there is no steady effort to reorganize medical education around primary health care" (p. 1872). Can the same be true for nursing education?

In learning any health profession, acquisition of knowledge and skills is essential to practice. Providing knowledge and skills requires a dedicated focus to include this content in the curriculum, including didactic and clinical experiences. With this experience, however, comes a greater responsibility to understand the many social determinants of health that impact those we care for in the world of primary care and make the connection with primary health care. In preparing students for the health disciplines, differentiating primary care and primary health care is imperative to addressing and meeting the needs of the nation's health. Helping students to understand this difference will allow them, when they are ready, to have their "aha! moment" and to embrace the larger context of practice. An education about primary care without primary health care is an incomplete education.

The second chapter of this text, written by Sandra B. Lewenson, is entitled *Public Health*

Figure 18-1 Health for all citizens.

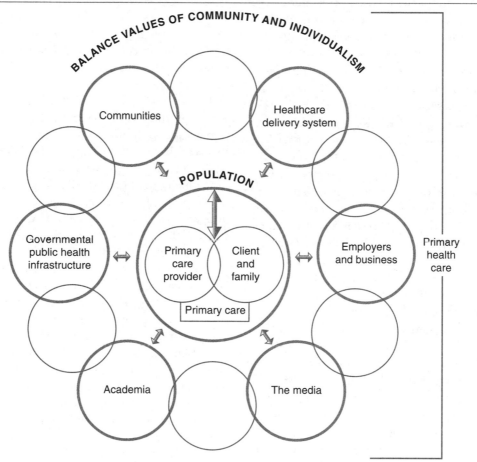

*This model facilitates a participatory approach and shared decision making

Source: Adapted from Institute of Medicine (2003). *The Intersectorial Public Health System: The Future of the Public's Health in the 21st Century.* Washington, DC: National Academy Press.

Nursing in the United States: A History. Reading this chapter informs us that nurses, particularly in public health nursing, have been practicing primary health care all along. As you read this chapter, point out the areas to which the Declaration of Alma-Ata refers. **Box 18-3** provides a more detailed example.

Take the time to read and reflect on how the conduct of these nurses emulated the principles of public health nursing and primary health care. Perhaps it is our professional heritage that facilitates our acceptance of these three words and a willingness to embrace all that primary health care has to offer. In fact, if one considers the 17 intervention strategies, these in and of themselves demonstrate the methods that nurses in general may use to practice primary health care. Furthermore, this chapter allows us to consider and articulate the connections between primary health care and the public health nursing interventions that we, as a profession, have always performed and will continue to perform. We in the profession of nursing are poised to meet the challenges in the recent Institute of Medicine report, *The Future of Nursing* (2011), specifically key message number three, which states, "Nurses should be full partners, with physicians and other health professionals, in redesigning health care in the United States" (p. 4).

BOX 18-3 PRIMARY HEALTH CARE AND PUBLIC HEALTH NURSING: AN EXAMPLE FROM HISTORY

The noted early 20th century public health nursing leader, Lillian Wald, believed in primary health care, even though the term itself was not yet used. Wald contributed to the health of populations living in urban centers as well as in rural communities. Not content to provide access to health care just to those living in New York City, Wald believed that those living in rural communities throughout the United States deserved the same kind of care. Wald's visionary leadership led to the establishment of the Red Cross Rural Nursing Service, which opened in 1912 and continued, under different names, until 1948. Wald saw the American Red Cross as a viable organization that could expand its wartime activities into peacetime initiatives that would bring public health nursing services into rural communities. Wald sought support from philanthropists, governmental officials, and nursing leaders to create a structure that supported public health nursing efforts in rural, isolated communities.

Each nurse who met the requirements for joining the American Red Cross and had a minimum of 4 months additional training as a public health nurse in rural communities could serve in this new capacity. These nurses would go into communities and work with various organizations within these communities, such as school boards, boards of health, or women's clubs, to bring health education, vaccinations, and other primary healthcare-type activities to the populations living within the communities. One of the later directors of this rural public health nursing service, Elizabeth Fox (1932) described the growth of this service throughout the first half of the 1900s as follows: "One by one, to the southern mountains, to mining camps, to farming counties, to small towns, to an industrial village, went Red Cross nurses, often the first to undertake rural work in a given State, and with them went a constant stream of wise advice and encouragement" (p. 173). These nurses provided bedside nursing when needed, set up well-baby clinics in rural settings, brought nursing into schools and industrial settings, arranged classes for mothers in home hygiene and care of the sick, and educated populations about how to stay healthy. Fox (1921) saw Red Cross public health nurses as the trailblazers: they tried to "fill the gaps in the health organization of the country and to blaze the trail in the unreached areas" (p. 108). Between 1912 and 1947, there were over "3,109 public health nursing services in about 1,800 counties under the sponsorship of some 2,100 chapters—a notable contribution to the health of America and an influence on many other agencies" (Kernodle, 1949, p. 469).

References

Beauchamp, D. E. (1985). Community: The neglected tradition of public health. *Hastings Center Report, 15*(6), 28–36.

Cueto, M. (2004). The origins of primary health care and selective primary health care. *American Journal of Public Health, 94*(11), 1864–1873.

DeVille, K., & Novick, L. (2011). Swimming upstream? Patient Protection and Affordable Care Act and the cultural ascendancy of public health. *Journal of Public Health Management and Practice, 17*(2), 102–109.

Dock, L., & Stewart, I. M. (1938). *A short history of nursing* (4th ed.). New York, NY: G. P. Putnam's Sons.

Edwards, J., Hicks, S., O'Neill, M., Corby, L., Kulkarni, L., Wiktorowicz, B., & Cooper, J. (2004). *A thousand points of light? Moving forward on primary health care.* A synthesis of key themes and ideas from the National Primary Health Care Conference, Winnipeg, Manitoba. Retrieved from http://www.eicp.ca/en/ resources/pdfs/PHC_Conference_Synthesis_Report.pdf

Feinsilver, J. (1993). *Healing the masses: Cuban health politics at home and abroad.* Berkeley, CA: University of California Press.

Gordon, E., & Plamping, D. (1996). Primary health care: Its characteristics and potential. In E. Gordon & J. Hadley (Eds.), *Extending primary care: Polyclinics, resource centers, hospitals-at-home* (pp. 1–15). Oxford, UK: Radcliffe.

Heard, G. C. (1990). *Basic values and ethical decision: An examination of individualism and community in American society.* Malabar, FL: Robert E. Krieger Publishing

Heggenhougen, H. (1993). PHC and anthropology: Challenges and opportunities (Review of the book *Anthropology and primary health care*). *Culture, Medicine and Psychiatry, 17*(2), 281–289.

Heggenhougen, H. K. (1984). Will primary health care efforts be allowed to succeed? *Social Sciences and Medicine, 19*(3), 217–224.

Institute of Medicine. (2011). *The future of nursing: Leading change, and advancing health.* Washington, DC: National Academies Press.

Keleher, H. (2001). Why primary health care offers a more comprehensive approach for tackling health inequities than primary care. *Australian Journal of Primary Health, 7*(2), 57–61.

Kernodle, P. B. (1949). *The Red Cross nurse in action 1882–1948.* New York, NY: Harper and Brothers.

Murray, L. R. (2011). Public health and primary care: Transforming the U.S. health system. *The Nation's Health, 41*(3), 1–35.

Rifkin, S., & Walt, G. (1986). Why health improves: Defining the issues concerning comprehensive primary health care. *Social Science Medicine, 23*(6), 559–566.

The University of New South Wales. (2010). *Primary Health Care Connect.* Retrieved from http://www. phcconnect.unsw.edu.au/

Wayland, C., & Crowder, J. (2002). Disparate views of community primary health care: Understanding how perceptions influence success. *Medical Anthropology Quarterly, 16*(2), 230–247.

Whiteford, L., & Branch, L. (2008). *Primary health care in Cuba: The other revolution.* Lanham, MD: Rowman & Littlefield.

World Health Organization. (WHO). (1978). *Declaration of Alma-Ata.* Retrieved from www.euro.who.int/__ data/assets/pdf_file/0009/113877/E93944.pdf

World Health Organization. (WHO). (2008). The world health report 2008: Primary health care now more than ever. Switzerland: Author.

World Health Organization. (WHO). (2011). *The Bulletin Series: Primary health care 30 years on.* Retrieved from http://www.who.int/bulletin/primary_health_care_series/en/

For a full suite of assignments and additional learning activities, use the access code located in the front of your book to visit this exclusive website: http://go.jblearning .com/londrigan. If you do not have an access code, you can obtain one at the site.

Appendix

Systematic Approach to Health Improvement

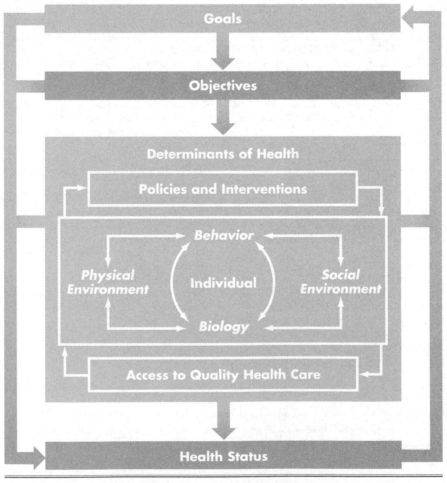

Source: U.S. Department of Health and Human Services. (2000).
Healthy People 2010 (Vol. 1). Washington, DC: U.S. Government Printing Office.

Glossary

advocacy: Acting on someone's behalf with the intention to ultimately build the capacity of the individual, family, community, or system so that they may ultimately support their own cause.

Affordable Care Act (ACA): Signed by President Obama in March 2010, this federal statute is intended to reform U.S. health care and provides for multiple healthcare changes and benefits.

agent: That which causes or contributes to a health problem or condition. The agent may be infectious, chemical, or physical, and is one of the parts of the epidemiological triangle.

age-specific rate: Provides information about a disease for a particular age group.

American Red Cross: The lead emergency response agency in United States, founded by Clara Barton in 1881.

analytical epidemiology: Illustrates the causal relationship between a risk factor and a specific disease or health condition. It seeks to answer the questions how and why with regard to the cause of a disease and the effects.

assessment: The process of gathering data from a wide variety of sources and critically analyzing the data to identify strengths and weaknesses and to prioritize the weaknesses.

assurance: Requires that public health agencies provide needed services and that the services are guaranteed for those unable to afford them.

attack rate: The incidence of a disease in a particular population over a period of time. This is important for the study of a single disease outbreak or epidemic during a short time period.

Black Death: The second recorded pandemic of the disease known as the bubonic plague swept across Europe from Central Asia in the 14th century, causing millions of deaths and devastating entire villages.

case finding: Actions and activities that help the healthcare professional locate individuals and families with identified risk factors and/or active disease and connect them with resources.

case management: Activities and actions that facilitate the seamlessness of a system's operation, thereby enhancing the capacity of the system. A system functioning at maximum capacity enhances the coordination and provision of services that optimize self-care of an individual and family.

chain of infection: Description of how an infectious disease results from the interaction between and among the agent, host, and environment. Transmission, direct or indirect, of an infectious agent takes place after the agent leaves its reservoir (host) by a portal of exit, such as the mouth when coughing. The agent then enters the susceptible host via a portal of entry, such as a skin wound, to infect the susceptible host.

coalition building: Promotes and develops partnerships among agencies and organizations for a common purpose. The coalition, via the partnership, serves to bring about change as all members work together toward the common vision and solve problems or enhance an already existing healthcare initiative.

collaboration: The working together of two or more individuals or organizations to achieve a common goal.

community health nurse: Any nurse who works in the community setting and focuses on the health of the community.

community organizing: Activities that bring together various community groups with a common goal and mobilize resources in the identified community to develop, implement, and evaluate the outcome of their initiative as they work collectively.

consultation: Interactive problem solving with a community, system, family, or individual that generates optimal and optional solutions to issues.

core functions of public health: Assessment, policy development, and assurance. Each of the functions requires a specific set of skills to ensure that the 10 essential services that fall under the three core functions are accomplished.

counseling: An interpersonal relationship between a health professional and a community, system, family, or individual with the intention to increase self-care and coping.

crude rates: Measure of the experience of an entire population in a specific area with the certain disease or condition being investigated.

cultural authority: Dictates specific behaviors and expectations within a group or society of respect and acceptance that confers authority, dominance, and influence for a particular idea, value, or belief over another.

culturally competent care: A healthcare provider's set of attitudes and behaviors that takes into account a client's or population's cultural beliefs, values, health practices, and ways of behaving in social interactions, which may differ widely from the expectations of the healthcare provider.

culture: The lifeways, folkways, rituals, taboos, and practices of a group of people who share symbols, values, and patterns of behavior.

data: Discrete elements or entities that are objective and that have not been interpreted.

database: A system or structure that allows for data to be stored in an organized way so that it may be easily accessed.

data mining: Discerning patterns and relationships from large aggregate data sources.

Declaration of Alma-Ata: Introduced in the 1978 World Health conference, which initiated the goal of primary health care for all.

delegation: Direct care tasks a registered professional nurse carries out under the authority of another healthcare practitioner as permitted by law. Delegation also includes any direct care tasks a registered professional nurse entrusts to other appropriate personnel to perform while still being responsible for that task.

descriptive epidemiology: The extent of an outbreak in terms of who gets the disease, where the disease occurs, and when the disease occurred. It is concerned with the acquisition of information about the occurrence of states of health, such as characteristics of person, place, and time. Descriptive epidemiology is essential for the description of the characteristics of disease occurrence and in the development of a hypothesis.

determinants of health: One of the four foundational health measures that serve as an indicator of progress toward achieving the goals of *Healthy People 2020*.

developmental and life-course perspective: The early life experiences of an individual which contribute to his or her susceptibility to disease later in life.

directly observed therapy: Administering or observing a patient as he or she self-administers prescribed medication to ensure that adherence and compliance with treatment are achieved.

disaster: A sudden, devastating occurrence within a community that demands a nursing and medical response.

discrimination: The process by which people are treated differently because they are members of a particular group. Particular -isms such as racism (bias against racial and ethnic groups), sexism (bias against women), ageism (bias against elders), heterosexism (bias against gays and lesbians), ableism (bias against disabled), and classism (bias against people of lower economic class) are forms of discrimination.

disease and health event investigation: The systematic collection and analysis of data about a threat to a population that ascertains the source of the threat, identifies cases and others at risk, determines strategic measures for action, and evaluates outcomes.

disparities: One of the four foundational health measures that serve as an indicator of progress toward achieving the goals of *Healthy People 2020*.

district nurse: A mid-nineteenth century English term that refers to a nurse whose main focus was caring for the sick poor in their homes.

economic policy: Set of rules or laws mandated by government to maintain financial growth and tax revenues, often influenced by political beliefs as well as the policies of parties.

education: One of the social determinants of health.

electronic health record: Individual and population health information that is collected and stored in a digital format with the potential of being shared across health settings.

emergency preparedness: Completion of the steps and actions to prepare for unexpected emergency situations and to be able to deal with the emergency as it is taking place, as well as in its aftermath.

environment: A factor that is considered extrinsic, which has an effect on the agent and the opportunity for exposure. It is one of the parts of the epidemiological triangle.

epidemic: Occurs when new cases of a particular disease, in a particular population, in a given time period is greater than expected.

epidemiological triad: The traditional model of infectious disease causation. The triad has thee components: the agent, the host, and the environment.

epidemiology: The scientific discipline that studies the distribution and determinants of diseases and injuries in human populations.

Essentials of Baccalaureate Nursing Education: A publication that identifies the framework for designing and assessing professional practice nursing education programs.

essentials of public health: The 10 essential public health services include responsibilities of local public health systems as well as strategies necessary for building a healthy, integrated public health system capable of facilitating the health of the public.

ethnocentrism: The interpretation of the world according to the norms of one's own culture.

evidence-based medicine: The application of research evidence as the best evidence to guide decision making. The term was first developed and used by medical professionals and was noted to be the new way of medical practice.

evidence-based practice: A systematic framework for decision making that uses the best available evidence in conjunction with the professional's expertise and the client's values and preferences to guide problem solving about how to best approach a situation.

general health status: One of the four foundational health measures that serve as an indicator of progress toward achieving the goals of *Healthy People 2020*.

health disparities: Gaps in health care related to the existence and the quality of health care for individuals, families, populations, communities, and systems.

health literacy: The degree to which individuals have the capacity to obtain, process, and understand basic health information and services needed to make appropriate health decisions.

health promotion: A primary level of prevention that includes strategies and behaviors that an individual engages in to enhance health. These strategies are not focused on any one particular disease, but rather focus on the individual, family, or population's overall health and optimal level of wellness.

health-related quality of life: One of the four foundational health measures that serve as an indicator of progress toward achieving the goals of *Healthy People 2020* health teaching: The communication of knowledge, facts, ideas, and skills that change competencies, attitudes, values, beliefs, behaviors, and practices of individuals, families, communities, and systems.

Healthy People 2010: A comprehensive, nationwide health promotion and disease prevention agenda that serves as a road map for improving the health of all people in the United States.

Healthy People 2020: A collaborative process that will build from the goals and objectives set forth in *Healthy People 2010*.

home care nurse: A nurse who provides care to individuals and families across the health continuum within their homes.

host: Individual affected by intrinsic factors and environmental exposure, susceptibility, and/or response to a causative agent. It is one part of the epidemiological triangle.

incidence rates: The number of new cases of a specified disease reported during a given time interval.

income: One of the social determinants of health.

income inequality: Describes where wealth is concentrated and who controls the wealth in society. Income inequality measures the degree of income variation in a population.

index case: The start of any investigation, which begins with an event, such as disease, that presents in an individual.

infection control: Is a discipline concerned with the prevention of infection within a health care setting and/or the factors and steps that need to be taken in the event of an infection to eliminate and control its spread.

influence: The ability to persuade an individual or group

informatics: Is an academic field that is concerned with the application of information science and technology to public health practice and research.

information: Data that are interpreted, organized, and structured.

information technology: The study, development, and implementation of computer-based technology that the healthcare professional can use to

access information; identify information for best practice; and apply technology in educational initiatives, communication, and in the support of research.

Institute of Medicine (IOM) Reports for Nursing Education: Publication based on the series of IOM reports aimed at improving the safety and overall quality of health care in the United States that addresses areas of interest to nurse educators in preparing students in public health.

knowledge: Information that is synthesized so that relationships are identified and formalized.

life course model: A model that suggests that the socioeconomic position of the family during childhood affects the child's health status, educational choices, and occupational choices in the future.

maintaining health: Engagement in activities that sustain an individual's present level of health.

Minnesota Department of Health Population-Based Public Health Nursing Practice Intervention Wheel Strategies: An organizing framework public health nurses use to guide their practice.

morbidity rate: The rate of illness, injury, or disability in a population (i.e., the number of people ill during a time period divided by the number of people in the total population).

mortality: A measure of the frequency of occurrence of death in a defined population during a specified interval.

multilevel analysis: An analysis necessary to understand all of the factors that contribute to disease. In a multilevel analysis, all factors are examined on an individual level and on an environmental level, such as a neighborhood, community, city, state, and so forth.

nursing history: Examining the social, political, and economic context in which nursing evolved over time.

nursing informatics: The integration of nursing science, computer science, and information science to manage and communicate data, information, knowledge, and wisdom in nursing practice.

outreach: The process of locating individuals, families, and/or populations of interest for the purpose of information dissemination and/or provision of service.

pandemic: An epidemic that spreads to a larger populations beyond to several countries or continents.

participant observation: A technique in which the nurse makes careful observations of specific processes, actions, or communications while providing care as a participant in the activity.

personal health record: Is the personal record related to a patient and the information pertaining to that patient.

policy development and enforcement: Actions and activities that place health issues on decision makers' agendas, acquire a plan of resolution, and determine needed resources. Policy development results in laws, rules, regulations, ordinances, and policies. Policy enforcement compels others to comply with the laws, rules, regulations, ordinances, and policies created in conjunction with policy development.

politics: The process of collective decision making performed by a group of people involved with government, religion, corporate, or academic issues.

population: A group of individuals who share specific characteristics such as social, physical, cultural, economic, or environmental characteristics.

population-focused care: Application of intervention wheel strategies that will access and provide care to a specific population.

population perspective: Viewpoint that suggests that an individual's risk for health problems cannot be isolated from the community in which he or she resides or from the population or society in which he or she belongs.

prevalence rate: A measure of the number of people in a given population who have a specific existing condition at a given point in time.

prevention/preventing disease: Engaging in an action or initiating an intervention to prevent the occurrence of a disease or an event.

primary care: Treatment of the patient based on a model of intermittent management of a person's specific condition, generally contained to a time-limited appointment, with or without follow-up, monitoring, or evaluation. Provider–client interaction beyond this visit may or may not take place.

primary health care: Bringing health care that is universally accessible to the people via their full participation.

primary prevention: Actions taken to prevent disease and/or injury and require strategies including health promotion and specific protection.

public health: Both a science and an art that ensures the public's health by engaging in interventions that promote health and prevent disease, prolonging life through organized community efforts.

public health informatics: The systematic application of information, computer science, and technology to public health practice and learning.

public health nurse: A term coined by Lillian Wald in the early 20th century that describes the work of the visiting nurse who cares for the sick at home and provides health promotion and disease prevention measures in the community. The work of the public health nurse is population focused and takes place on three practice levels: individual/family, community, and system.

public policy: Encompasses the choices that a government makes regarding goals and priorities and the way it allocates resources to attain those goals.

pull POD model: The administering of mass prophylaxis or vaccines to employees who report to a specific central location.

push POD model: Utilizes mobile teams to physically bring prophylaxis to the employees, decreasing the amount of time spent away from work.

quarantine: The isolation of a contagious individual from the remainder of the population.

rate: The primary measurement used to describe the occurrence of a health problem. It is a measure of the frequency of a health-related event in a specific population within a given period of time.

A rate consists of a numerator and a denominator and calculated by dividing the number of conditions or events by time, and multiplying by a base multiple of 10.

referral and follow-up: Actions and activities that serve to assist individuals, families, and/or populations by connecting them to needed services for possible treatments and other resources, including follow-up to identify outcomes.

regional health information exchanges: Organizations established to electronically collect and organize a core set of data from multiple organizations within a community or region.

risk: The probability that an event will occur within a specific time period.

risk reduction: Completion of specific strategies designed to reduce risk or the probability that an event will occur.

ritual: An act often associated with key life events. It may enhance joy, as in the case of celebratory traditions such as weddings and holidays; provide a sense of comfort, as in the case of death and dying; or promote a gracious lifestyle, as exemplified by table manners and the offering of food to guests.

screening: A strategy of the Intervention Wheel that serves to identify individuals with disease who are asymptomatic or those individuals with health risk factors.

secondary prevention: Strategies that facilitate early detection of disease, thus resulting in early diagnosis, early treatment, and prevention of spread to others and long-term disability. An example of secondary prevention would be screening.

service learning: A hands-on approach to education where community service, instruction, and reflection serve as a meaningful learning experience.

social capital: Social resources such as parks, medical facilities, schools, and economic investments that are needed to ensure that communities have the resources to maintain health.

social context: A guiding concept of social epidemiology. The social context of behavior addresses individual behavioral risk factors such as smoking and drinking and examines these behaviors in a larger social context, or examines the social influences or conditions that contribute to specific behaviors.

social epidemiology: The study of epidemiology that deals with social distribution and social determinants of health and disease. Social epidemiology makes the case that social determinants of health, which consist of socioeconomic status (income, occupation, and education), socioeconomic position, and discrimination, can influence health outcomes.

social justice: Justice as it is considered and applied to every aspect of society and to every member of society.

social legitimacy: Popular acceptance of a prevailing idea, value, or belief.

social marketing: Actions and activities that operationalize social marketing principles and the application of appropriate technology for program design with the expressed purpose of influencing the knowledge, attitudes, values, beliefs, behaviors, and practices of a population of interest.

social policy: Guidelines for the creation of positive living conditions for the people's welfare, such as in regards to housing, education, and health.

socioeconomic position: Determined by an individual's socioeconomic status. How much money an individual has, his or her educational attainment, and his or her occupation have a bearing on and reflect the individual's socioeconomic position, or standing in society.

socioeconomic status: Consists of family income, educational level, and occupation.

Spanish Influenza: An epidemic of 1918–1919 (caused by the virus H1N1) that developed toward the end of World War I and was estimated to have caused a global mortality of between 50 and 100 million.

specific protection: Considered in the primary level of prevention, it focuses on a particular disease and/or injury and the prevention of those situations before they take form by stopping the causal event. Examples of these actions include immunizations, environmental sanitation, and nutrition.

state-sanctioned control measures: Government-implemented measures to control the spread of a disease. During the Black Death, Italian city-states were at particular risk. These states were the first to introduce systematic measures to protect their populations from plague.

surveillance: The monitoring of health events and the facilitation of the ongoing systematic collection, analysis, interpretation, and evaluation of data for the purpose of planning, implementing, and evaluating public health initiatives.

teaching–learning strategy: Method of education to meet the needs of and enhance the learning of a specific individual, family, community, population, or system.

tertiary prevention: Strategies that stop a disease from progressing and prevent further disability. An example of tertiary prevention is rehabilitation and education on maximum use of an individual's capabilities, thus supporting his or her human capital.

the 5 A's: A framework for the healthcare practitioner to use when working with populations at the individual/family, community, and systems levels of practice to assess how well the population can gain entry into needed resources and use those resources with ultimate positive outcomes.

tobacco use: Is the leading preventable cause of premature death in the United States. The majority of tobacco users smoke cigarettes, with a smaller number smoking cigars and pipes. Smokeless tobacco is the smallest user group, which includes snuff and chewing tobacco. Passive smoking is a process where nonsmokers inhale smoke.

visiting nurse: A term used interchangeably with district nursing in the United States, this term refers to the trained nurse who provided care for the sick public in their homes.

vulnerable populations: A group of individuals who are at greater risk than other populations and who also share specific characteristics such as social, physical, cultural, economic, or environmental characteristics.

xenophobia: The conscious fear of foreigners.

Index

Boxes, figures, and tables are indicated by b, f, and t following the page number.

A

AARP, 307
Abuse
  domestic violence, 181, 188,
    192–193, 193b, 225
  elder, 269
  sexual assault, 279–280
  substance, 188, 281
ACA. *See* Affordable Care Act of 2010
Access to care, 93
Accountable Care Organization (ACO),
  209
Action research, 183
Action step for surveillance data,
  233–235
Active Living Research, American
    Association for Cardiovascular
    and Pulmonary Rehabilitation,
    307
Active surveillance
  defined, 233
  of rabies exposure, 243
  of tuberculosis, 240, 244
Acute care in the home, 43, 87
Acute pulmonary tuberculosis, 239
Adaptation mechanisms, 123
Adolescents
  juvenile offender intervention
    programs, 188–189
  overweight and obesity, 316–320
  as parents, 183, 286
  physical activity guidelines, 303, 304b
  sexual assault, 279–280
  smokadiabesity and, 299
  tobacco use, 142–144

Advanced practice public health nurses,
  49
Advocacy in shaping health and public
  policy, 193, 203, 217–219,
  320–324, 323b
Affordable Care Act of 2010 (ACA)
  government branches involved in,
    205, 212
  healthcare coverage, increase access
    to, 137
  impact of, 210–211
  Medicaid expansion, 212
  nurse's expand role, 204
  problems addressed in, 208–210
  scope of, 400
  state response to, 216–217
  survival of, 214–216
  tobacco use regulation, 141
African Americans
  nurses, 32, 42
  stereotyping and, 180, 181
  women using cocaine and, 183–184
Agency for Healthcare Research and
  Quality, 231
Agent, in epidemiological triad, 115f,
  116
Age-specific rates (diseases), 111, 112t
AIDS. *See* HIV/AIDS
Airborne diseases, 239–240
Alaska earthquake (1964), 362–365
Alma-Ata International Conference
  (1978), 9, 400–404,
  401–403b
American Academy of Nursing, 185
American Academy of Pediatrics, 307

American Alliance for Health, Physical
  Education, Recreation, and
  Dance, 307
American Association of Colleges of
  Nursing, 49, 300
American Association of Retired
  Persons, 307
American Cancer Society, 307
  Guidelines on Nutrition and Physical
    Activity for Cancer Prevention,
    303, 304b
American College of Sports Medicine,
  303, 304b, 307
American Diabetes Association, 194,
  285
American Heart Association
  Council on Nutrition, Physical
    Activity, and Metabolism, 302
  national physical activity coalition, 307
  physical activity guidelines, 303, 304b
American Legacy Foundation, 143
American Medical Association, 303
American Nurses Association (ANA)
  Code of Ethics for Nurses, 322
  delegation and, 267
  National Association of Colored
    Graduate Nurses and, 32, 42
  Nurses Associated Alumnae of the
    United States and Canada
    and, 31
  Public Health Nursing: Scope &
    Standards of Practice, 322
American Nurses Association
    Political Action Committee
    (ANA-PAC), 218

American Recovery and Reinvestment
    Act of 2009 (ARRA), 212–214
American Red Cross, 354. *See also*
    Disaster nursing
American Red Cross Public Health
    Nursing Service, 38–39
American Society of Superintendents
    for Nurses, 31
AmeriCorps, 290
ANA. *See* American Nurses Association
Analysis of health status, 62, 97
Analytical epidemiology, 113–115
ANA-PAC (American Nurses
    Association Political Action
    Committee), 218
Anthrax bioterrorism event (2001), 370
Apomediation, defined, 163
ARRA (American Recovery and
    Reinvestment Act of 2009),
    212–214
Arthritis, 318
Assessments. *See also* Public Health
    Nursing Assessment Tool
    as core function of public health, 12
    defined, 54
    epidemiology and, 108–109
    on-site, 245
    screenings, 225, 383
    self-assessments, 383
    Seven A's, assessment tool, 60–61,
        93, 285
Assistive living, 90
Associate degree programs, 48, 49
Association of Community Health
    Nursing Educators, 162
Assurance, core function, 12, 13*f*
Attack rates (disease), 111, 112*t*
Awareness-raising campaigns, 346–347

B
Baccalaureate degree programs, 48, 49
Barriers
    in culturally diverse projects, 196
    physical, 86
    to referrals and follow-up, 254,
        259–260
Behavioral change, 325
Behavioral theory, health promotion
    model, 325–326

Behaviors
    epidemiology and, 109
    gender-appropriate, 181
    health determinant assessment and,
        61–62, 69–74, 96
    individual, 284
    social context of, 118–120
Bias
    culturally competent care and,
        180–181
    in making referrals, 256
    as social determinant of health, 104,
        124–126, 125–126*f*
Biology, health determinant assessment
    and, 59, 73, 282
Bioterrorism, 370
Black Death, 336–341
Body mass index (BMI), 317, 318
Boston University School of Public
    Health, 144
Breast cancer survival rate, 118
Bridges Out of Poverty (Payne, DeVol, &
    Smith), 388
Bubonic plague, 336–341
Built environment, 85, 302

C
Cancer
    breast cancer survival rate, 118
    cervical cancer screening, 227
    colorectal cancer screening, 231
    prevention programs, 303, 304*b*
    screening tests for women, 227, 229
Cardiovascular disease, 318. *See also*
    American Heart Association
Cardiovascular-specific genogram, 229
Case definitions, 110
Case findings, 223–249. *See also*
    Intervention programs and
    strategies
    case study application, 244–246
    Minnesota Department of Health
        Population-Based Public Health
        Nursing Practice Intervention
        Wheel, 224–236
        disease and health event investi-
            gation, 236–237, 236*b*
        effectiveness/technology, 235–236
        levels of practice, 246–247

    outreach, 225–228, 228*t*
    overview, 224–225
    screening, 228–231
    surveillance, 232–235
    overview, 223–224
    public health issues in practice,
        237–244
Case management, 263–266, 270–272
Case studies
    advocacy, 321
    clinical research, 172–173
    community projects, cultural issues
        in, 195–196
    computerized scheduling system, 165
    databases, 156–157
    database tracking, 158–159
    genetics, 270–271
    geriatric medicine, 270–271, 271*b*
    home care, 169–170
    home care nurse, 174–175
    migrant farm workers and their
        families, 190–191, 191*b*
    physical activity, 309–310, 309*b*
    Project IDEAL, 193–195, 195*b*
    rural domestic violence project,
        192–193, 193*b*
    student health services, 167–168
    technology in home care, 166
    tobacco use, 138–139
    tuberculosis, 239–240, 244–246
    visiting nurses, 171–172
Causal relationships, 109–110
CBO (Congressional Budget Office),
    209
Center for Medicare and Medicaid
    Innovation (CMI), 209
Centers for Disease Control and
    Prevention (CDC)
    data collection and, 154
    National Environmental Public
        Health Tracking Network, 161
    National Environmental Public
        Health Tracking Program,
        160–161
    smallpox status, 370
Centers for Medicare and Medicaid
    Services, 170
Cerebrovascular disease, risk of, 229
Cervical cancer screening, 227

Chain of infection, 116–117, 117*f*
Childhood Obesity Demonstration
  Project, 211
Children. *See also* Adolescents
  early childhood programs, 280
  health education, 282
  health screenings, 389
  immunization program, 227
  overweight and obesity, 211,
    316–320
  physical activity guidelines, 303,
    304*b*
  safe routes to school program, 308
Children's Health Fund, 230
Cholera investigation, 237, 237–238*b*
Cigarette Labeling and Advertising Act
  of 1965, 139
Cigarette smoking. *See* Tobacco use
Circumcision, 185–186
Classification standardization, 175–176
Cleansing data, 158
Client acceptance of referrals, 258,
  259–260
Client utilization of resources, 259
Clinical domain of health literacy, 135
Clinical experiences, 382–389, 384*f*.
    See also Case studies
  faith-based clinics, 388–389
  immunization clinics, 387–388
  overview, 382–3383
  school health screenings, 389
  service learning, 388
  simulation experiences, 386–387
  wellness screening, 383–385
Clinical judgment model, 383
Clinical nursing, 105, 105*b*
Clinical research, 156–157, 171,
  172–173
CMI (Center for Medicare and Medicaid
  Innovation), 209
Coalition building, 305–307, 306*f*,
  307*b*
Coalitions to promote health, 281–282,
  283*t*
COBRA (Consolidated Omnibus
  Budget Reconciliation Act of
  1985), 212–214
Code of Ethics for Nurses (ANA), 322
Cognitive case-finding instrument, 225

Cohort studies, 115
Collaboration, 300–305, 301*b*, 373.
    See also Partnership programs
Collection of surveillance data,
  232–233
Colorectal cancer screening, 231
Commonwealth Fund Commission,
  216
Communicable diseases, 116
Communication. *See also* Internet
  assessment of, 81
  barriers in culturally diverse projects,
    196
  disaster situations and, 361–362
  health literacy and, 137–138
  media and, 143
  outreach programs and, 227
  social media and, 144
  technology and, 168–169
Communities
  composition of neighborhoods, 319
  in context of human relationships,
    408
  cultural issues in community
    projects, 195–196
  Healthy People 2020 and, 18–21
  Henry Street Settlement, 287–288
  history of, 84
  neighborhood clinics, 406
  organizational structure of, 94
  participation of, 407–408
  political issues in, 95
Community boards of health, 40–41
Community-focused practices
  advocacy, 323–324, 323*b*
  case management, 266
  collaboration, 305
  community organizing, 308
  referrals and follow-up, 262–263
Community Health Centers, 211
Community health nurses, 44–45
Community organizing, 307–308
Community Transformation Grants
  (CTG), 210
Competencies for public health work
  force, 173–174
Comprehensive Smoking Education Act
  of 1984, 139
Computerized scheduling systems, 165

Computers. *See also* Informatics;
    Internet
  nurse's cases studies using, 158–159,
    165–168, 171–174
  senior services educational program,
    293
Confirmed foodborne cases, 241
Conflicts
  cultural competence and, 185–186
  in referrals and follow-up, 261–262
Congressional Budget Office (CBO),
  209
Connectivity of information systems,
  165–167
Consolidated Omnibus Budget
  Reconciliation Act of 1985
  (COBRA), 212–214
Consultation
  collective considerations, 285–286
  Minnesota Department of Health
    Population-Based Public Health
    Nursing Practices Intervention
    Wheel, 280–281
  partnerships, 290–291
Contacts identification and investigation
  for TB case, 245–246
Contagion theory, 337
Conversation Map Kits (diabetes
  education), 285
Core functions of public health, 12, 13*f*
Coronary heart disease, 318
Cost containment, 264–265
Cost of healthcare in U.S., 208, 209
Council on Cardiovascular Disease in
  the Young, 302
Council on Cardiovascular Nursing, 302
Council on Nutrition, Physical Activity,
  and Metabolism (American
  Heart Association), 302
Counseling
  collaborative partnerships and,
    291–292
  collective considerations, 285–286
  domestic abuse, 193
  Minnesota Department of Health
    Population-Based Public Health
    Nursing Practices Intervention
    Wheel, 278–280
  partnerships and, 290–291

Crude rates (diseases), 111, 112*t*
Cuban American adolescents, risky behaviors, 189
Cuban National Health System, 406
Cultural rituals, 180, 181–182
Culture, 179–199. *See also* Global worldview
  Alma-Ata Declaration, 403
  case studies
    community projects, cultural issues in, 195–196
    migrant farm workers and their families, 190–191
    overview, 189–190
    Project IDEAL, 193–195, 195*b*
    rural domestic violence project, 192–193, 193*b*
  culturally competent care, 184–187, 187*b*
    conflicts and, 185–186
    learning process for, 186–187, 187*b*
    overview, 184–185
    sensitivity and, 185
  overview, 179–182
  participant observations, 182–184, 184*b*
  public health nursing, 187–189
Culture of poverty, 188–189, 391
Curriculum improvements, 137–138, 300, 380–381, 380–381*t*

D

Data. *See also* Surveillance
  defined, 154
  used to leverage gaps in healthcare quality, 218–219
Databases, 57, 58*b*, 154–158, 155*b*
Data cleansing, 158
Data collection, 58, 154, 232–233
Data mining, 158–160
Data tracking, 157–158
Death rituals, 182
Debriefing, 392–393
Declaration of Alma-Ata International Conference (1978), 9, 400–404, 401–403*b*
Degree programs for nursing, 48, 49
Delegated functions, 266–269
Dementia identification, 225

Dental care, 92
Descriptive epidemiology, 109, 113, 114*t*
Determinants of health. *See also* Public Health Nursing Assessment Tool
  behaviors, 61–62, 69–74, 96, 284
  biology, 59, 73, 282
  education, 123–124
  environmental, 86
  genetics, 59, 73, 282
  health services, 60–61, 87–93
  income, 122–123
  occupation, 124
  physical environment, 59–60, 84–86, 284, 285*b*
  social factors, 59–60, 75–83, 104, 124–126, 125–126*f*
Developmental and life-course perspective, 118, 119*f*
Diabetes
  education, 193–195, 285
  prevalence of, 289, 299, 299*f*, 317–318
Diabetes Prevention Program, 320
Digital disparity, 164
Directly observed therapy (DOT), 240
Direct transmission of diseases, 116
Disaster drills, 386–387
Disaster nursing, 353–367. *See also* Emergency preparedness
  Alaska earthquake (1964), 362–365
  Galveston hurricane (1900), 355–356
  influenza pandemic (1918–1919), 356–358
  Johnstown flood (1889), 354–355
  overview, 353–354
  Texas City ship explosion (1947), 358–362
  yellow fever, 354–355
Disaster Research Group of the National Academy of Sciences, 360
Discretionary federal spending, 214–215
Discrimination
  bias in making referrals, 256
  culturally competent care and, 180–181
  as social determinant of health, 104, 124–126, 125–126*f*

Diseases. *See also specific diseases*
  airborne, 239–240
  cardiovascular, 318
  cerebrovascular, 229
  communicable, 116
  coronary heart, 318
  epidemic, 336
  foodborne cases of, 241
  indirect transmission of, 116–117
  infectious, 107*t*, 108, 233, 234*b*, 247
  investigation of, 236–237, 236*b*
  noninfectious, 107*t*, 108, 116, 298–299
  notifiable, 233, 234*b*, 247
  prevention of. *See* Prevention programs and health services
  screening programs, 228–231
  transmission of, 116–117
Disparities
  in digital information access, 164
  in health care, 55, 62, 97, 207
  health literacy and, 136
  health outcomes impact and, 124–126, 289, 407, 407*b*
Dissemination of surveillance data, 233
Distance learning, 231, 386–387
District nurses, 27–30
Doctoral degree programs, 48
Document literacy, 135
Domestic violence, 181, 188, 192–193, 193*b*, 225
DOT (directly observed therapy), 240
Drug abuse prevention program, 281
Drug therapies for AIDS, 346

E

Early childhood programs, 280
Economic conditions affecting health care, 204, 213–216, 284, 288–289
Ecosocial theory, 124–125
Education. *See also* Health teaching
  Alma-Ata Declaration and, 403
  bioterrorism, 373
  curricula changes in, 137–138, 300, 380–381, 380–381*t*
  diabetes, 193–195, 285
  integrated learning, 381–382
  media-based, 227

nutrition program, 228, 291–292
of public health nurses, 47–49
smallpox vaccinations, 371
as social determinant of health, 78, 123–124
Educational attainment
health literacy and, 136
of people over 25 years, 83
Elder population
arthritis and, 318
computer training for, 293
geriatric medicine, 269–272, 271*b*
health education programs for men, 282
physical activity guidelines, 303, 304*b*
physical activity programs, 308
senior housing outreach project, 226
senior nutritional education program, 228
senior services, 239–240
Transitional Care Model, 286
Electronic Health Records (EHRs), 162
Emergency preparedness, 369–375. *See also* Disaster nursing
disaster response and, 354
influenza vaccine initiative, 372–373
lessons learned, 373–374
overview, 370
pull point of dispensing care delivery, 370
push point of dispensing care delivery, 370
smallpox initiative, 370–372
Employer-based health insurance coverage, 207
Employment as social determinant of health, 82
Ending the Tobacco Epidemic (DHHS), 145
Ending the Tobacco Problem (IOM), 141
Entitlement programs, 214–215
Environment
in epidemiological triad, 115*f*, 116
health determinant assessment and, 59–60, 84–86, 284
Henry Street Settlement, 289–290
Environmental hazards, tracking of, 160–161

Epidemic diseases, 335–351
AIDS in Britain, 344–347
bubonic plague in Italy, 336–341
influenza in U.S., 341–344
overview, 336
Epidemiological triad, 115–116, 115*f*
Epidemiologic surveillance, 117, 232
Epidemiology, 104–117. *See also* Social epidemiology
approach to, 110–115, 114*t*
history of, 106–108, 106–107*t*
overview, 104–106, 105*b*
public health surveillance data, 117
uses of, 108–110
Epinephrine injections, 267
Essentials of Baccalaureate Nursing Education for Entry Level Community/Public Health Nurses, 381
Essentials of public health, 12, 12*b*
Ethics
Code of Ethics for Nurses (ANA), 322
data collection, 58
ranking of nursing profession on, 203
referral and follow-up interventions, 261–262
screening and case finding interventions, 253
Ethnocentrism, 180–181
Evaluating assessments, 63–64
Evaluation of referrals, 259
Evidence-based medicine, 132
Evidence-based practice, 131–149
Healthy People 2020 and, 134–145
health literacy, 134–139
tobacco dependence, 139–145, 139*f*
overview, 131–132
population-based health issues, 132–134, 133*b*
Exchanges for health insurance markets, 212
Exercise is Medicine program, 303
Exercise prescriptions, 303–305
Experimental studies, 113
Eye contact in Latino groups, 194

F

Faith-based institutions and programs, 183, 280, 388–389

False positive or negative testing results, 230–231
Family level of practice. *See* Individual/family level of practice
Family Smoking Prevention and Tobacco Control Act of 2009, 140
Farm Worker Family Health Program (FWFHP), 190–191
Fast-food consumption, 320
FDA (Food and Drug Administration), 140
Federal Emergency Management Agency (FEMA), 387
Federal government's public health role, 9–10, 12, 211–213, 408
Federal policy, 202–206
Federal spending, 214–215
Feedback and feedback loops, 168–169, 392–393
FEMA (Federal Emergency Management Agency), 387
Female circumcision, 185, 186
Financial cost management, 44
Fire department assessments, 81
First responders immunization programs, 371–373
Flu. *See* Influenza
Focus groups, 186, 326
Follow-up programs. *See* Referrals
Food and Drug Administration (FDA), 140
Foodborne illnesses, 240–242
Food pantries, 290
Food production and marketing, 319, 320
Formal resource networks, 254–255
Foundational health measures
Healthy People 2020, 18, 55, 62
PHNAT, 58–62
behaviors, individual and population, 61–62, 69–74, 96
biology and genetics, 59
disparities, 55, 97
general health status, 55, 58, 68–72, 97
health services, 60–61, 87–93
policymaking, 61, 94
social factors, 59–60, 75–83

Four Ps of marketing, 325
Framingham Study, 115
Fry formula, 138
Future of Nursing (IOM report), 132, 203, 411
FWFHP (Farm Worker Family Health Program), 190–191

G

Galveston hurricane (1900), 355–356
Gender-appropriate behavior, 181
Gender distribution worksheet, 74
General health status, 55, 58, 68–72, 97
Genetics, health determinant assessment and, 59, 73, 282
Genital mutilation, 185
Genograms, 229
Geriatric medicine, 270–272, 271*b*
Global worldview, 389–393
   culture of poverty, 391
   debriefing, 392–393
   global learning, 391–392
   healthcare missions, 390–391
   overview, 389
   social justice, 389–390
   systems thinking, 392
Good Friday Earthquake (1964), 362–365
Google Flu Trends, 163
Government-funded healthcare programs, 39–40
Government's public health role, 9–10, 12, 211–213, 408
Grand Army of the Republic, 356
Graphic Model for *Healthy People 2020*, 14, 15*f*, 282

H

Head Start programs, 288
Health and Human Services Department, U.S.
   Ending the Tobacco Epidemic, 145
   health literacy and, 137, 138
   Healthy People in Healthy Communities, 19
   physical activity guidelines, 303, 304*b*, 320, 321*b*
   Prevention and Public Health Fund, 210

Public Health Functions Steering Committee, 12
Health Care and Education Reconciliation Act of 2010, 208
Healthcare missions, 390–391
Healthcare policy and politics, 201–221
   Affordable Care Act. *See* Affordable Care Act of 2010
   federal government's role in society, 211–213
   federal policy and, 202–206
   history shaping health care, 213–214, 411, 412*b*
   overview, 201–202
   policy making, 217
   political engagement of nurses, 217–219
   U.S. healthcare system, 206–208
Health community, defined, 19
Health event investigation, 236–237, 236*b*
Health information exchange (HIE), 217
Health information technology (HIT), 217
Health Information Technology for Economic and Clinical Health Act of 2009 (HITECH), 162
Health insurance exchanges, 212
Health Insurance Portability and Accountability Act of 1996 (HIPAA), 168
Health Knowledge: Screening (online tutorial), 231
Health literacy, 134–139
Health Literacy Innovations (software), 137
Health maintenance, 7
Health on the Net Foundation logo, 167
Health policies, 95
Health promotion, 7
Health promotion model, behavioral theory, 326
Health-related conditions attributed to overweight and obesity, 317–318

Health-related quality of life and well-being, 55, 58, 72, 265
Health services, determinant of health, 60–61, 87–93
Health teaching, 5, 6*t*, 281–286, 283*t*, 290–291
Healthy life expectancy analysis worksheet, 71
Healthy People 2020, 134–145
   communities application of, 18–21
   disparities in health care, 62
   foundational health measures, 18, 55
   Graphic Model for, 14, 15*f*, 282
   health literacy, 134–139
   HIV intervention recommendations, 260
   model of, 54–55, 54*f*
   overarching goals, 14–16, 16*b*
   overview, 13–14, 15*f*
   physical activity, 303, 320
   physical environment examples, 60
   technology and, 236
   tobacco dependence, 139–145, 139*f*
   topics and objectives, 16–18, 17–20*f*
   vision and mission, 14, 16*b*
Healthy People in Healthy Communities (DHHS), 19
Healthy Professions Education (IOM), 132
Heart Awareness for Women Program, 183
Heart disease, 318. *See also* American Heart Association
Helplines for support, 346
Henry Street Settlement (New York City)
   beginning of, 10, 29, 30, 32–33
   community of, 287–288
   economics, 288–289
   environmental characteristics, 289–290
   partnerships, 290–291
   population and programs, 288
   social and health systems, 289
Hepatitis A, 111, 111*b*, 113
HIEs (Health information exchanges), 162, 217
HIPAA (Health Insurance Portability and Accountability Act of 1996), 168

Hispanic population. *See* Latino populations
Hispanic youth programs, 188–189
HIT (Health information technology), 217
HITECH (Health Information Technology for Economic and Clinical Health Act of 2009), 162
HIV/AIDS
    AIDS in Britain, 344–347
    epidemiologists and, 109–110
    intervention recommendations, 260
    outreach programs, 225
Home care assessment, 88
Home care nurses, 43, 158–159, 166, 169–170, 357
Home health nursing, 43–44
Homeless population, 227, 228, 292
Hospitals, origin of, 340–341
Host, in epidemiological triad, 115*f*, 116
Housing conditions, 75
Hurricane Katrina evacuees survey, 5

I

Identification of contacts for TB case, 245–246
IHI (Institute for Healthcare Improvement), 216
Illegal drug programs, 286
Immersion programs, 186, 190–191, 195, 391
Immigrants, undocumented, 186, 226
Immigration services, 181, 193, 288
Immunization clinics, 387–388
Immunization programs, 227, 371–373
Incidence rates (diseases), 111, 112*t*
Incident Command System online course (FEMA), 387
Inclusiveness of health care, 403
Income as social determinant of health, 122–123
Income inequality, 104, 123
Income of family, 83
Independent Payment Advisory Board (IPAB), 209
Index case, 236
Indirect transmission of diseases, 116–117

Individual and population, behaviors of, 61–62, 69–74, 96, 284
Individual/family level of practice
    advocacy, 323*b*, 324
    analysis worksheet, 69, 72
    case findings, 224
    case management, 265–266
    client relationship, 247
    collaboration, 303–305
    referrals and follow-up, 262, 264
Individualism, 407–408, 410*f*
Individual mandate for healthcare insurance, 212
Industrial accidents, 359
Industries in community, 82
Infection control, 344
Infectious diseases, 107*t*, 108, 233, 234*b*, 247
Influence, political, 203–204
Influenza
    Google Flu Trends, 163
    push POD initiative, 372–373
    in U.S. (1918–1919), 341–344, 356–358
Infodemiology, 163
Informal resource networks, 255
Informatics, 151–177
    case studies
        clinical research, 172–173
        computerized scheduling system, 165
        databases, 156–157
        database tracking, 158–159
        home care, 169–170
        home care nurses, 174–175
        student health services, 167–168
        technology in home care, 166
        visiting nurses, 171–172
    information technology (generally)
        data, 154
        databases, 154–158, 155*b*
        data mining, 158–160
        information, knowledge, and wisdom, 160–161
    information technology in public health nursing, 161–176
        access and adaptability, 163–165
        applying to public health, 170–171
        challenges, 173–176

communication technology, 168–169
    connections, 165–167
    definition and goals, 162–163
    infrastructure, 161–162
overview, 151–153
technology role, 153–154, 235–236
Information, defined, 160, 161*f*
Information technology. *See* Informatics
Innovative case findings techniques, 226
Innovative information technology
    case studies, 164–165, 166, 169–170
Insite (medically supervised injection facility), 286
Institute for Healthcare Advancement (California), 138
Institute for Healthcare Improvement (IHI), 216
Institute of Medicine (IOM)
    curricula change recommendations, 300
    Ending the Tobacco Problem, 141
    To Err Is Human, 131
    The Future of Nursing, 132, 203, 411
    government's responsibility, 9, 12
    Healthy Professions Education, 132
    information science and, 160
    multi-discipline approach, 7–9, 9*f*
    nursing education reports, 379
    public health defined by, 4
    public health priorities, 379, 379*b*
    Quality Initiative, 209
Institutionalized racism, 126
Insulin administration, 267
Integrated learning, 381–382
Internalized racism, 126
International Council of Nurses, 32
International experiences, 391–392. *See also* Global worldview
International Honor Society, 182
Internet. *See also* Communication
    advantages and disadvantages, 166–167
    case study of use, 167–168
    educational programs, 231
    intervention programs, 144
    resources, 57, 58*b*, 169
    usage statistics, 144

Interprofessional Education Collaborative report, 300
Intervention programs and strategies. *See also* Case findings; Minnesota Department of Health Population-Based Public Health Nursing Practice Intervention Wheel
adolescent juvenile offenders, 188–189
educational, 5, 6*t*
in foodborne disease cases, 241
health literacy, 137
Internet-based, 144
PHNAT and, 63
policy interventions, 137
population-focused, 137–138, 141–142
rehabilitation, 7, 8*f*
Intimate partner violence (IPV), 225. *See also* Domestic violence
Investigation of health events, 236–237, 236*b*
IOM. *See* Institute of Medicine
IPAB (Independent Payment Advisory Board), 209
Isolating communities, 339–340, 344

J

Japanese women's breast cancer survival rate, 118
Jewish cultural expectations, 180
John Sealy Hospital (Galveston, Texas), 359, 360
Johnstown flood (1889), 354–355
The Joint Commission (TJC), 137
Joint Committee on Community Nursing Service, 41
Join Together, smoking cessation program, 144

K

Keepin' it REAL, drug abuse prevention program, 281
Kennesaw State University, WellStar School of Nursing, 193
Knowledge, defined, 160, 161*f*

L

Language standardization, 158–159, 174–176

Latino populations
adolescent risky behaviors, 189
diabetes education, 193–195, 285
domestic violence, 188, 192
outreach programs, 226
Law enforcement, 80
Legal advocacy services, 193
Legal interventions in foodborne cases, 241
Legally required referrals, 262
Let's Move campaign, 320
Leveling schemes, 133*b*, 134
Library services, 80
Lienhard School of Nursing, 290, 293
Life course model or perspective, 121
Life expectancy, 15, 71
Long-term care, 89
Lyme disease
descriptive epidemiology and, 113
epidemiological triad and, 116
tracking of, 157–158

M

Male circumcision, 185
Mandated referrals, 262
Mantoux tuberculin skin testing (TST), 239
MAPIT (mobilize, assess, plan, implement, track) process, 19–21, 57
Marketing
food production and, 319, 320
social marketing, 324–328
Mass screening programs, 229–230
Master's degree programs, 48, 49
Media-based education, 227
Media communications, 143, 346, 382
Medical errors, 209
Medical surveillance, 232
Medicare and Medicaid legislation, 43, 210–212, 215
Men
circumcision, 185
health education programs for, 282
overweight and obesity, 316–320
smokadiabesity and, 299, 299*f*
Mental health, 72, 90, 318–319
Metabolic syndrome, 318

Metropolitan Life Insurance Company, 37–38
Mexican-born immigrants. *See* Latino populations
Microparasites, 336
Migrant farm workers, 187, 190–191, 191*b*
Minnesota Department of Health Population-Based Public Health Nursing Practice Intervention Wheel
advocacy, 320–323
coalition building, 305–307, 306*f*, 307*b*
collaboration, 291–292, 300–305, 301*b*
collective action, 309–310, 309*b*
community organizing, 307–308
consultation, 280–281
counseling, 278–280
disease and health event investigation, 236–237
effectiveness/technology, 235–236
health teaching, 281–286
intervention strategies, 10, 62–63, 290
levels of practice, 246–247, 252–263
outcomes, 292–293
outreach, 225–228, 228*t*
partnerships, 290–291
PHNAT and, 54–55, 62–63
plan and implementation, 62–63, 99–100
practice, 269–272, 271*b*
public health nursing defined by, 46–47
screening, 228–231
surveillance, 163, 232–235
Mission statements, 306, 306*f*, 307*b*
Mobile vans or healthcare units, 226, 230, 405
Monsanto Chemical Plant, 359
Montefiore Medical Center (New York City), 371–373
Morbidity and mortality, 70, 136, 140–141
Multidisciplinary collaborations, 7–9, 9*f*, 373
Multilevel analysis, 118, 120–121

Multilevel approaches to social determinants of health, 121–126
Muslim cultural expectations, 180
Mycobacterium tuberculosis, 239

N

National Academy of Sciences, Disaster Research Group, 360
National Action Plan to Improve Healthy Literacy, 137
National Assessment of Adult Literacy, 135
National Association for Home Care, 43
National Association of Colored Graduate Nurses, 32, 42
National Center for Education Statistics, 135
National Coalition for Promoting Physical Activity, 307, 307*b*
National Council Licensure Examination, 380
National Council of State Boards of Nursing, 266
National Environmental Public Health Tracking Network, 161
National Environmental Public Health Tracking Program, 160–161
National Health and Nutrition Examination Survey, 316, 318
National healthcare system, 210
National Health Service Corp, 211
National Institutes of Health, 137
National League for Nursing, 31
National League of Nursing Education, 31
Nationally Notifiable Infectious Diseases list, 233, 234*b*, 247
National Organization for Public Health Nursing, 33–37
National Prevention Strategy, 210
National Primary Health Care Conference of 2004, 408–409
National Youth Tobacco Survey, 143
Native Americans, 188
Natural disasters. *See* Disaster nursing
Natural environment, 85
Navigation of health system, 135–136
Needle exchange programs, 345

Needs assessment for referrals, 257–258
Neighborhoods. *See* Communities
New Jersey Department of Health and Senior Services (NJDHSS), 239–240
New York City Housing Authority, 288
NFP (Nurse Family Partnership), 286
Noninfectious diseases, 107*t,* 108, 116, 298–299
North American Nursing Diagnosis Association, 175, 176
Nurse-client relationships, 262, 279
Nurse educators, 378–379, 379*b,* 393–394
Nurse Family Partnership (NFP), 286
Nurses Associated Alumnae of the United States and Canada, 31
Nurses' Emergency Council, 358
Nurses' Health Study, 111
Nursing education, 377–397
   clinical experiences, 382–389, 384*f*
      faith-based clinics, 388–389
      immunization clinics, 387–388
      overview, 382–3383
      school health screenings, 389
      service learning, 388
      simulation experiences, 386–387
      wellness screening, 383–385
   educators, 378–379, 379*b,* 393–394
   global worldview, 389–393
      culture of poverty, 391
      debriefing, 392–393
      global learning, 391–392
      healthcare missions, 390–391
      overview, 389
      social justice, 389–390
      systems thinking, 392
   overview, 377–378
   responding to public health needs, 379–381, 380–381*t*
   teaching-learning strategies, 381–382
Nursing history, 353
Nursing informatics, 162
Nursing Intervention Classifications, 175
Nursing Outcome Classifications, 175
Nutrition education program, 228, 291–292

O

Obesity. *See* Overweight and obesity
Occupation, as social determinant of health, 124
Occupational assessment, 91
Omaha Classification System, 175
Online courses, 231, 386–387
Online databases, 57, 58*b. See also* Internet
On-site assessment for TB case, 245
Osteoarthritis, 318
Outcome and Assessment Information Set (OASIS), 170
Outcome-based quality improvement (OBQI), 170
Outreach, 225–228, 228*t,* 266, 268
Overweight and obesity, 316–320
   health related conditions, 317–318
   mental health and, 318–319
   overview, 316–317
   physical activity and, 320
   reasons for increase in, 319
   schools contribution to, 319–320
   smokadiabesity, 299, 299*f*

P

Pace University Lienhard School of Nursing, 290, 293
PACs (political action committees), 218
Palliative care, 92
Pandemics, 336, 345
Participant observations, 182–184, 184*b,* 196
Participation measures, 58, 72
Participatory action research (PAR), 281
Partnership programs, 290–293, 403–404. *See also* Collaboration
Passive surveillance
   defined, 233
   foodborne illnesses, 240
   rabies exposure, 243
   tuberculosis, 240
Pasteur Institute (Paris), 345
Patient-Centered Outcomes Research Institute (PCORI), 209
Patient information privacy, 168

Patient Protection and Affordable Care Act (PPACA). *See* Affordable Care Act of 2010
Patient-reported outcomes measurement information system (PROMIS), 58, 72
PEP (postexposure prophylaxis), 242, 244
Personal Health Records (PHRs), 162
Personally mediated racism, 126
Pest houses, 339–340
Philosophy of teaching primary health care, 409–411, 412*b*
PHNAT. *See* Public Health Nursing Assessment Tool
PHRs (Personal Health Records), 162
Physical activity
  case studies, 309–310, 309*b*
  guidelines, 303, 304*b*, 320, 321*b*
  programs for elder population, 308
  promoting, 307, 307*b*
  social support and, 305
Physical Activity Committee (American Heart Association), 302
Physical barriers or boundaries, 86
Physical environment determinants, 59–60, 84–86, 284, 285*b*
Physical inactivity, 298, 299*f*
Physically unhealthy days analysis worksheet, 72
Plain Writing Act of 2010, 137
Plan and implementation assessment, 62–63, 99–100
Pneumonic plague, 337
POD (point of dispensing) methods, 370–372
Policy and policymaking
  advocacy and, 217
  defining, 204–205
  development and enforcement, 328–330, 329*f*
  as foundational health measure, 61, 94
  healthy teaching and, 284–285
  interventions, 137
  issues, 203
  values and, 205–206
Political action committees (PACs), 218

Political engagement of nurses, 202–204, 217–219
Political issues in communities, 95
Politics, defined, 206
Population. *See also specific demographic groups*
  assessment worksheet, 69–74
  defined, 5–7, 6*t*
  race distribution worksheet, 74
  in U.S., 26
Population-based behavior, 61–62
Population-based health issues, 132–134, 133*b*
Population-focused interventions, 137–138, 141–142, 382
Population perspective, 118
Poster presentations, 388
Postexposure prophylaxis (PEP), 242, 244
Post-stroke depression, 225
Poverty
  blamed for plague, 340–341
  culture of, 188–189, 391
Pre-exposure vaccination for rabies, 242
Pregnancy, cultural expectations about, 180
Prepathogenesis period of disease prevention, 7
Presumptive diagnosis of TB, 239
Prevalence rates (diseases), 111, 112*t*
Prevention and Public Health Fund, 141, 210
Prevention domain of health literacy, 135
Prevention Institute, 302
Prevention programs and health services
  Affordable Care Act and, 210–211
  cancer, 303, 304*b*
  diabetes, 320
  diseases, 7
  drug abuse, 281
  policymaking and, 217
  public health role of, 7, 8*f*
  rabies, 242–244
  referrals and, 256
  wellness screening and, 383–385
Price component of marketing model, 325

Primary care, 408–409
Primary care assessment, 88
Primary disease prevention, 7
Primary health care, 399–413
  Alma-Ata Declaration (1978), 9, 400–404, 401–403*b*
  challenges, 407–409, 410*f*
  defined, 400, 403–404
  overview, 399–400
  progress in, 404–407, 404*b*, 405–406*t*
  teaching philosophy, 409–411, 412*b*
Prioritization of issues, 62, 98
Privacy of patient information, 168
Private duty nurses, 31, 33
Private sector's contribution to healthcare system, 207
Probable diagnosis
  foodborne case, 241
  tuberculosis case, 244
Process Model for *Healthy People 2020,* 14, 19, 57
Product component of marketing model, 325
Project IDEAL, 193–195, 195*b*
PROMIS (patient-reported outcomes measurement information system), 58, 72
Promotion component of marketing model, 325
Prose literacy, 135
Prospective studies, 115
Providence Hospital (Anchorage, Alaska), 362–363
Public health
  assessments. *See* Assessments
  culture and. *See* Culture
  defined, 4–10, 10*b*
  disease prevention and health maintenance, 7, 8*f*
  emergency preparedness. *See* Emergency preparedness
  ensuring public's health, 9–10
  epidemics. *See* Epidemic diseases
  epidemiology. *See* Epidemiology
  evidence-based practice. *See* Evidence-based practice
  informatics. *See* Informatics
  multi-discipline approach, 7–9, 9*f*

policy and policymaking. *See* Policy and policymaking
populations, 5–7, 6t
primary health care. *See* Primary health care
service, 10
surveillance. *See* Surveillance
Public Health Action Support Team, 231
Public health informatics, defined, 162
Public health nurses
culture and, 187–189
defined, 10–11, 26–27, 40
as delegatee, 268–269
as delegator, 267–268
education of, 47–49
in England, 27–30
evolution of, 27–49
1930s era, 39–41
20th century, second half of, 41–45
21st century, 45–47
district nurses, 27–30
early experiments in, 37–39
emergence of, 32–33
modern nursing movement, 31–32
National Organization for Public Health Nursing, 33–37
visiting nurses, 30–31
expanded role of, 34, 37, 40, 45–46, 204
funding for, 36
standardizing requirements, 35
in U.S., 26
Public Health Nursing: Scope & Standards of Practice (ANA), 322
Public Health Nursing Assessment Tool (PHNAT), 53–101
analysis of health, 62
foundational health measures, 58–62
behaviors, individual and population, 61–62, 69–74, 96
biology and genetics, 59, 73
disparities, 55, 62, 97
general health status, 55, 58, 68–72, 97
health services, 60–61, 87–93
policymaking, 61, 94
social factors, 59–60, 75–83

Minnesota Intervention Wheel Strategies, 54–55, 62–63
overview, 53–58, 55–57b
prioritization of issues, 62, 98
reflection, 64, 101
tracking and evaluation, 63–64
Public Health Service
Framingham Study, 115
tobacco use guidelines, 142
Public Health Work Force Competencies, 173
Push POD model, 370

Q

Quality and Safety Education for Nurses (QSEN), 132
Quality healthcare initiatives, 209
Quality Initiative (IOM), 209
Quality of life, 55, 58, 72, 265
Quality ratings, 133, 133b
Quantitative literacy, 135
Quarantine, 344
QuitNet, smoking cessation program, 144

R

Rabies prevention, 242–244
Race distribution worksheet, 74
Race relations during disaster response, 361
Racism, 126, 126f, 180–181. *See also* Discrimination
Rate of disease
definitions, 110–111, 112t
infectious diseases, 108
specific calculations, 11, 11b
Recreational facilities, 78
Red Cross Rural Nursing Service, 412b
Referrals, 252–263
barriers to, 254, 259–260
ethics of, 261–262
follow-up programs, 230
follow-up strategies, 260–261
formal resources, 254–255
needs identification, 255–256
overview, 252–253
receivers of, 253–254
senders of, 253–254
steps to conducting, 256–259

systems and community practice levels, 262–263
Regional Health Information Exchanges, 162
Rehabilitation intervention strategies, 7, 8f
Rehabilitative care assessment, 89
Relationship status with clients, 257
Relative income inequality, 123
Research. *See also* Case studies
action, 183
clinical, 156–157, 171, 172–173
Residential shelter nutrition program, 292
Resources
Internet, 57, 58b, 169
linking individuals and families to, 252–253
search for and availability of, 254, 258
Retrospective studies, 115
Rights of delegation, 267
Risk reduction, 7
Rituals, cultural, 180, 181–182
Robert Wood Johnson Foundation (RWJF)
The Future of Nursing, 203
Initiative of the Future of Nursing, 204
Quality and Safety Education for Nurses, 132
Roy Adaptation Model, 123
Rural communities
emergence of public health care in, 38–39
vulnerable populations in, 189
Rural Domestic Violence Project, 192–193, 193b

S

Safe Routes to School (SRTS) program, 308
St. Mary's Hospital (Galveston, Texas), 360
Salvation Army, 354
SAM (Suitability of Assessment Materials), 138
Sandhills Fever Hospital (Jacksonville, Florida), 355
Sanitarians, 241

Sanitary legislation, 337
Sanitation, 86
Scheduling systems, 165
School-based programs, 91, 143, 281, 321
School health screenings, 389
School nurses, 267, 321
Schools' contribution to overweight and obesity, 319–320
Screenings
  assessments, 225, 383
  cancer, 227, 229, 231
  ethics of, 253
  programs, 228–231, 280
  school health, 389
  wellness, 383–385
Scrubbing data, 158
Secondary disease prevention, 7
Self-assessments, 383
Self-reflection, 64
Senders of referrals, 253–254
Senior population. See Elder population
Sensibility of testing techniques, 230
Service learning, 388
SES (socioeconomic status), 115, 116
SESPAN (Southeast Senior Physical Activity Network), 308
Seven A's, assessment tool, 60–61, 93, 285
Seven-minute screen, cognitive case-finding instrument, 225
Shigellosis, 241–242
Sigma Theta Tau, 182
Simplified Measure of Gobbledygook, 138
Simulation experiences, 386–387
Sisters of Charity of the Incarnate Word, 360
Slogans, effectiveness of, 326
Smallpox initiative, 370–372
Smokadiabesity (smoking, diabetes, and obesity), 299, 299f
Smoking cigarettes. See Tobacco use
SNAP (Supplemental Nutrition Assistance Program), 290
Social capital, 120, 123
Social context of behavior, 118–120
Social determinants of health, 121–126
  assessment of, 59–60, 75–83

defined, 121
  health education, 282–284
  Henry Street Settlement, 289
  multilevel approaches to
    discrimination, disparity and health, 124–126, 125–126f
    education, 123–124
    income, 122–123
    income inequality, 123
    occupation, 124
    socioeconomic position and status, 115, 116, 122
    overview, 121–122
Social epidemiology, 117–126
  defined, 117
  developmental and life-course perspective, 118, 119f
  guiding perspective in, 118, 119t
  life course model or perspective, 121
  multilevel analysis, 118, 120–121
  multilevel approaches to social determinants of health, 121–126
  overview, 117–118, 119t
  population perspective, 118
  social context of behavior, 118–120
Social justice, 388, 389–390
Social marketing, 324–328, 327f
Social media, 144
Social policy, 204
Social services, 79
Socioeconomic status (SES), 115, 116, 121
Soup kitchens, 358
Southeast Senior Physical Activity Network (SESPAN), 308
Spanish influenza, 342
Specificity of testing techniques, 230
Specific rates (diseases), 111, 112t
Spousal abuse, 181, 193
SRTS (Safe Routes to School) program, 308
Standardized language and classifications, 158–159, 174–176
Standards of Performance for Local Boards of Health, 239
State Action on Avoidable Rehospitalizations (STAAR), 216

State HIE Cooperative Agreement Program, 217
State response to ACA, 216–217
State Scorecard on U.S. Health System Performance, 2009 (Commonwealth Fund Commission), 216
State-Trait Anxiety Inventory, 182
Stressors, individuals response to, 123
Student health services nursing, 167–168
Substance abuse programs, 188, 281
Suitability of Assessment Materials (SAM), 138
Summer Showdown softball tournament (rabies exposure case), 243–244
Supplemental Nutrition Assistance Program (SNAP), 290
Support groups
  African American women who used cocaine, 184
  Latino population, 192, 194
  online resources for, 169
Supreme Court and ACA legislation, 212
Surveillance
  active, 233, 240, 243, 244
  data, 117, 154, 232–235
  epidemiologic, 117, 232
  factors for effective systems, 235–236
  medical, 232
  passive, 233, 240, 243
  process, 232–235, 235f
  systems, 163, 232–235
Systematic reviews, 133
System-focused practices
  advocacy, 323b, 324
  case management, 266
  coalition building, 306–307, 306f, 307b
  collaboration, 305
  community organizing, 308
  referrals and follow-up, 262–263
Systems thinking, 392

T
Taiwanese studies
  of immigrant youth, 181
  of nurses, 182
TANF (Temporary Assistance for Needy Families), 265

Task Force on Community Preventive Services, 260
TB (tuberculosis) control, case study, 239–240, 244–246
TCM (Transitional Care Model), 286
Teaching IOM: Implications of the Institute of Medicine Reports for Nursing Education (IOM), 379
Teaching-learning strategies, 381–382
Teaching philosophy of primary health care, 409–411, 412b
Technology. *See* Informatics; Internet
TeleHealth and virtual home visits, 171–172, 293
Telephone helplines for support, 254, 346
Temporary Assistance for Needy Families (TANF), 265
Terence Higgins Trust (UK), 345
Tertiary disease prevention, 7
Texas City ship explosion (1947), 358–362
Thailand's Primary Health Care, 405
TJC (The Joint Commission), 137
Tobacco use
    case studies, 138–139
    as public health condition, 139–145, 139f, 299, 299f
    smokadiabesity, 299, 299f
To Err Is Human (IOM), 131
Toxic substances, 86
Tracking assessments, 63–64
Tracking data, 157–158
Transitional Care Model (TCM), 286
Transitional housing, 193
Transmission of diseases, 116–117
Transportation, 76
Trust relationships, 120, 246, 279
TST (Mantoux tuberculin skin testing), 239
Tuberculosis (TB) control, case study, 239–240, 244–246
211 switchboards (community resources), 254

U

UK National Screening Committee, 230

Undocumented immigrants, 186, 226
United Nations, 185, 298
Universal precautions approach to health literacy, 137
University of Medicine and Dentistry of New Jersey's Mobile Health Care Project, 230
University of Texas Medical Branch (UTMB), 359, 360
University of Texas School of Nursing (Galveston, Texas), 358
Urban sprawl, 319
U.S. Diabetes Conversation Map Kits, 285
U.S. Preventive Services Task Force, 231, 232b

V

Vaccinations. *See* Immunization programs
Values
    of community, 407–408, 410f
    public policy and, 205–206
Vector transmission of foodborne illnesses, 240
Vietnamese American women, 227
Virtual home visits and TeleHealth, 171–172, 293
Visiting Nurse Associations of America, 43
Visiting nurses, 26, 30–31
Visiting Nurse Service of New York, 287
Vital statistics analysis worksheet, 69
Voluntary referrals, 262
Vulnerable populations, 279–280. *See also specific populations groups*

W

Welfare Transition Program (WTP), 265
Well-being measures, 58, 72
Wellness screening, 383–385. *See also* Prevention programs and health services

WellStar School of Nursing, Kennesaw State University, 193
"What if" questioning technique, 393
Who Will Keep the Public Healthy? (IOM report), 131
Wilder Research Center, 300–301
Windshield survey, 60, 84
Women
    cancer screening, 227, 229
    domestic violence and, 181, 188, 192–193, 193b, 225
    female circumcision and, 185, 186
    heart awareness program, 183
    improving health outcomes for, 265–266, 286, 288
    overweight and obesity, 316–320
    pregnancy, 180
    schizophrenics and BMI, 299, 299f, 318
Women's Christian Temperance Union, 356
Women's Relief Corps, 356
Workplace assessments, 77
World Health Organization
    childhood obesity, 317
    data collection and, 154
    factors for effective surveillance systems, 235–236
    female circumcision, 185
    "Health for All," 400
    learning activities, 390–391
    physical inactivity and, 298
    World AIDS Day, 346
    World Health Report 2000, 207
Worldview. *See* Global worldview
Worship places, 79
WTP (Welfare Transition Program), 265

X

Xenophobia, 181–182

Y

Years of potential life lost (YPLL) analysis worksheet, 71
Yellow fever, 354–355
Youth Risk Behavioral Surveillance System, 302